SOUND SLEEP AND SECURE ATTACHMENT WITH AWARE PARENTING

Many parents have questions about sleep and are often confused by conflicting advice. Should they hold their babies until they fall asleep or put them down when they are still awake? How can they help their babies and toddlers sleep through the night? When should a child move out of the family bed? What's the best approach to use with children who resist bedtime? And what about teenagers who stay up all night? In this book, Marion Rose answers all these questions, and many more, from an Aware Parenting perspective, which involves deep trust in children's natural body wisdom. Parents will learn loving and effective solutions to common sleep issues while enhancing their children's emotional well-being and strengthening attachment. I highly recommend this book for all parents, especially those who yearn for a good night's sleep!

– Aletha Solter, PhD, Founder of Aware Parenting

In a world filled with conflicting sleep advice, Marion Rose's book stands out like a beacon of light. It offers an unparalleled level of compassion for parents while also providing clear, practical guidance on how to achieve better sleep for the whole family.

Aware Parenting, as Marion explains so beautifully, is one of the few, if not the only, parenting paradigms that truly recognises babies' and children's physiological sleep needs, while also addressing the cultural expectations and conditioning that often cloud our understanding. Aware Parenting deeply understands our innate human capacity to heal from stress and trauma, which is key to achieving restful sleep – and Marion adds the missing piece with her beautiful explanations, filled with examples and empathy.

What I love most is Marion's view of babies and children as whole beings – not just deserving of our care and kindness, but also of our deep trust. Her approach brings reassurance and clarity, offering parents a profoundly different yet nurturing way to meet their children's needs, as well as their own, when it comes to sleep.

– Maru Rojas, Aware Parenting instructor

This book is a powerful resource for all exhausted parents. It is a deeply compassionate and informative book that beautifully describes what we need as babies, children, and teens in order to fall asleep when tired, to stay asleep and to feel safe, connected, and relaxed for deep, restorative sleep. Marion Rose shares in detail the Aware Parenting perspective on supporting babies, children, and teens to relax through emotional release, connection, and safety.

She describes the effect of stress on sleep, how babies and children experience stress at bedtime, what their bodies do in response to stress, and how we can support them to no longer need to go into hyper-arousal or to dissociate in order to sleep. She illustrates in powerful language how to distinguish between true relaxation and dissociation, so that even the most sleep-deprived parent can quickly bring changes to their family and get the restful sleep they need.

Marion challenges the cultural conditioning about sleep, so that it is no longer a frustrating, exhausting struggle and instead becomes an opportunity for deep connection and healing. There is wisdom and gold on every page and Marion invites parents to tune in to what resonates for them, not telling them what to do but empowering them to make an informed choice for their family.

The structure of the book is perfect to support parents to find exactly the right information they need with whatever challenges they are facing, whether their child is a baby, a toddler, or a teen. She shares powerful stories from parents and Aware Parenting instructors, provides detailed descriptions of supporting the most common challenges parents face with sleep and answers frequent questions about children at all ages.

It is a compassionate guide to bring trust and deep connection and plentiful sleep for everyone in the family. I highly recommend this book for all parents.

— Joss Goulden, Level 2 Aware Parenting instructor

Marion, you have put the most beautiful words together in this book for parents to truly understand sleep.

My understanding of sleep (before I was introduced to Aware Parenting) was that children needed to be taught how to sleep. I remember so well having someone come in to our home to teach me how to teach my daughter how to sleep. It felt so wrong. Being told to not pick her up, or if I felt I must – to pat her through the cot sides. My body ached as I tried so hard to get her to sleep in a dark room.

We were so disconnected already after the traumatic birth and separations that occurred. I can see that this 'sleep training way' was devastating to our attachment. It left me feeling unable to trust myself and my daughter's natural ability to sleep.

Four and a bit years later and after lot of learning about attachment theory, I had my son. We co-slept, I offered so much closeness and connection. He would make a peep and I would feed him, sing, gently rock – all to stop him crying. Well, this did not allow for the beautiful sleep I was hoping for. Rather, he was a little tornado in the night, constantly rolling, and so very restless. It didn't make sense that he wasn't sleeping, I was meeting all of his needs!

I soon learned through completing Marion's sleep course that I was missing a very important need… to express his feelings to me!!

This book reflects the beautiful natural ability we all have to sleep with loving support! Marion's beautiful pauses for self compassion are moments of pure gold. They invite you to see a bigger picture and to hold yourself and your life journey with much needed compassion.

To know there is a third way to get sleep, and that that way includes all family members' needs also being met, brings so much hope and healing to many families.

– Kimberley Cousins – Aware Parenting instructor, Perinatal Registered Nurse

Marion has done it again! This beautiful book – the third in her trilogy of books about Aware Parenting – offers an incredibly detailed, comprehensive, and clear explanation of how the philosophy of Aware Parenting applies to sleep. And it is so easy and enjoyable to read – I literally couldn't put it down!

In *Sound Sleep and Secure Attachment with Aware Parenting*, Marion offers the bigger picture and cultural context, inviting readers to consider how we've been conditioned to misinterpret or ignore our children's innate needs and biological wisdom when it comes to sleep. She outlines how many common sleep practices actually work against children's innate wisdom, leading us as parents to inadvertently get in the way of natural relaxation processes that ultimately result in peaceful sleep.

Marion clearly articulates how it really is possible to have secure attachment with our children AND decent sleep – that we really don't need to sacrifice one for the other. This information is offered in a non-judgmental and compassionate way, inviting us to see sleep as a barometer of our child's emotional AND physiological state. Readers will walk away feeling empowered to understand what's actually going on for children by looking behind their sleep-related challenges, so we can address root causes in a supportive and holistic way.

I wish I could go back in time and give this book to myself as an exhausted and bewildered first-time mum. While I had a basic understanding of Aware Parenting at the time, I experimented with schedules/wake windows, lured by the promise of restful sleep, and also breastfed my baby all night long, believing that was the only way to remain connected with her. This book would've been a game changer for me in those early months – I love how it centres parents as the researcher of our own children, inviting us to attune, observe and ultimately TRUST! And it's absolutely jam-packed with practical and specific tips for parents to experiment with.

I highly recommend *Sound Sleep and Secure Attachment with Aware Parenting* to everyone and truly believe it has the power to change the world.

– Meg Rankin, Aware Parenting instructor, Social Worker

In this book, Marion is gentle and thorough in her discussion on sleep and Aware Parenting. These pages are steeped in deep compassion and an unwavering dedication to find the most helpful ways to be with our little ones and to understand ourselves as human beings. I am so grateful this book is here for my growing family, and for all the families I am sure will find and turn to Marion's words for reassurance and guidance.

– Jasmine Prescott, Psychotherapist specialising in attachment and trauma

Sleep. One of our basic needs and skills, too. No one needs to be taught how to sleep. But our society has made it another issue for parents to be stressed about, to not trust their children with.

Marion Rose invites us to look at sleep from another perspective. To trust that our children want to sleep and will do so, when their needs are met and they are relaxed and tired enough.

She offers compassion for every feeling and thought that may arise for us while reading this book, and empowers us to choose connection with our children. Another amazing book, which has deeply touched me and made me change the way I parent my child.

Thank you, Marion.

– Eirini Anagnostopoulou – Parent Coach

I'm Here and I'm Listening is an absolutely fantastic deep dive into the practice of Aware Parenting. I would highly recommend it to anyone interested in learning more about themselves and any children in their lives. Marion has a lot of compassion and empathy which absolutely shines through in this book! I couldn't put it down!!! Thank you for putting such a beautiful offering out into the world Marion, we are all better off for it.

– Anna Haberfield

I love the structure of *I'm Here and I'm Listening*. The way that Marion Rose offers an overview and returns later for more details and depth makes it easy to read and to comprehend. I love the clarity of it all! And of course, the richness; there is so much without being overwhelming. I would just highlight the entire book, it is all so important. I just can't put it down! The way it is formulated means it's really such a pleasure to read!

– Linde Lambrechts, Psychotherapist and Aware Parenting instructor

I'm Here and I'm Listening is not an ordinary parenting book. I could describe it more as a guide for personal growth, which at the same time gives us the ultimate motivation for it: our children's wellbeing, and a harmonious life. Even from the title I could feel its power, and wondered how the world will be when we start being present, and truly listening to the people we love, especially our children. Marion Rose invites us to deeply trust our children's innate wisdom and ability to heal from stress and trauma, if we give them the chance to express themselves. She offers us an invaluable change of perspective on tantrums, rage, and aggression. She gives us the tools we can use to connect with our children and give them the space to show us all their feelings. With so much compassion, she allows us to reflect on our conditioning from the society we live in, our experiences, thoughts, and beliefs, and to grow from our realisations. She reminds us of the significance of taking care of our needs, so we can be present and support our children in feeling their feelings. It's a book that I will definitely read again and again, and use as a resource for my practice. Thank you, Marion. Thank you for this book, and the motivation to be a part of this new generation of parents who will change the world!

– Eirini Anagnostopoulou – Parent Coach

I just finished *The Emotional Life of Babies* for the second time since buying it a couple of months ago. That's how good it is!!! There's dog ears, highlighted sections, and asterisks from front to back.

I love how this book centres parents as the researcher of our own baby, inviting us to put aside preconceived ideas about things like crying, feeding, and sleep; attune to our baby's needs, experiment with Aware Parenting approaches right from birth and observe our baby's responses... and then decide for ourselves whether this is the right fit for our family. It is not at all prescriptive (as many other baby books are!) – in fact it's quite the opposite – above all, this book encourages us to trust ourselves and to trust babies.

– Meg Rankin, Aware Parenting instructor, Social Worker, Counsellor

I began reading this book on a whim, my son had been crying and I wasn't sure why. HOLY MOLY what I wasn't prepared for was the complete revolution to our lives that comes with understanding the knowledge Marion shares in *The Emotional Life of Babies*.

I feel like I had been walking through motherhood blindly and this book has given me sight; I now understand my baby's every move with so much more ease. And even better, I am assured that I am raising him in the most compassionate way possible. The conclusion of the book sums it up very eloquently; the way we respond to our baby's feelings and needs will affect how they respond to their own when they're older; the way we talk to them will determine their own internal dialogue; the more empathy we share the more empathy they will be able to share (with themselves and others)... the list goes on. Read this book if you want to raise a child who is emotionally aware and knows how to move through their own feelings with grace and ease.

This book has also facilitated my own healing as I began to acknowledge my own needs and suppressed feelings. The compassion Marion shows to parents throughout the book with her writing style makes this book a deeply enjoyable read. The book offers continual reminders of the concepts/practices of Aware Parenting and is written in a compassionate and easy to absorb way (which my 'mum brain' really appreciated). It's been a long time since I've sponged up information with such enthusiasm and joy! This book has made me a deep believer in the Aware Parenting philosophy – if only the whole world could read it we would raise the next generation of humans to be much more peaceful, connected and kind to one another! Bless you Marion for sharing your wisdom, my baby's life is going to be so much better for it!!!

– Sara

I'm so thankful for Marion Rose's book *The Emotional Life of Babies*! She has such a sensitively attuned way of writing and knows her field tangibly... you can tell she lives Aware Parenting without the beliefs coming off as imposing (that notion is as far away as can be!), with respectful acknowledgment towards the reader's intuition... It is such a privilege to read these fitting words that resonate so much with my intuition.

Despite my passion for attachment theory, neuroscience, and trauma pedagogy (as an avid early childhood educator), I've seldom read a book like this, that mirrors these branches so harmoniously and close to heart and of course also integrated with her own experiences and transparent learning path. Thank you so much, Marion... I feel your book is already enriching the relationship between my daughter and me. How fortunate I am to be able to read this book during this time of expecting her!"

– Ebru Ingvarsson, Early Childhood Educator

Published in Australia by
Loving Being Publishing
PO Box 256, Doreen, VIC 3754
marion@marionrose.net
www.marionrose.net

First published in Australia 2024
Copyright © Marion Rose 2024

National Library of Australia Cataloguing–in–Publication entry

A catalogue record for this book is available from the National Library of Australia

ISBN: 978-0-6459985-5-9 (paperback)
ISBN: 978-0-6459985-6-6 (hardback)
ISBN: 978-0-6459985-7-3 (epub)

Cover photography by Michael Rose
Cover layout and design by Jelena Mirkovic
Typesetting by Sophie White Design

Printed by Ingram Spark

Disclaimer: All care has been taken in the preparation of the information herein, but no responsibility can be accepted by the publisher or author for any damages resulting from the misinterpretation of this work. All contact details given in this book were current at the time of publication, but are subject to change.

The advice given in this book is based on the experience of the individuals. Professionals should be consulted for individual problems. The author and publisher shall not be responsible for any person with regard to any loss or damage caused directly or indirectly by the information in this book.

Today, and every day, I acknowledge the Traditional Custodians of this land where I live and work, which include the Arakwal people, the Minjungbal people, the Widjabul people, and the Bundjalung people. I pay my respects to elders past, present and emerging. I acknowledge and recognise them as the original storytellers and wisdom keepers.

Sound Sleep and Secure Attachment

WITH AWARE PARENTING

Transform sleep for your baby, child, or teen
with this compassionate, trauma-informed
approach to deep relaxation

MARION ROSE, PHD

To Aletha Solter, with such gratitude for teaching me to deeply trust in the innate wisdom of children.

ABOUT THE AUTHOR

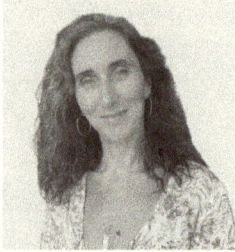

When I was pregnant for the first time in 2001, I was searching online for a parenting approach that fitted with all that I had learnt in my previous 14 years being immersed in developmental psychology and psychotherapy. I had a PhD from The Winnicott Research Unit at Cambridge University, where I researched the mother-infant relationship and infant development in the context of postnatal depression. I'd also been a Post-Doctoral Research Fellow in infant development, as well as a University Lecturer and Psychotherapist in private practice.

When I found Aware Parenting, the approach developed by Aletha Solter, PhD, it was a match with all that I'd been looking for.

I saw that Aware Parenting was based on attachment theory. It was trauma-informed (before that term was well-known). It recognised that babies and children are deeply affected by what they experience in utero and during their birth. It matched all that I'd learnt in my psychotherapy training and practice, about the importance of presence, attunement, and listening to feelings.

It deeply resonated with me, and I knew straight away that this was what I would practice with my daughter.

In addition, I was astounded to learn that Aware Parenting had a magic extra element that had not been recognised by any of the previous modalities I had trained in.

The missing piece was that babies and children have inbuilt processes to heal from stress and trauma, right from birth. Babies and children continue to try to evoke these intrinsic healing responses, even though we live in a culture which does not recognise them, and often teaches us to actively work against them.

I was to discover that this innate wisdom we're all born with – which when supported, brings about life-changing effects to emotional wellbeing, behaviour, relaxation, and sleep – isn't recognised, understood, or taught, in most psychology departments, psychotherapy trainings, or in the majority of parenting paradigms (yet!).

When I started practicing Aware Parenting with my baby daughter, I did so because I believed (and still do) that it was the most helpful parenting paradigm for her emotional and psychological development. With it, I wanted to help her be deeply connected with herself, and for her to feel deeply relaxed, aware, and present. I wanted her to know that all her feelings were welcome and that she was unconditionally loved, however she felt. I was willing to help her heal from anything that happened to her that was stressful or traumatic.

I wasn't thinking about what Aware Parenting would mean for her sleep.

However, what I experienced with her, and also with my son, who was born four and a half years later, is that Aware Parenting helps babies, children, and teens feel both deeply connected and profoundly relaxed. Those two elements lead to restful, restorative, and easeful sleep.

In my first 17 years of parenting, I didn't lose any sleep (!) over nighttime sleep. I didn't worry about sleep or focus much on sleep, because I knew that if I focussed on practicing the three elements of Aware Parenting[1], relaxed sleep was the result. And it was. My daughter and son generally slept easily and restfully at night. That made a huge difference to how I felt in the daytime, and how much energy and compassion I felt in my parenting. When we're tired, we're less able to suppress our feelings. As a result, our big emotions bubbling over as parents can make the days long and hard, and we're way more likely to react in harsh ways towards our children. Having plenty of restful sleep was such a supportive foundation for me in my mothering.

---

1   Which I will share about soon!

We co-slept for plenty of years and they both breastfed for two years. We all slept peacefully the majority of the time. That didn't mean breastfeeding them lots throughout the night. Nor did they move all around the bed as toddlers. Their muscles were usually deeply relaxed while they slept. They generally woke up feeling refreshed and happy.

I love telling parents that they really don't need to choose between seemingly only two options of secure attachment or sound sleep. With Aware Parenting, we really can have both!

With full transparency, there were two times in my children's lives where I didn't find the sleep journey as easy. One was with naps when my daughter was a toddler, and the other was in my son's early teenage years. Those situations were both because at those times I didn't understand some of the relevant nuances in Aware Parenting – and I had some of my own inner work to do. I came to comprehend exactly *why* those two times were challenging for me, and *what* I could have done to prevent them. I'd love to support you in not having those challenges that I did!

I believe that the gifts that come from when we find something hard can be as valuable to share with others as those that arrive because of what is easy for us. I'm so willing for the learnings I received to save you from lots of angst yourself.

I want to share something else with you that is very important to me, and central to the understandings I share in this book. To do that, I invite you to come back in time with me, to a decade before my daughter was born.

Back in 1992, when I was doing my PhD, I used to love visiting a little dusty old secondhand bookshop. I still remember the exact moment when I went in there one day, looking – as I frequently did – for books about babies, and one jumped out at me from the shelf. I still have that exact copy on my own bookshelf today. It was entitled *The Continuum Concept*, by a woman called Jean Liedloff, who wrote about what she had learnt from living with the Indigenous Yequana people in South America. The book evoked a strong desire in me that continues to this day, more than 30 years later. That is – to understand more about – and share about – two powerful pieces of information:

1. Babies and young children have intrinsic needs for plenty of closeness.

2. Each culture has different beliefs about the most helpful ways to respond to babies and children, which profoundly affect how they feel, and the core beliefs that they acquire.

Over the ensuing years, my fascination with these two elements – which we could call *closeness* and *culture* – has deeply affected both my personal and professional journeys.

When I first read *The Aware Baby*, nearly a decade later, I saw how Aletha Solter's research also included the importance of attachment needs, including *closeness*. However, I also discovered that Aletha Solter understood the effects of *cultural* beliefs on child-rearing practices from an even wider perspective than the one I had learnt up until that time.

In *Sound Sleep and Secure Attachment with Aware Parenting*, you'll see these two threads of *closeness* and *culture* running throughout the book.

You'll read about how closeness powerfully affects sleep. I will also share lots about sleep and attachment practices of both our ancestors and other present-day cultures including Indigenous ones. I'll explain how Aware Parenting helps us understand what's going on for a baby or child when they go to sleep with closeness or without it. I'll also talk about the developmental trajectory of attachment, and what that means for older children and teens as they become increasingly independent. I'll include research about Indigenous cultures to highlight this process.

I'll also give you lots of details about the missing puzzle piece that Aware Parenting offers – the one I was so surprised to first learn about all those years ago – and why it has such a huge effect on sleep.

I'd love to share another part of my journey with you. Back in 2002, when my daughter was nine months old, I became passionate about language, which was ignited by starting to learn Nonviolent Communication, by Marshall Rosenberg. You'll see my passion for the power of language woven throughout this book.

I discovered that language is one of the key ways that cultural beliefs are passed down. That's why I'll also be inviting you to look at the language you use with – and about – your child, and also towards yourself. This is part of the reparenting and re-culturing process I've created called *The Marion Method*, which is devoted to us getting free from *Disconnected Domination Culture[2] (DDC)* beliefs and conditioning.

All of the parenting theory and practice in this book is based on Aware Parenting. The reparenting and language elements are from *The Marion Method* (these are inspired by Aware Parenting and are akin to practicing Aware Parenting with yourself!).

Aware Parenting isn't only influenced by studying the parenting methodologies of our ancestors and of existing traditional cultures. Research on attachment theory, non-punitive discipline, trauma, and healing from trauma also directly influences the principles and practices of this approach.

I've been an Aware Parenting instructor since 2005, and I've been a Level 2 instructor for many years. I've worked with thousands of families. Although not every parent who practices Aware Parenting has an easy journey with sleep, I have seen so many transformational experiences happen for families when they put this philosophy into practice.

As the Regional Coordinator for Australia, New Zealand, and Indonesia, I love supporting people to become Aware Parenting instructors and to help other families with this beautiful approach. In *The Aware Parenting Podcast*, in my courses and mentoring sessions, workshops and books, I love sharing about Aware Parenting. I see the huge effect it has had on my own son and daughter, who are deeply connected with themselves as young adults. Every day I hear from parents about the differences they observe from practicing Aware Parenting with their babies and children.

This is the third book in my trilogy of Aware Parenting books. The first, called *The Emotional Life of Babies*, is for parents of babies. The second, *I'm Here and I'm Listening*, is for parents of children aged 1-8. If you want to dive in deeper into Aware Parenting after reading *Sound Sleep*

---

2   This is a term I've created and use in *The Marion Method* to describe cultures where disconnection and domination are core to the beliefs and practices of the culture.

and Secure Attachment with Aware Parenting, I invite you to read these, as well as all of Aletha Solter's books. My books are designed to complement Aletha Solter's, which are full of deeply clear and concise information about all aspects of Aware Parenting.

Aware Parenting helped me deeply understand my children and what they needed. With it, their dad and I supported them to heal from many of the daily stresses that all babies and children experience, as well as some unique traumas, and helped them to stay deeply connected with themselves. As a result, they were generally deeply present and relaxed. They were able to concentrate for long periods and loved to learn. They were deeply aware of their physical environment and noticed details. They were naturally gentle with each other, with other children, and with animals.

As young adults now, all of these qualities continue. They still concentrate for long periods on what they love, and trust their own interests and callings. They think in clear and creative ways and follow their own paths. They enjoy thinking deeply about the world.

I see all of those as innate capacities which children are born with, and which Aware Parenting helps them stay connected with.

Practicing Aware Parenting has also helped me transform my beliefs and behaviours in profound ways that extend beyond parenting. It invited me to see all humans in a different light. I have questioned and released lots of cultural beliefs. My own life has transformed. It has inspired me to develop my own reparenting modality to support parents in their parallel healing journey alongside parenting their children.

By now, you've probably noticed my passion for authenticity and transparency. I'd also love to share with you that I experienced some very painful challenges in my parenting at times (as well as with naps with my daughter as a toddler and conflicts around my son going to sleep when he was a young teen). Those challenges happened after my children's dad and I separated. We all felt so many painful feelings. The effects of that required years of healing for my children and me. With Aware Parenting, profound healing from ruptures with our children is also possible. Even – and especially – with all the challenges, I can clearly see what a huge difference Aware Parenting has made for us all.

So, with first-hand experience, I can share with you that we don't need to do Aware Parenting 'perfectly' for it to make a huge difference.

In fact, I will argue that it isn't possible to do it 'perfectly', and that there is no such thing as 'perfect'! I was (and still am) on a learning and healing journey – as we will all be with Aware Parenting, given that it is so different to what most of us grew up experiencing, and to what the *DDC* teaches now.

I am so happy to be sharing with you about what I've learnt through my own experiences, both as a mother and Aware Parenting instructor.

I'm so willing for this book to help you even more deeply understand your baby, child, or teen, and how to help them both release stress and heal from trauma, and feel deeply relaxed in their body, so they can have restful and restorative sleep.

I'm incredibly grateful to Aware Parenting, and to Aletha Solter for creating it. I'm so honoured to share elements of it here with you. And if what you read here resonates with you too, I am so willing for you to experience beautiful transformations in your life as a result!

Much love,
Marion
xoxox

October 2024

AUTHOR'S NOTE

This book is an educational resource focusing on the emotional needs of babies, children, and teens; it is not intended to be a substitute for medical advice or treatment. Many of the behaviours and symptoms discussed can be an indication of serious emotional or physical issues in babies, children, and teens.

Readers are advised to consult with a competent health care provider whenever babies, children, or teens display behavioural or emotional challenges, a sudden change in sleep, eating, or crying patterns, or when pain or illness are suspected. Furthermore, some of the suggested practices in this book may not be suitable under all conditions or with babies, children, or teens suffering from certain physical or emotional challenges.

If you are ever concerned when your baby, child, or teen is crying, or if their crying is suddenly high pitched, please seek advice from your health care provider. One of the reasons that babies, children, and teens cry is when they are in physical pain, so please trust yourself if you are ever worried.

If you choose to co-sleep, please make sure you do so safely, including researching the most up-to-date information about co-sleeping and sleep positioning.

I ask that you don't do anything just because you read it in this book; rather, I invite you to always view yourself as your own authority in parenting – and to first listen in to whether what you read resonates with you, and if you do, to try it out – and observe the behaviour of your baby, child, or teen afterwards. You are the researcher here. I will be talking about this process of you claiming your authority as a parent in more detail in the following pages.

Most of all, please listen to yourself. If you are concerned, please listen to that concern. You know your baby, child, or teen the most. I invite you to deeply trust your perceptions and intuition.

CONTENTS

Introduction

WELCOME

Hello and a big warm welcome to you!

Are you new to Aware Parenting? If so, what you read in the following pages may turn your understanding of sleep on its head. If you're already familiar with this approach, I'm so willing for this book to bring you even deeper clarity and more understanding about sleep from an Aware Parenting perspective.

Whether you're reading this to understand more about sleep for your baby, your child[3], or your teen, I will be inviting you to see sleep from a very different perspective to what is generally shared in this culture (which I call the *Disconnected Domination Culture*, or *DDC*[4]).

Changing our cultural beliefs can be a big and powerful process, and I'm sending you love if this book invites you to change your acquired ways of thinking.

I have a passion for compassion. I love to help parents be more compassionate with their children and themselves with whatever their own unique next steps are.

---

3   Please note that sometimes I will collectively refer to babies, children, and teens as 'children'. Please always adjust this to fit the age of your baby, child, or teen!

4   The Glossary shows which terms are from Aware Parenting, and which are from *The Marion Method*, like this one is.

What I won't be doing in this book

I don't have any 'shoulds' about parents practicing Aware Parenting, and I am unwilling to judge any parent.

- I **won't** tell you that you've been doing something *'wrong'*.
- I **won't** be *judging* you or *shaming* you.
- I **won't** be telling you that there are things that you *'should'* or *'shouldn't'* do.
- I **won't** be telling you *what to do.*

And in terms of theory and practice, there are also things I won't be telling you to do:

- I **won't** be suggesting you use concepts such as *sleep windows, sleep schedules, fighting sleep,* or *sleep regressions.*
- I **won't** be saying sleep is something to be s*chooled, trained, or learned.*
- I **won't** be suggesting that you *put up with* years of broken sleep.
- I **won't** be inviting you to teach your baby to *'self-soothe'* to go to sleep.
- I **won't** be teaching you to say, *"Calm down!"* when your child is playful before bed.
- I **won't** be telling you to *punish* your tween if they don't go to bed when you would like them to.
- I **won't** be suggesting you *threaten* your teen with 'consequences' if they want to stay up later than you.

Self-Compassion Moment

If you've done any or many of those things in the list above, I invite you to drop what I call the guilt stick. This is a part of reparenting yourself with The Marion Method[5]. Guilt is another form of cultural conditioning. I'll be talking lots about the guilt, shame, and self-judgment sticks, and I'll be inviting you to put them down!

How might you do that? Well, every time you notice yourself feeling guilty, or you become aware of judgmental thoughts about yourself, I invite you to say to yourself something like, "I'm not willing to judge myself." You might choose to think, "I am willing to be compassionate with myself instead."

If, after realising that we have done things that have been painful for our child, we stop judging ourselves, and are compassionate with ourselves instead, we may then feel sadness. Sharing our grief through crying with a loving listener can be an important part of our own process of healing. Feeling and expressing those feelings brings about a very different experience, compared to judging ourselves for what we did or didn't do.

When we acknowledge the effects that our actions and choices have made on our children, we can feel a lot of emotional pain, and if you connect with that as you're reading, I'm sending so much love to you. I know that mourning the results of my actions on my children has been really painful, so I understand if you experience that too.

Although this book is about sleep, I'm so willing for it to also support you on a path of getting free from guilt, shame, and self-judgment, and becoming deeply compassionate with yourself and your feelings as a parent. You might find that not only do you see the beauty of your child's crying, but you also find yourself welcoming your own tears. I'm here with you while you understand even more about your child's experiences, feelings, and needs, and the powerful influence you have on them, as well as gaining even more clarity about your own childhood experiences and their effects on you and your parenting.

---

5   *The Marion Method* is distinct from Aware Parenting. It includes reparenting and was influenced by Aware Parenting as well as other modalities.

What I will be doing in this book

I *will* be inviting you to:

- *listen in* to yourself and your sensations, feelings and thoughts as you read this book, and whether what you are reading *resonates* with *you*;

- gradually *drop cultural beliefs and assumptions* about sleep that you've learnt growing up in the *DDC* that *don't* actually *resonate* with you;

- *observe* your child to see what is *really* going on for them in relation to sleep;

- *see* your child's innate body wisdom for sleep that your cultural conditioning may have prevented you from seeing before, and which may have even been fighting against;

- *refrain* from *judging* or *shaming* yourself when you reflect on your past parenting;

- *learn* about the *two* core *elements* children need to feel relaxed enough to fall asleep;

- *understand* the *three ingredients* for relaxed and restful sleep;

- *work out which* of these three ingredients your child might be needing;

- get *clear* about what *you need* to be able to support them with what *they need*;

- take *action* in ways that bring about more sleep; and

- learn to *trust* your baby, child, or teen's body wisdom in relation to sleep.

Along the way, I'll also help you see how supporting your child with sleep will also mean that you're cooperating with their innate wisdom to heal from daily stresses and larger traumas. This is likely to have wonderful and far-reaching effects that *go way beyond* their sleep.

Most of all, I'm here to support you to deeply connect with yourself and your child and the innate wisdom you both have for profound relaxation and healing.

I imagine you might find that the outcome
is also more restful sleep.

Sleep is a sign. It's an emotional and physiological
barometer. Most of all, it's a reflection of the degree of
deep relaxation that is felt.

In this book, I'll offer ways to help you understand what your child's sleep-related behaviours are likely to be communicating, and how to create deep change that results in restful, relaxed, and restorative sleep.

I will also be repeating information throughout the book, for two reasons.

1. I assume that many people reading this might not be getting the sleep they need, and may not have much time or concentration to read an entire section of the book. So, I have made each chapter somewhat complete in itself.

This means that if you do have plenty of time and concentration, and you read a section or even the whole book from cover to cover, you will probably notice plenty of repetition. I'm sending love if you have feelings in response to this.

2. Much of this information is very different from what is commonly available to parents, and invites you as the reader to change your core beliefs. Because of that, I'm offering the repetition to support the process of you changing your ways of thinking about sleep (if what you read resonates and you are willing to change your thoughts about sleep).

What called you to read this?

I wonder what called you to pick up this book?

Becoming a parent?

- *Maybe you're going to become a parent soon, and you want to get more restful sleep than you see your parent friends getting, but you don't want to do 'controlled crying', or to leave your baby to 'cry-it-out', or to try to get them to 'self-soothe'?*

Do you have a baby?

- *Is your baby taking a long time to go to sleep, and you're spending longer and longer every evening jiggling them, or rocking them, or bouncing them while sitting on a fit ball, or pushing them in a stroller, or taking them out in the car, or feeding them? And are you thinking that there is surely something else going on here – and something you could be doing differently?*

- *Does your baby wake at the slightest sound, and you're at your wits' end, walking around on eggshells?*

- *Have you learnt about 'sleep windows', 'sleep regressions', and babies being 'overtired', and you're feeling confused and overwhelmed by the information? Maybe it doesn't quite make sense? Perhaps you're doing everything suggested, but something just doesn't feel right to you? Or are you feeling somewhat disconnected from your baby in this process?*

- *Are you on the verge of doing some form of 'controlled crying' because you're so desperate for sleep, but you're longing for there to be another way that doesn't involve leaving your baby alone with their feelings?*

- *Or have you already been doing some form of 'controlled crying' or 'cry-it-out', and you really don't want to be doing it anymore, but you just can't face going back to such broken nights?*

- *Perhaps you're co-sleeping and breastfeeding your older baby and you're wondering if it really is possible for you and your baby to have more restful sleep while continuing to co-sleep and breastfeed?*

Are you already into Aware Parenting?

- *Are you already practicing Aware Parenting and want to understand more nuances about how it applies to sleep?*

Are you the parent of a toddler?

- *Perhaps you've been practicing attachment parenting with your toddler and they're now waking up more and more frequently as the night goes on?*

- *Is your toddler wriggling around in bed for ages before sleep, and it really seems as though they just don't want to go to sleep, and you're confused or frustrated?*

- *Or maybe your co-sleeping toddler is restless through the night, moving all around the bed, and you're not getting much sleep at all, and you're thinking that putting them in their own bed in their own room is the only solution?*

- *Are you breastfeeding your toddler repeatedly throughout the night and wondering if it's what they really need? Does the feeding become more frequent as the night wears on? Are you feeling resentful, exhausted, or frustrated? Do you want to find a loving way to stop breastfeeding at night while continuing to co-sleep – and to breastfeed during the day?*

Are you the parent of a child?

- *Maybe your child experienced birth trauma or separation after birth, and you think that these experiences are affecting their sleep, but you don't know what you can do to help them heal (and sleep more restfully too!).*

- *Has your partner been sleeping in a separate bed for years while you co-sleep with your child, because you don't know how everyone can get their needs met – and it's affecting your relationship?*

- *Does your child get playful every evening before bed, and you've had enough of cajoling them into calming down?*

- *Does your child ask for a 'million' things before bed, and you get really frustrated – but don't know what to do except keep saying yes (and staying up half the night), or getting harsh with them (and feeling guilty afterwards)?*

- *Is your child going to bed later and later, and you're not getting enough sleep yourself as a result?*

- *Do you want to know whether your child is truly ready to go to sleep on their own without any harmful consequences?*

- *Does your child keep coming in to your room at night and you're confused about whether that is helpful for them and what you can do?*

- *Maybe your five-year-old seems to wake up feeling tired and grumpy and you're sure that they can sleep for longer, but you don't know how to help them?*

- *Or perhaps your seven-year-old still wants to co-sleep, you're worried about what your friends and family would say if they knew, and you want to understand if it's healthy for your child.*

- *Does your nine-year-old find it hard to go to sleep and you just don't know what to do?*

- *Do you want to know what age you can start trusting your child to choose what time they go to sleep – and what might happen as a result?*

Do you have a teen?

- *Is your teen wanting to chat with you every evening before sleep and you're feeling fed up because you just want to get some time for yourself, or even to go to bed earlier?*

- *Or is your teen coming to wake you up in the middle of the night to talk through things and you keep feeling really frustrated and reacting harshly?*

- *Is your teen staying up super late most nights and you've had enough with fighting with them to get them to go to bed earlier, but you just don't know what else to do?*

- *Or perhaps your teen is on screens and you keep feeling concerned about them – and worried about what other parents would think about you and your parenting if they knew?*

Are you a grandparent, health-care professional, or a carer of children?

- *Are you wanting to understand the Aware Parenting approach to sleep, and how and why it is so different from other paradigms?*

Love and compassion to you

Whatever called you here to be reading this, I welcome you here and send you lots of love. I'm passionate about compassion. Whatever brings you here, and however you're feeling right now, I welcome all your feelings. I'm here to share with you that it really is possible to stay deeply connected with your child (or to reconnect with them) and for you both to experience restful and restorative sleep most of the time.

How are you feeling as you read this? I'm here with you, and I'm sending compassion to your feelings, whatever they are.

I'm sending so much love to any tiredness or exhaustion you might feel because your:

- *baby* is taking 'forever' to get to sleep, or is waking up multiple times at night;
- co-sleeping *toddler* moves around in the bed all night;
- older *child* is wanting to play or talk for hours in the evening;
- *teen* and you are often fighting because they're not going to bed when you want them to.

My heart goes out to you if you're feeling physically uncomfortable because:

- your *baby* is breastfeeding all night long and you're waking up with a sore neck;
- your co-sleeping *toddler* is taking up all the space in the bed, and your back is painful;
- your *child* keeps on coming into your bed at night and needs to be glued to you to be able to sleep, and you're waking up with a sore shoulder;
- your *older child* or *teen* wants to play rough games before bed and you sometimes get physically hurt.

I'm offering empathy to your feelings if you're feeling powerless or frustrated because:

- you don't know how to help your *baby* sleep for longer stretches at night while staying true to your parenting values;

- your *toddler* always gets really rambunctious in the evening, and you don't seem to be able to get them to calm down;

- you want your *child* to go to bed at a particular time and you're having battles about it;

- your *teen* wants to be chatting to their friends all evening and is glued to the screen before bed, and you want them to be spending their evenings in a different way.

If you're feeling chronically tired, my heart goes out to you.

Parenting can be so much harder if we're tired, for three main reasons:

1. We may *feel uncomfortable physical sensations of tiredness* that are communicating that we need more sleep. This can make it hard to focus on all the things we need to do in our day-to-day lives;

2. We might *not have as much energy to respond* to our baby or child's needs and feelings, which might lead to disconnection and more challenging behaviour; and

3. When we're tired, *we are less able to suppress our painful feelings,* and so they're more likely to bubble up and out. If we're not having regular spaces and practices to feel and express our feelings in healing ways, those feelings can come out as harshness towards our children.

Self-Compassion Moment

I wonder if you're experiencing any or all of these? If so, I'm sending you so much compassion. If you're finding sleep challenging, my heart goes out to you.

BACKGROUND

Aware Parenting

This book is based upon Aware Parenting, a philosophy and set of parenting practices that were developed by Aletha Solter, PhD, a Swiss-American developmental psychologist who is an expert on attachment, non-punitive discipline, trauma, and healing from trauma.

Aware Parenting aims to see beyond cultural conditioning, to clearly identify the most helpful practices for babies, children, and teens to thrive physically, emotionally, mentally, and spiritually.

I'm incredibly grateful to Aletha Solter for her powerful and life-changing work and for her ongoing support and guidance. If what you read in these pages resonates with you, I invite you to read her beautiful, clear, and concise books, which you can find at the Aware Parenting Institute website: **www.awareparenting.com**.

How sleep challenges arise

A core cause of sleep challenges is the conflict between our innate body wisdom and the culture we live in.

Most sleep challenges for babies, children and teens arise because their bodies are adapted for when we were were hunter-gatherers, yet they live in the *Disconnected Domination Culture.*

Every culture has different beliefs about child-rearing, and has specific requirements for what is needed to survive and thrive in that particular society and climate. Those beliefs and parenting practices become deeply embedded during childhood, since each culture requires the people who live in it to continue the cultural practices and traditions into the next generation.

When we grow up in that culture, we believe that those thoughts and practices are the truth, rather than seeing them as culturally determined.

I will share about how so many of the parenting practices taught to parents at this time, particularly in relation to sleep, are set up to serve the culture we live in, but aren't actually the most beneficial or optimal for children's emotional, intellectual, and spiritual development.

In this book, I will be inviting you to clearly see your conditioning, as well as your child's innate needs and biological wisdom.

In this de-conditioning and relearning process, I will invite you to really understand, observe, and trust your child's innate body wisdom.

I'll be inviting you to be compassionate with yourself as you more clearly see your own conditioned beliefs.

I'm here to offer a deep understanding of *how* you can parent in ways that are *more* of a match for what children's bodies expect – and are capable of – in relation to sleep, *while* living in the *DDC*.

I'll also offer you information and opportunities to reflect on how your own childhood experiences of sleep may be getting in the way of you supporting your child to be able to sleep soundly and be securely attached.

I'll also explain how natural it is for our own beliefs, feelings, and past experiences to get in the way of our child's sleep, given that we are living in a culture where there is no recognition of the innate wisdom of babies, children, teens, and adults to feel deeply relaxed, and where that process is often actively worked against.

I'm so willing for this book to help you understand the *real* reasons why your child is doing whatever it is that they are doing regarding sleep. Not only that, I'm also willing for it to support you to know exactly *how* you can both get more restful sleep, as well as more of your other needs met too.

My background and experience

Before becoming a mother back in 2002, I was a Researcher in developmental psychology. Infant observation was key to both my Doctoral and Post-Doctoral work. These experiences have deeply influenced my passion to support parents in learning how to observe their children and be researchers themselves. I also had my own psychotherapy practice, where my clients consistently told me about the effects that not having their feelings welcomed as children was having on their adult lives. The practice of Aware Parenting welcomes children's feelings, which is one of the reasons why I'm so passionate about it.

I've worked with thousands of parents in the 19 years that I've been an Aware Parenting instructor.

However, so much of what I learnt about babies, children, teens, and sleep came from my experiences as a mother. I'm a mother of two, and as of October 2024, my daughter is 22 and my son is 18. I practiced all the elements of Aware Parenting with my daughter from when she was three months old (and the attachment-style parenting aspects of it from the beginning), and my son right from birth. As a result, they were both securely attached *and* slept restfully and soundly. Sleep during the night was never an issue in our home throughout their childhoods. They slept peacefully, restfully, and for long periods.

I did experience two challenging periods in relation to sleep, because at those times, I didn't understand all the relevant nuances of Aware Parenting, and because some of my own childhood experiences were affecting both my feelings and my responses. The first challenging time was when my daughter was 18 months old, and I was finding it increasingly hard to help her have a daytime nap. Later in the book, I explain that challenge from an Aware Parenting perspective, and how you can make it less likely that happens for you, if you have a baby or toddler. When my son was born, I knew exactly what to do so that the nap issue didn't happen with him. As a result, he continued to nap easily, until he naturally dropped his daytime nap once he no longer needed it.

The second time that things got challenging was when my son was

13. I will tell you more about exactly what happened in the section on teenagers. I wish I'd known then what I know now about teens and sleep from an Aware Parenting perspective. I'm so willing for what I learnt to be helpful for you when you are parenting a teen.

In fact, it was through Aletha Solter's edits of the initial draft of this book that I had a simple yet powerful insight into the exact causes of the challenges I experienced in my son's early teenage years. I'll be sharing that information with you in the section on teens. I wish I had made an appointment to have a consultation with her back then, as I had done when my children were younger.

It's something I often hear parents say. They wish that they had reached out for support from an Aware Parenting instructor earlier in their journey. They realise that this could have had a huge effect in speeding up the process of them learning and embodying Aware Parenting, and could have prevented them from experiencing unnecessary painful challenges. I invite you to hold this in mind as you read this book, knowing that there are many Aware Parenting instructors all over the world who can help you with implementing and embodying Aware Parenting.

The two apparent sleep options in this culture

In the past several decades in this culture, it has seemed that there are only two general and broad options with sleep with babies and young children, either:

1. to meet a baby's attachment needs with co-sleeping and breastfeeding, while believing that frequent night-waking is biologically normal and necessary for the first several years of a child's life, *or*

2. to help a baby sleep alone in a cot, either with swaddling, or a dummy, soft toy, or thumb-sucking, with various methods with titles such as 'controlled crying' or 'cry-it-out', or what's often called teaching them to 'self-soothe' or 'self-settle'.

In the first option, a baby's attachment needs are fulfilled, but sleep needs for baby and parent/s tend to be met less.

In the second option, parents often get much more sleep, but a baby's attachment needs are not met before and during sleep.

> ### Self-Compassion Moment
>
> I won't be judging you at any point in this book, and I'll be frequently inviting you to refrain from judging yourself! Here's a loving invitation from me. Whatever you have done, and whatever you are doing in your parenting, I invite you to be unwilling to judge yourself. You might say to yourself, "I'm not willing to judge myself or my parenting." I invite you to be deeply compassionate with yourself in your parenting journey. You have always had important reasons for doing what you did.
>
> When we understand the causes of our choices, and are unwilling to judge ourselves for what we did or didn't do in the past, we will be more able to welcome any mourning and sadness that we are invited to feel in relation the past. Then, we will be more able to parent in ways that are most a fit with our values now.

Aware Parenting offers 'the third way', which supports both secure attachment and restful sleep. It is significantly different from both of the other approaches. I will explain how in detail in this book.

I'll also explain what is going on physiologically in the three different approaches, and how that is related to the biological imperative that babies and children can go to sleep in whatever climate and culture they're born into.

The three main ideas underpinning this book

1. Sleep is so essential that there are *many* ways that babies and children *can* sleep.

Sleep is essential for survival, and given that humans can live in such different climates with such different requirements to survive in those environments, their biological wisdom means that there are many ways for babies, children, and teens to go to sleep and stay asleep. Sleep is more important than many other needs, so it is prioritised by the body.

There are two main outcomes that arise from the differences in sleep practices:

- The *quality* and *quantity* of sleep.
- The *effects* on emotional, intellectual, and spiritual development.

In this book, I will explain in detail what those outcomes are.

I will also share how Aware Parenting offers a way to help children to sleep restfully which also supports their optimal emotional, intellectual, and spiritual development.

2. There are three ingredients for relaxed, restful and restorative sleep.

These include both **intrinsic needs** and **innate body wisdom**. As parents, we often work against *one* or *both* of these. This is because we've commonly been given information that neither recognises nor understands the intrinsic needs babies and children have, nor the innate relaxation process that they are born with.

I will suggest specific and tangible actions that you can take that are in harmony with these three ingredients, to support your child to have restful and relaxed sleep.

The more you understand these three requirements, and the more you see evidence for them, the more you will be able to trust that your child innately knows how to sleep in a relaxed, restful, and restorative way.

You will probably see how your child has been inviting you to support them in that process, but because of other parenting beliefs, you may have been working against their intrinsic needs and/or innate relaxation processes.

This really turns around the belief that children often 'fight sleep', and replaces it with the understanding that it is often we as parents who are fighting against those natural processes.

Our long-term context with Aware Parenting is to support our baby and child so that they become a teen and then an adult who remains deeply connected with their innate body wisdom with these three ingredients, so that they can also sleep restfully at these older ages.

3. Modern day beliefs and parenting practices work against *some* - and sometimes *all* - of the three requirements for restful sleep.

The culture of most industrialised countries, the *Disconnected Domination Culture,* works *against* much of both our children's innate needs *and* their intrinsic biological wisdom (as well as our own). It does so through the thoughts and beliefs we acquire about sleep, and many of the sleep practices that are seen as normal.

We are born with intrinsic body wisdom, which, when supported, leads to deep relaxation.

I will be offering different ways of looking at and understanding sleep, based on what we can see in existing traditional cultures, as well as in modern research on attachment, trauma, and healing. I'll be repeatedly inviting you to listen in to what resonates with you as you read, and to be your own researcher in your parenting.

Aware Parenting invites us to return to a
deep trust in the wisdom of our bodies, a wisdom that
shines through whether we're talking about a baby,
child, teen, or adult.

INVITATIONS

I will repeatedly offer you two main invitations as you read this book:

1. To be unwilling to feel guilty (and to choose self-compassion instead).

I will be inviting you to be deeply compassionate with yourself and to drop what I call the '*emotional sticks*[6]', which are the guilt and shame sticks that we learn to metaphorically hit ourselves with, growing up in the *DDC*.

Guilt is a form – and result – of cultural conditioning, and as such, is something we can get free from (I know this, because I've done that for myself and have supported many other parents to do so, too).

I would love to support you in being much more compassionate with yourself as a parent. Parenting in the *DDC* is innately hard, for reasons I will go into in the book. I love supporting parents to be deeply compassionate with themselves, and to get free from shame and guilt. This is why I created *The Marion Method*. This is another part of freeing ourselves from harsh cultural conditioning.

Most of us were taught information that is set against our innate wisdom. Let's all be deeply compassionate with the younger parts of ourselves who needed to believe what we were told was true, as well as with our here and now selves who are living with the effects of that.

We were all once babies who came into the world with these intrinsic needs and wild wisdom.

We learnt to judge and guilt ourselves. Guilt and self-judgment are not innate to being human. They are cultural constructs[7]. However, it is

---

6 This is another *Marion Method* term.
7 I'm so grateful to Marshall Rosenberg for Nonviolent Communication, which is where I learnt this information.

absolutely possible to get free from guilt and self-judgment, and this is what I love supporting parents to do with *The Marion Method*.

It is also possible to look back and see what we didn't know in the past, without judging or shaming ourselves for what we did or didn't do.

Getting freer from those guilt, shame and other self-judgment sticks can also help us support our children with their innate biological wisdom even more. When we're compassionately listening to our feelings and needs and the true causes of our challenging parenting moments instead, we're more likely to be able to parent in alignment with our values.

You being more compassionate with yourself will also help your child.

I also invite you to imagine me walking beside you as you read this, offering you compassion and empathy, hearing your feelings and thoughts, and supporting you to have both more sleep, and more compassionate connection with yourself and your child. You might like to imagine me reaching out my hand to you, offering you my presence, letting you know that you're not alone as you take in this information. I'm right here with you.

2. To listen to whether you are willing to keep reading.

I invite you to check in with yourself regularly about whether you are willing to keep reading this book. Your willingness is your full-body yes[8]. Listening to our yeses and noes is key to *The Marion Method* work.

You might want to imagine me asking you every now and again:

- *Do you want to keep reading?*
- *Do you want to pause, be present with yourself, and mull over what you've read?*
- *Do you want to throw this book across the room!?* (I invite you *not* to do that if you're reading it on an iPad, tablet, or e-reader!)

---

8   Another *Marion Method* term

- *Would you like to do some journalling about your feelings and thoughts?*
- *Do you want to reach out to share your thoughts and feelings with an empathic listener?*

This is a huge journey. You might already be feeling exhausted. Taking in new information can be challenging, and can be even harder when we're tired. Finding the time to read this might in itself be a huge stretch for you. If that's the case, I'm sending you lots of loving compassion.

Although Aware Parenting can help us support our child to have more restful and restorative sleep, it also requires a lot from us, not only in the work of changing old beliefs, but also through putting it into practice, because that invites us to be with the uncomfortable feelings in us it will inevitably evoke at times.

It is certainly not a quick fix approach to sleep, but it can have incredibly transformative and long-term effects in *all* areas of a child's life, including sleep, as well as in the relationship between us and our child.

I deeply acknowledge your willingness to keep reading. And I support your no, if you want to stop at any time. I'm also sending love to every feeling that comes up in you as you take in these words.

You are the researcher

You might love evidence-based information. As you read this book, you might be wondering, "Is there any research about sleep and Aware Parenting?" To answer that question, there *aren't* any official studies about sleep and Aware Parenting at the time of writing this book. However, there is *anecdotal* evidence from many parents around the world who have transformed their children's sleep with the Aware Parenting approach.

I also have a radical suggestion for you, from my experience having been trained in infant and child observational research at Cambridge and Oxford Universities[9].

I invite you to be your own researcher.

You can find your own evidence during your own parenting journey!

The *first* part of the research involves listening in to yourself and to whether the information you read resonates with you.

If it *does*, the *next* part of the experiment is to try out whichever practice you've read about and resonate with.

Then, I invite you to observe your child, and compare what you see in them now with what you saw before, when you responded to them in the previous ways.

In the book, I'll suggest markers that you can look out for in your child which indicate an increase in relaxation – and a decrease in tension caused by stress and trauma.

I'll show you how to differentiate true relaxation from mild dissociation (and why that's so important in terms of sleep).

I'll explain about what you might observe, and how you can make sense of what you see.

You are the researcher.

You are there with your baby, child, or teen. I'm not there, seeing what you see.

Only through observing them clearly will you receive reassurance that what you're doing is helpful and is making a difference.

---

9   I did my PhD at Cambridge, and one of my PhD supervisors was at Oxford University, where I learnt some of the observation system that I used in my PhD.

In the *DDC*, we're taught to give away our power to outside authorities and to do what we're told to do. In contrast, I invite you to do the opposite – to *trust* yourself, to listen within, to do what resonates with you, and to trust your own observations of your child and what *they* show *you*.

I'm here to offer you information about sleep. You are the one who has the power to:

- *Listen in* to whether it *resonates* with you;
- *Experiment* with the practices that *do resonate*;
- *Make* your *own choices* about *your* parenting practices.

Trust yourself

I invite you to trust yourself in terms of whether any of this information calls you to explore more. Your intuition is powerful and you also have deep innate wisdom.

The most important question to keep asking yourself as you read this book is, "Does this resonate with me?"

I'm here with you. I trust your inner knowing.

A note on physiological causes of sleep issues

This book describes children's innate needs and intrinsic body wisdom in regards to sleep, with a focus on emotional needs.

There are many physiological causes of sleep issues.

Please see the Appendix for a partial list of possible physiological factors to check for first, as well as some recommendations for addressing these.

However, this book does not offer medical advice. Please see a trusted health practitioner if your child has physical pain or other health issues.

I invite you to check out whether there might be any physiological stressors or challenges which might be preventing your child from feeling deeply relaxed in their body – and thus to be able to sleep restfully and restoratively.

Once you've checked these possibilities off your list, you'll probably be more confident to support your child with both their innate needs and their intrinsic relaxation process for sleep.

One of the core aspects of Aware Parenting is to make sure that a child's needs are met. This is because the first aspect of Aware Parenting is attachment-style parenting, which includes prompt and attuned responsiveness to needs. Aware Parenting deeply values honouring children's intrinsic needs. The list in the Appendix – in addition to what you will read in the book – will help you to ensure you're meeting all of your child's needs in relation to sleep.

In addition, each child is unique in terms of what they are affected by, in their sensitivity levels, and in their own individual physiology.

In Aware Parenting, we invite parents to deeply understand the particularities of each individual child.

CHAPTER SUMMARY

There are three main ideas underpinning this book:

1. Sleep is so essential that there are *many* ways that babies and children *can* sleep.

2. There are *three* ingredients for relaxed, restful and restorative sleep.

3. *DDC* beliefs and parenting practices work *against* some (or at times, all) of the three ingredients for restful sleep.

I will repeatedly offer you two main invitations as you read this book:

1. To be *unwilling* to feel guilty (and to choose self-compassion instead).

2. To listen to whether you are *willing* to keep reading.

There are two main outcomes that arise from the differences in sleep practices:

1. The *quality* and *quan*tity of sleep.

2. The *effects* on emotional, intellectual, and spiritual development.

I invite you to check through the list of other physiological causes of sleep issues if you are ever concerned that there is something else going on, and to always trust your intuitive sense of what is going on for your child.

I trust your innate wisdom
and your intuition.

THE LAYOUT OF THIS BOOK AND SUGGESTIONS FOR HOW TO READ IT

The book is divided into five main parts:

- The first is about *general principles* of Aware Parenting and sleep.
- The second is about babies, (0-2 year olds).
- The third is about children, (2-12 year olds).
- The fourth is about teens, (13-19 year olds).
- The fifth section includes a concluding chapter plus a summary and glossary.

Suggestions and invitations for how to read the book:

- I invite you to start with the general principles *first*, and *then* either go through the rest of the book in order, or skip to the section that's most relevant to you.
- *I invite you to trust yourself and what you're called to read.*
- Or, after reading the first section, you might just use the book more like a dictionary or manual, reading the parts that are most relevant to you.
- Or perhaps you'd like to refer to it more like you would an oracle, opening it at random and reading the page that you turn to.
- *I trust you and the way you are called to both read this book, and to respond to what you read.*
- If you have a teen, you might still like to read the sections about babies and children, to help you understand your teen's early experiences even more.
- If you have a baby or child, you might enjoy reading about the older age group too, so you know what may be helpful in preparation for the years in the future.
- **I invite you to *trust* the exact way *you* feel called to read it.**

Lots of love xoxo

PART 1

General Principles

1. Biology, culture, and parenting

The Continuum Concept

In the *'About the author'* chapter, I shared about the dramatic effect that reading *The Continuum Concept* had on me in 1992, when I was doing my PhD at Cambridge University. I'd love to share more about my *aha* moment with you and why that is so relevant to this book.

After that, I'll talk more about why I think that understanding the effects of both biology and culture on parenting is so important, especially in regard to sleep.

On the day I found The Continuum Concept *in that little old secondhand bookshop, I went back to my post-graduate student room, and sat in the bay window, with the dappled sunshine shining through the light green leaves. As I read about the Yequana people, my previous 24 years of cultural conditioning about babies was swept away. I cried and cried, reading about all the closeness that babies received in the Yequana community.*

This grief was particularly deep for me. I experienced the usual separation and disconnection of babies born in the late 60s and early 70s in England, where cots were standard, and co-sleeping was rare. However, I also experienced much more isolation, because I was born prematurely and was in an incubator for the first five weeks after my birth.

Reading about babies' innate expectations and needs for closeness in The Continuum Concept *struck a deep chord within me. Finally, what I'd felt in my body for the previous 24 years – but had not yet understood – was being articulated. Deep loss and sadness poured out of me, in the form of tears and sobbing.*

As a baby, I hadn't experienced the closeness that I innately expected to experience, and the effects on me had been profound. In fact, it was those early experiences – and the deep grief and terror that I carried around with me as a result – that had called me to study psychology in the first place, followed by researching the mother-baby relationship for my PhD.

The phrase 'the continuum concept' is based on the idea that babies innately need experiences that have helped human beings to survive. These experiences have been universal for babies over millennia. They are thus expectations that all babies come into the world having, called 'continuum expectations'. In Western industrialised cultures, they are often neither understood nor met.

Many modern parenting practices that are required for the culture to continue are very different to what babies and children actually need to thrive emotionally, intellectually, and spiritually.

For millennia, babies experienced natural birth, breastfeeding, co-sleeping, plenty of closeness, responsive care, and expectations that they innately wanted to connect, cooperate, and become competent members of the culture.

When I first read *The Aware Baby* by Aletha Solter, PhD, nearly a decade after I read *The Continuum Concept*, I saw how Aletha Solter's theories about the innate needs of babies and children included an even deeper understanding of cultural contexts than I'd learnt about up until then.

Aletha Solter wrote, *"All over the world, parents raise their children to become productive members of their specific cultures. Parenting fosters the development of different values depending on their religious or cultural beliefs, as well as the requirements for survival, whether these are cooperation or obedience, dependence or independence, creativity or conformity, sharing or ownership, humility or pride. Parents also emphasize the development of social, motor, memory, language, or reasoning skills depending on what will best serve the child later on in life. Parents transmit their cultural values, expectations, and skills to their babies in a myriad of ways: by how the parents respond to crying, how much they hold their babies, what kinds of stimulation they offer, how often they feed them, where the babies sleep, and how they set limits. In most cultures, these traditions are assumed to be the "natural" and correct way to treat babies......*

*However, no culture is perfect. In most cases, **the cultural values and economic constraints force parents to impose certain restrictions on their children and ignore legitimate needs, such as the need to express emotions, to be fully accepted, or to explore freely in a safe environment.** The fact that infants survive and grow up able to carry on the culture and reproduce **does not imply that their basic human needs have been met, or that they have attained their human potential for intellectual, emotional, or spiritual development.** (The Aware Baby, pages 1-2). [emphasis mine].*

Later on, she wrote:

*"This new approach [Aware Parenting] is not based only on the requirements of our particular culture. **It also recognizes deep and universal human needs that must be met if babies are to grow up emotionally healthy in any culture.**" (The Aware Baby, page 3). [emphasis mine].*

Aware Parenting differentiates between parenting practices that are designed to meet children's innate needs that help them thrive, and those that are in place to help children to fit into – and continue recreating – the specific culture they are born into.

Reading *The Aware Baby* intensified my already strong calling to understand more about these differences.

Humans are incredibly adaptable to the conditions we find ourselves in, including the climate, geography, and available resources. Each culture has parenting practices that are relevant to their own time and place, but which don't necessarily generalise to other cultures, times, and places. Parenting practices also change over time *within* cultures.

Because humans are both highly adaptable, and deeply affected by cultural parenting beliefs and practices, I believe that it's important for us to understand the cultural contexts of parenting practices, particularly in relation to sleep.

However, in the *Disconnected Domination Culture*, part of our conditioning teaches us to *extract* information and practices from other cultures *without* understanding the importance of the wider context, including cultural beliefs, climate, geography, resources, society, and economy.

Sleep is so vital that babies, children and teens are able to sleep, whatever the climate or culture, through many different methods. However, these different approaches lead to a great variety in both the quality and quantity of that sleep. They also have profound effects on other aspects of a child's development.

In this book, I will explain how the capacity of children to sleep in every climate and culture is reflected in the multitude of sleep practices we see, both around the world and within the *Disconnected Domination Culture (DDC)*.

I will explain how, in industrialised cultures, many of us have been influenced by what other cultures do regarding parenting and sleep, but often without understanding the full cultural context in which these practices originally came about.

I'll talk about the three main categories of parenting that are practiced in industrialised countries, and how one of them was affected by observing practices of traditional cultures in very hot climates.

In very cold climates, *many* Indigenous cultures had different parenting practices. Later, I'll explain why understanding this is important in terms of the sleep practices which exist in the society that we live in.

Having hunter-gatherer bodies in the *Disconnected Domination Culture*

Most sleep challenges with babies and children occur because their bodies are still adapted to a hunter-gatherer lifestyle.

Parenting (including in relation to sleep) is so hard for many parents because of two core effects of the *DDC*:

- The nuclear family set up, which makes it hard for both parents and children to get their needs met.
- The cultural beliefs and parenting practices which aren't in accordance with the innate wisdom of children's hunter-gatherer bodies.

We know that for hundreds of thousands of years, humans lived in multigenerational groups with familial and tribal bonds. One or two parents caring for children for long periods is very different to what happened for millennia. Living in communities – where many people shared the care of the children – supported both parents' and children's needs for closeness and support.

Many sleep practices that are taught to parents are based on cultural beliefs, rather than on children's biological needs and inbuilt wisdom.

In contrast, Aware Parenting both supports the meeting of children's intrinsic needs and trusts the innate wisdom of their bodies – within this modern society. It also invites parents to find ways to meet their own needs alongside their children's.

Having our needs met and our feelings heard as parents is central to being able to parent in this way.

Children's bodies are very similar to those of our ancient ancestors. However, sleep beliefs and practices in Western industrialised nations have radically changed.

I believe that it's important that we understand our innate body wisdom and learn from both our hunter-gatherer past and present-day Indigenous cultures as well as non-Western cultures. This helps us clearly know what children need for secure attachment and sound sleep, so we can adapt what we do as parents to support their innate sleep processes, while still living in the modern world. Thus, we are more likely to be able to offer our children what they *really* need to grow up and flourish as deeply self-connected beings.

Learning about other cultures and sleep can help us see our own cultural beliefs more clearly.

When my children were young, I would regularly think about the Mediterranean approach to sleep, where children often stayed up late to have dinner along with the rest of the family. I would also recall documentaries I'd watched, of Indigenous cultures in hot climates where children slept in hammocks with the rest of the community. This helped me see how I had been affected by the place and time of my own upbringing. In the UK in the seventies, babies slept in cots in nurseries and children were often 'put to bed' alone in their own rooms at the same time every night, whether it was summer or winter, and regardless of whether they were tired or not. Thinking about the sleep practices in other cultures helped me feel much more comfortable to do things differently with my family's sleeping arrangements, compared to my own past experiences, as well as to what I saw parents around me doing.

In the *Disconnected Domination Culture*, there is an emphasis on early independence, which is reflected in many present-day parenting practices. The cultural beliefs are that it's important for babies and toddlers to become independent early on, including for sleep.

From an Aware Parenting perspective, we see that this is a reflection of what the culture needs in order to continue, rather than being in service of the most optimal emotional development of the child.

Self-Compassion Moment

I want to remind you that I'm not judging you, and I invite you to be unwilling to judge yourself. We are meant to be deeply affected by the culture we grow up in and live in. When we were growing up, we needed to believe that the things we saw around us were just the way things were. Seeing things differently to our cultural conditioning naturally requires a lot from us. For the survival of a society, cultural conditioning is strong and hard to change. Changing the beliefs and practices that were passed down to us can lead us to feel overwhelmed, uncomfortable, or confused. I'm sending so much love to you, however you're feeling when you read this.

I will be inviting you to keep enquiring into your cultural conditioning throughout this book – and I'm sending you loving compassion if you take up my offer to do so, because this can be an uncomfortable process at times, particularly when we discover that what we thought was true isn't actually the case.

In addition, if we want to avoid feeling guilty as parents, it's vital that we differentiate between taking in new information, and judging ourselves for not knowing what we are now learning. If you want to keep growing as a parent, you will keep learning new things that you didn't know before. This is likely to happen even more if you're wanting to practice Aware Parenting, which has many beliefs and practices that are different to those that you may have grown up with and probably see all around you still.

I invite you to be deeply compassionate with yourself for not knowing earlier what you know now, or are learning now. Just as we wouldn't be willing to judge a toddler who doesn't yet know how to write, we can be unwilling to judge ourselves for what we didn't know in the past. You might say to yourself something like, "I'm not willing to judge myself for not knowing this information before. I am willing to be compassionate with myself, to feel my sadness and mourn that I didn't know this before, and even to celebrate myself for being willing to learn new things and change old beliefs." I wonder how you feel in your body if you experiment with a phrase like that?

Comparing traditional parenting practices in very hot and very cold climates

In many cultures with very *hot* climates, babies are (or were) generally carried most of the time, with skin-to-skin contact, often by the mother (for easy and quick access to breastfeeding to prevent dehydration), but also by other members of the community[10], often grandmothers and fathers. Babies generally sleep in the daytime while being carried and while the mother or others go about their day-to-day activities. During the night, babies and children sleep close with their family or wider community.

In some very *cold* climates before modern housing and efficient heating systems (and in traditional cultures still existing today), babies were wrapped warmly and sometimes swaddled before being carried next to the mother's body, or were carried naked within their mother's big coat. In *some* cultures, at *some* times, there would have been more separation during the *daytime*, such as with the use of a wooden carrier (sometimes called a cradleboard), carried on the adult's back, which meant less experience of closeness for the baby[11]. In yet other cultures, there may have been even more distance between parents and babies, with the baby being attached to a sled. Babies have less of a need for frequent breastfeeding in colder climates because there is a lower risk of dehydration. In addition, less frequent, but longer feedings allow babies to get more of the hind milk, which is rich in fat and takes longer to digest. However, *at night*, babies and children slept close with their siblings and parents and perhaps their wider community, depending on the size of housing structures they were sleeping in.

Aradia Wyndham[12] explains the effects of different climates and geographical regions on carrying infants. In Northern Europe, hard carriers created a microclimate of warm moist air. They were used to

---

10 "40 out of 48 cultures studied in the tropics had close and frequent physical contact", Whiting: Hewlett, Barry S. (2017). Hunter-Gatherer Childhoods: Evolutionary, Developmental, and Cultural Perspectives

11 In the same study, Whiting found that 29 out of 37 societies outside the tropics used heavy swaddling or cradleboards. Two exceptions are the Eskimo and the Yahgan of Patagonia, which both kept babies in close contact.

12 The Baby Historian: https://thebabyhistorian.com/

keep babies away from cold surfaces and could be either carried or propped up. Geographical climates would determine whether carriers were made of wood or textiles.

For time immemorial, babies have been carried while adults were working and would sleep whenever they needed. However, in some cultures, these attachment practices stopped many centuries ago. As cultures changed from hunter-gatherer to agricultural to industrialist to technological to the information age, parenting practices, particularly in relation to closeness, sleep, and feeding, changed too.

We could also hypothesise that increased physical distance between babies and mothers, including for sleep – such as with cribs then cots, prams, and strollers – began in some colder climates and spread around the world with colonisation and industrialisation.

In later chapters I will talk about these cultural differences in more detail, and why knowing about them is important if we are to truly understand present-day sleep practices.

Swaddling and other constraints

Swaddling, where babies are wrapped and are unable to move, has been common in many cultures for hundreds of years. Swaddling was practiced by the ancient Greeks, Romans, and Jews, and was still used in the Middle Ages in Europe. It was also practiced in areas of Eastern Europe and Japan.

In *some* traditional cultures in very *cold* climates, babies were often swaddled for warmth and then *also* carried, such as in the hood of their mother's coat. However, in *warmer* climates (*but not in very hot areas*, where swaddling would present a risk of overheating), swaddling was used in some cultures during post-hunter-gatherer eras to keep a baby immobile and separate from adults, who then engaged in their daily tasks away from their babies.

As Robin Grille shares in his book *Parenting for a Peaceful World*, in England and America until the 18th century and France and Germany until the 19th century, swaddled babies were tied to wooden boards and hung up on hooks where they were left alone for hours. Hundreds-of-years-old traditions in places such as Tajikistan include keeping babies bound within a special cradle called a Gahvora, in some cases for the majority of the day and night. This not only freed up parents to complete tasks without carrying infants, but was seen as important to help babies develop the qualities that were important to the culture.

In the next few chapters, I will explain why infants who were swaddled past early infancy – or who were left alone in cradles – stop crying, and what this tells us about what's going on for babies in modern-day sleep practices of ongoing swaddling and cots.

Self-Compassion Moment

I'm sending you lots of loving compassion if you're feeling any painful feelings when you read this. I invite you to put down any guilt sticks you might be tempted to pick up!

When the cultural sleep practices fit with the culture

In most traditional cultures, there is a fit between core survival needs and the parenting practices.

For example, in traditional cultures in *very hot* climates, babies are carried everywhere by their mother and a variety of adults, such as grandmothers and fathers, and sometimes by children. They are frequently fed to sleep or carried while the mother is working, and they fall asleep while being carried. That sleeping arrangement is a fit, because there are many people to help with the carrying, and because the cultural expectations are that people's bodies are inherently strong enough to carry babies and toddlers. In the evening, where babies fall asleep while co-sleeping and breastfeeding, feeding and night waking also fits in with cultural expectations, especially in places where everyone is somewhat wakeful during the night, because of all the possible dangers from predators or other possible perils.

In *very cold* climates in traditional cultures, babies might be carried bare within their mother's furs, but are more commonly swaddled on their mother's back or on a cradleboard or sled. They will often fall into a deep sleep because of the combination of the movement, being swaddled or within warm coverings while it's very cold, as well as the greater consumption of hind milk high in fat. At night, they may wake less frequently, again because of this combination of cold temperature and heavy clothing and coverings. Those practices work in that culture, because the babies are prepared for the hardship of living in such a cold climate, and to keep warm, and in some cultures, for separation[13].

There may be emotional costs to the baby in each case, but for the parents, and for the babies who grow up to become adults who continue those cultures, the practices are a fit.

In Indigenous cultures, parents don't generally wait until babies and children go to sleep to do what they want or need to do, because the culture is set up for everyone to live and work together.

There are usually plenty of people around to support everyone to get their needs met.

We can imagine that in many traditional cultures where there is community-based living, children might roam around in the evening, playing, dancing around a fire if there is one, or joining in with any music or drumming that the community created. We can see how they might easily release some pent up feelings and tension through vigorous play.

In many traditional cultures, when children are older, are no longer breastfeeding, and don't need as much closeness, they have freedom to choose when they go to sleep in the evening. They also have responsibility for the consequences of their sleep choices.

This is also a fit within the cultures they live in, where children are perceived to be learning to be competent members of that culture.

---

13 As an aside, we can see how modern-day baby carriers have evolved from these different types of carriers in different climates and cultures, with more recent versions of both soft wraps, slings, Asian-style (Meh Dai) carriers, and more structured back carriers with metal frames.

Why do so many children and adults have sleep challenges in the *DDC*?

What has happened in the **DDC** *that sleep challenges are so common in families? Why are the practices no longer a fit between the children, the parents, and the culture?*

One of the reasons why certain practices and their 'effects' are no longer a fit is because of newer inventions which now meet basic needs, such as using houses, cots, and baby monitors to keep babies safe. From the parents' perspective, the baby or young child is safe at night, sleeping alone in their own cot in their own room. However, babies and young children don't *experience* the same physiological sense of safety as they would when sleeping close to their family.

The parents know that their baby is safe, but the sense of safety is not felt by the baby.

This is why I am so passionate about seeing the world through a child's eyes. For a parent, knowing that their baby is in a cot – and cannot move anywhere, with a baby monitor – and having infomation about whether the baby is awake or asleep, can meet their needs for reassurance that the baby is safe. However, for a baby, if they cannot feel the presence of others, their survival system is on alert. Once a baby becomes mobile, being unable to get out of the cot might also be experienced by them as not safe, because they cannot flee if they need to.

From a mother: My baby is all snug and safe, swaddled up and cosy in the beautiful cot I bought for her. I love her so much. I put her in the cot, and I have the baby monitor on. I would love to just hold her and gaze at her, but everyone has been telling me that it's important that she becomes independent. I guess it's just my needs to be close and she doesn't need me. I do also have so much to do, anyway, when she's asleep. She is safe, I know that, because I can see her and hear her on this video monitor I bought. She clearly doesn't need me, because she's fallen asleep now.

From a baby: Where is everyone? What is going on? When will Mummy come back to me? There are all kinds of shapes and shadows. I can't hear a heartbeat, or voices. There is no-one here but me. Am I safe? My mouth makes this shape and movement. Mummy said I was yawning. Is it safe for me to sleep? I love being with Mummy. Where is she? I love how she smells and feels. I am one with her. We are one together. I call out but she doesn't come. I try to move but nothing happens. I don't even really know how to make different parts of my body move yet. I don't know what all the parts of my body are called, but I try again. Usually that makes the parts move, but this time, nothing happens. It's so strange, because the more I cannot move, the more fuzzy I feel. I'm staring at the shadow on the bars for eternity. Staring but not really seeing. I am falling asleep.

Self-Compassion Moment

I'm sending so much love to you, however you feel when you read this. As you will hear from me many times in this book, it's so normal for our feelings to bubble up at times like this. I invite you to notice what you're feeling. If it's guilt, I'm sending loving compassion to you and all the parts of you who learnt to judge yourself. I invite you to drop the guilt stick. I'm not judging you and I invite you to be unwilling to judge yourself. You might say, "I'm not willing to judge myself." If you're feeling sad, perhaps because either your baby was or is in a cot, or you're thinking of yourself in a cot, I'm sending so much love to your sadness. You might feel outrage or fear or some other feeling, and my heart goes out to you. It's part of our own wise healing system for our own painful feelings to bubble up from the past. Or you might feel a bit numb or dissociated. I'm sending you loving compassion. I invite you to do some journalling or reach out to a loving listener to have your feelings heard.

Another reason for the mismatch is the changes in the structure of society. When there are many people to care for babies and young children, where there are no fixed work hours, and where there's flexibility for parents to have naps, frequent night waking can be manageable and comfortable for all.

In contrast, when there is just a single parent or two parents doing much of the care for babies and young children, often also including work schedules to earn money, frequent night waking can become a challenge for the parent/s getting their own sleep needs and other needs met.

In very cold countries, teaching babies to get used to the hardship of a cold climate and independence may no longer be needed, such as with the technology of efficient heating and more indoor and sedentary lifestyles, so parents may be left wondering whether swaddling and separation are necessary for babies.

In modern nuclear families, it's often harder for parents to get their needs met while their babies and children are awake, so having a set bedtime, so that the parent/s know that they have time 'for themselves' each evening, is a direct result of a lack of community. Set bedtimes can often bring huge stress into families.

Other cultural developments have brought in new challenges, including beliefs about the importance of early independence, as well as separate sleeping areas for babies and young children, fixed bedtimes, school and work schedules, books, and screens.

Without community support, nor community gatherings with music and dancing, children often don't have the freedom to release tension through wild movement and play during the evening, and are often encouraged to 'calm down'.

In present-day 'modern' cultures, older children and teens are often not trusted in their desire to become competent members of society. So, rather than believing in their innate wisdom to make choices about their sleep, parents are taught to control their bedtimes, leading to friction with a teen's innate desire for competence, autonomy, and self-determination.

There have also been changes in perceptions of the emotional needs of babies, children, and teens that have entered the cultural consciousness with research into infant and child development and understandings from child and adult psychotherapy. This means that practices that may have been seen as acceptable in the past may no longer be seen that way.

The combination of the availability of new inventions, plus changes in social structures, expectations, and perceptions, all lead to parents finding certain elements of sleep that might previously have been accepted and acceptable, as challenging and stressful, particularly:

- babies, children, and teens going to sleep *late*;
- babies and toddlers *waking frequently* throughout the night;
- babies and children *wanting to be close* throughout the night; and
- children and teens *wanting to choose when* they go to sleep.

In this chapter, I have not included much infomation about the extra element in Aware Parenting that babies, children and teens all have innate body wisdom to deeply relax rather than dissociate before sleep. This deep relaxation can profoundly affect points one and two in the list above: the lateness when children go to sleep, and frequent night waking. I will talk about this more in the next chapter.

> When we practice Aware Parenting, we become detectives and experimenters, ready to discover exactly how our child (from infancy to young adulthood) is inviting us to support them to experience relaxed sleep *and* optimal emotional wellbeing, *within* the culture we live in (while also getting our own needs met, including for sleep).

Self-Compassion Moment

I wonder how you're feeling now? I'm sending so much love to you, however you're feeling, and whatever you're thinking. I want to remind you that it's so natural for us to feel uncomfortable when we are invited to see our core beliefs as beliefs rather than 'the truth'. If that's going on for you right now, my heart goes out to you, and to whatever feelings you might be feeling.

Repeatedly throughout this book, I will invite you to: connect in with yourself; notice what resonates with you; try out the practices; and observe your child.

Through observing your child, then experimenting with practices that resonate with you, and observing your child again, you will understand what is really going on for them. When you increasingly *trust* yourself and your child, and know *how* to observe, *how* you can experiment, and *what* to look for, you really can bring about significant change, not only in sleep, but in many other areas of how your child *feels* and *behaves*.

In this way, I'm inviting you to look beyond cultural beliefs and dictates, to what your own **unique** *baby, child or teen needs, and how you can most support them to flourish* **within** *the culture you live in (while also honouring your own needs and feelings).*

CHAPTER SUMMARY

Many modern parenting practices are very different to what babies and children actually need to thrive emotionally, intellectually, and spiritually.

Aware Parenting differentiates between parenting practices that are designed to meet innate needs, and those that are in place to help children to fit into – and continue creating – the specific culture they live in.

Different sleep approaches lead to a great variety in both the quality and quantity of children's sleep. They also have profound effects on other aspects of their development.

In many traditional cultures, there is a fit between the core survival/ economic needs and beliefs – and the parenting practices.

In many industrialised cultures, the combination of the availability of new inventions, plus a change in social structures, expectations, and perceptions, all lead to parents finding certain elements of sleep that might previously have been accepted and acceptable, as challenging and stressful.

Changing our ways of seeing things can be very uncomfortable. I'm here with you if you're in the middle of changing old beliefs right now.

2. Aware Parenting, sleep, and our hunter–gatherer ancestors

The three aspects of Aware Parenting and how they relate to sleep

I'd love to start by explaining more about the three core aspects of Aware Parenting, and how they relate to trusting children's innate body wisdom in relation to sleep.

I'll also explain how knowing about the lives of our hunter-gatherer ancestors helps us understand what's really going on with children's sleep today.

The three aspects of Aware Parenting are:

1. Attachment-style parenting.
2. Non-punitive discipline.
3. The *prevention* of stress and trauma – and supporting the *healing* from those when they do occur – through children's innate healing processes of crying, raging, and vigorous movement, as well as play and laughter, in the context of a loving parent-child relationship.

1. Attachment-style parenting

Attachment-style parenting has been influenced by:

- attachment research since the middle of the 20th century[14];
- observations of Indigenous cultures, as well as other societies around the world; and
- information about our likely heritage from our hunter-gatherer ancestors.

One of the main tenets of attachment-style parenting is offering plenty

---

14 Bowlby proposed that the attachment-forming processes of human infants evolved in a context of hunting and gathering.

of closeness and responsiveness to babies and young children, both day and night.

This is a match with the needs of babies and children since hunter-gatherer times, where closeness would have been required for safety (before houses and baby monitors), as well as warmth in colder climates (before efficient heating).

In *The Aware Baby*, Aletha Solter says:

*"The strong desire of human babies to sleep near their mothers may have its basis in our evolutionary history. During the hunter-gatherer stage of our species' existence babies would have been extremely vulnerable to predators and cold weather, especially at night. **Infants who feared the dark and who refused to sleep alone had a much better chance of surviving than those infants who did not complain when put down.** So there was strong selective pressure in favor of such fears. **Although predators are no longer a threat, and we have heated homes, modern human infants' reflexes, instincts, and needs are still geared to the hunter-gatherer way of life.** "* (page 99). [emphasis mine].

During the night, it's likely that whatever the weather or work that happened during the day, babies and young children in *all* cultures and climates would have slept close to their mother and other family members at night. This was for *safety*, as well as for access to *breastfeeding* for younger babies (particularly in warm climates), and for warmth in cold climates.

Babies and young children sleeping alone in rooms separate from adults is a relatively recent phenomenon in human history. Inventions such as houses, baby monitors, and efficient heating have presented new ways of offering safety and warmth.

But biologically, babies and children's bodies are still adapted to living in the wild.

This knowledge has profound implications for sleep.

The results of attachment-style parenting are not only safety and secure attachment. They include independence (or more accurately, interdependence) at a child's own timing and pace. The outcome of secure attachment is a child who knows that they are safe to explore their world, while also knowing that support is there if and when they need it. This is relevant to sleep for older children and teens, as I'll talk about later in the book.

> ### Self-Compassion Moment
> I'm sending you so much love if you didn't know about attachment theory or attachment-style parenting, and if you're now wishing you had known about it. Whatever the age of your child, you can always offer them more connection, closeness, and responsiveness, and you can support them to be more securely attached. If you're tempted to hit yourself with a guilt stick right now, I invite you to put that down, with a phrase such as, "I'm not willing to hit myself with a guilt stick." Instead, I invite you to have compassionate thoughts towards yourself as you continue to read. You might find that you feel sadness if you are learning things that you didn't know before. Being with the sadness we feel, although painful, is a very different experience to judging ourselves. If you're feeling sad, I'm sending compassion to your sadness, and invite you to express it to a loving listener.

2. Non-punitive discipline

When practicing Aware Parenting, one of our aims is to search for – and attend to – the underlying causes of any challenging behaviours, including those related to sleep. In Aware Parenting, these reasons fall into one of three categories:

i. a need for information;

ii. present moment needs; or

iii. unexpressed pent-up painful feelings from past stressful or traumatic experiences.

When we are responding at this causal level, we don't need to turn to punishments or rewards, bribing, shaming, coercing, forcing, or guilting children into doing things. Those methods all have non-optimal effects on a child's emotional wellbeing.

Non-punitive discipline is particularly relevant when we're talking about sleep for older children and teens. I'll be talking more about this later in the book.

This approach to understanding – and responding to – children, is very different from what is taught to parents in the *Disconnected Domination Culture*. It's thus normal for this to be new information for many parents. We are invited to change our core beliefs about human nature and the causes of behaviour, including sleep. This process can be uncomfortable and can take some time.

Self-Compassion Moment

I'm sending so much love to you if you've felt frustrated or powerless when your child wasn't going to bed – or wasn't falling asleep – when you wanted them to, and if you've tried to bribe, punish, or reward them to make them go to bed. Our own feelings of powerlessness (including from our childhood) can easily bubble up at times like this, especially if we're tired, or we're waiting for our child to go to sleep before we meet our own needs – including for sleep – or attend to our long list of things to do. At times like this, understanding the importance of our own needs and feelings is also vital if we're to avoid using punishments and rewards.

I wonder if you've found yourself resorting to threats, bribes, punishments, or rewards when you are desperate for some time for yourself in the evening, and are longing for your child to go to sleep or to go back to sleep? If so, I'm sending you so much compassion. Or perhaps you've felt powerless when you're tired and want to go to sleep and your older child or teen wants to stay up? Maybe, in that powerlessness, you've turned to power-over, or have been tempted to harshly threaten or punish them? If so, my heart goes out to you as you recall those times.

In later sections, I'll be talking about supporting and trusting older children and teens in relation to when they go to sleep. That can be transformative for us as parents!

The more we *understand* the *true* reasons for sleep challenges, the more we can address them at that *causal* level.

3. The prevention and healing of stress and trauma

From an Aware Parenting perspective, we understand that despite everything we might do to protect our children from stress and trauma, *all* babies, children, and teens *do* experience stress and minor traumas, and *many also* experience bigger traumas.

We also recognise that children from birth onwards have an innate way to heal from stress and trauma, and will inherently keep searching for opportunities to do so – through special forms of play and laughter, as well as crying and raging while moving vigorously – in the context of a loving parent-child relationship.

For *pre-crawling babies*, this always means crying in arms.

For *toddlers* and *young children*, this means crying, raging, and playing with our loving support.

Older children and *teens* talk to express and share their painful feelings, although they may still need to cry with us, or express outrage, or be playful and laugh after stressful experiences.

Understanding the effects of stress and trauma – and children's innate healing processes – is central to knowing why so many babies and children take a long time to go to sleep, wake up frequently at night, and wake up very early in the morning, and why so many teens have sleep challenges.

This clarity gives us specific practices to support children to naturally sleep more restfully and peacefully. I'll be sharing these with you later in the book.

Modern life has sources of stress and trauma which weren't present in the lives of our hunter-gatherer ancestors, such as disconnection from community living, the land, the seasons, meaningful traditions, and rites of passage. There's also all the extra stimulation, such as the noise and speed of cars and other machines, such as phones and computers, as well as the stresses and time pressure of school, jobs, productivity, competition, and so on.

There would have been stressful and traumatic events in our hunter-gatherer ancestors' lives, such as tribal or territorial fighting, disease, and predators, as well as accidents and natural disasters. However, it is possible that some of the effects were ameliorated by the degree of community support people experienced during times of stress.

We don't really know the extent to which the innate healing processes were understood or utilised in hunter-gatherer times, and there are few, if any, reports of this understanding in current traditional cultures.

The cultural beliefs of anthropologists – and their lack of recognition of the innate healing process of crying and raging – means that it's likely that any crying and raging they did observe in other cultures would *not* be perceived as a healing process. This is the case with reports where children in some traditional cultures cry a lot (sometimes for weeks or months) when mothers are no longer willing to breastfeed them, or when adults aren't willing to carry them anymore.

Anthropologists have interpreted that the crying indicates that the stopping of breast-feeding or carrying is traumatic. The researchers didn't understand that the children were probably catching up on expressing accumulated painful feelings that they hadn't had the opportunity to release earlier.[15]

---

15 As described in *The Aware Baby* by Aletha Solter, PhD.

However, these anthropologists' reports suggest that some of those cultures didn't actively prevent crying after infancy.

In the next chapter, I'll talk more about what we can ascertain from these cultural patterns.

Babies, children, and teens have innate processes to feel relaxed enough to sleep restfully. Those processes are also the ways they heal from stress and trauma. The more relaxed they feel, the more restfully they sleep.

Hannah's quote below is one of my favourite (and most vibrant) descriptions of children's innate wisdom for relaxing before bed. She said:

"When there's squealing laughter and silly games as we put on PJs and brush teeth, I'm so glad that I don't share the cultural belief that we have to get children to 'wind down' at bedtime! That would be like trying to squeeze an octopus into a sandwich box... fighting their nature! But with rough and tumble, laughter, and tears if they need them, bedtimes are much more relaxing for all of us."

Self-Compassion Moment

This aspect of Aware Parenting is often the part that can help us connect with our biggest and most painful feelings, for several reasons. It's the element of Aware Parenting that is most different to our present-day cultural beliefs, so we might feel uncomfortable, confused, or overwhelmed when we're new to these ideas. If you're feeling any of those emotions as you read, I'm sending you lots of love and compassion.

We may also connect with feelings of sadness, overwhelm, or anger, thinking about the ways in which our own crying and other expressions of feelings were responded to when we were a baby, child, or teen. If you're feeling any of those, I'm sending love to all your emotions. It's so natural to have lots of big feelings when we take in this information.

In addition, your own cultural conditioning might mean you're tempted *to hit yourself with a guilt stick or other self-judgments such as about 'doing it wrong' or 'failing'. If you notice those, I invite you to put the sticks down. I want to remind you that they won't actually help you, your child, or your parenting. You might state to yourself, "I'm not willing to judge myself for what I did or didn't do. I am willing to be compassionate with myself." You might find that you feel sad instead. I invite you to welcome any mourning you might need to do if you didn't know about this earlier in your child's life.*

Aware Parenting, trust, and the four basic assumptions

In Aware Parenting, we deeply trust babies, children, and teens. We trust their intrinsic wisdom, and that they innately know what they need in terms of sleep, attachment, relaxation, nourishment, learning, and how to heal from stress and trauma.

Trusting children's innate biological wisdom corresponds to recognising the ancient needs and instincts that have supported us to survive since hunter-gatherer times.

In *The Aware Baby*, Aletha Solter outlines the four basic assumptions of Aware Parenting, which I include here:

1. Human beings are *born knowing what they need* for both survival, and for optimal physical, emotional, and intellectual development;

2. *How* babies and children are *treated determines how they act*. Aggressive actions are caused by unhealed trauma.

3. *Early life experiences* – including unmet needs and unhealed trauma – can have a *profound and lasting effect on feelings and behaviour* patterns later in life.

4. When *optimal conditions* are present, babies and children *can heal* from many of the *effects of stress and trauma*.

Let's revisit points one and four, which are two key elements that I'll be returning to throughout the book, because of their relationship with sleep. Those are: trusting their intrinsic wisdom regarding their needs, and trusting their innate body wisdom for healing.

Trusting their intrinsic wisdom about their needs:

Aletha Solter continues, in *The Aware Baby*, "*...babies know and indicate what they need, and we can therefore trust them to be in charge of their own lives as much as they are physically able.*" (pages 4-5)

Trusting their innate body wisdom for healing and homeostasis:

She goes on to say, "*Babies' natural biological tendency is to strive for health and physiological balance (homeostasis).*" (page 6)

Our intrinsic wisdom is meant to support us not only to survive, but also flourish, including in terms of the quality and quantity of sleep we experience.

Aware Parenting invites us to get freer from our cultural conditioning, so we can more clearly see how our baby or child keeps on inviting us to support them – both in being securely attached (because their needs are promptly met) – and in having restful sleep (because they feel connected, safe, and deeply relaxed).

In Aware Parenting, our invitation with sleep is to:

• *understand* what our child really needs and to meet those needs;

• *trust* their innate wisdom in relation to sleep; and

• *support* their intrinsic relaxation processes.

Aware Parenting invites us to release our cultural conditioning when we might be tempted to use power over them, for example by coercing them to go to bed when *we* want them to. Instead, we are invited to support them and then trust them to be deeply connected to:

• the sensations in their bodies;

• what they need to feel relaxed;

- when they want to go to sleep; and
- how much sleep they need.

As they grow older and become more independent, they will know how to trust their innate body wisdom in relation to sleep, because we have shown them how to do this.

However, if we are coming to Aware Parenting later, and we didn't trust their innate wisdom when they were younger, or our own unhealed trauma made that hard even if we were practicing Aware Parenting, I am here to reassure you that this healthy and growing independence can still be supported. It really is possible for us to help them reconnect with their body's intrinsic knowledge about deep relaxation and sleep, even in later childhood or their teen years.

In other words, both *attachment* and *relaxation* are most relevant to sleep. Meeting intrinsic attachment needs leads to secure attachment and relaxation. Cooperating with their innate body wisdom for healing and homeostasis leads to *deep* relaxation. Together, they create the quality of relaxation that leads to restful and restorative sleep.

Self-Compassion Moment

I wonder how you feel when you read about trusting babies, children, and teens? Trusting them can be hard for us, because in this culture, children aren't generally trusted or seen as wise. Often, the opposite is the case, and they are seen as defective or lacking. Learning to trust our children can be a big journey. This process often happens alongside us becoming aware of the ways our own sleep wisdom wasn't trusted, and how we are being invited to reclaim that for ourselves. I'm sending love to you and however you are feeling right now.

CHAPTER SUMMARY

There are three aspects of Aware Parenting:

1. Attachment-style parenting.
2. Non-punitive discipline.
3. The prevention and healing of stress and trauma.

Understanding the effects of stress and trauma – and children's innate healing processes – is central to understanding why so many babies and children take a long time to go to sleep, wake up frequently at night, and wake up very early in the morning, and why so many teens have sleep challenges.

Aware Parenting deeply trusts babies, children and teens. We trust their intrinsic wisdom and that they innately know what they need in terms of sleep, attachment, relaxation, nourishment, learning, and how to heal from stress and trauma.

Both attachment and relaxation are most relevant to sleep. Meeting intrinsic attachment needs leads to secure attachment and relaxation. Cooperating with their innate body wisdom for healing and homeostasis leads to deep relaxation. Together, they create the quality of relaxation that leads to restful and restorative sleep.

I trust you and your innate wisdom, and I trust in the innate wisdom of your child/ren. I'm here to support you in reclaiming that trust for yourself.

3. The Disconnected Domination Culture and sleep

Let's look at what sleep practices are common in the *Disconnected Domination Culture,* and how those practices might *not* support the most optimal development for children.

Schedules

A lot of mainstream sleep advice, particularly for babies, shows the effects of the industrial revolution and *DDC* consciousness. There's a lot of talk about schedules, timing, windows, counting clocks, and routines. This can continue into childhood and the teen years, such as if there is a required and fixed 'bedtime'. Those practices are helpful for the *DDC* – since they encourage children to become adults who are used to schedules and routines.

However, this isn't the most supportive approach in helping a child become an adult who is deeply connected with their own inner barometer and innate wisdom, and who knows when they are tired and need to sleep because of what their body tells them, rather than from looking at the clock.

The focus on calculating the timing and amount of sleep babies and children have was also deeply influenced by behaviourism and the medicalisation of infant sleep that happened in the 20th century. Parents were increasingly told what to do by paediatricians and psychologists, rather than relying on their own intuition, observing their child, or following their own regional, cultural, or familial practices.

These influences continued into parenting of older children and teens, rather than supporting them to listen to their own bodies and trusting them to go to sleep when they felt tired, as is the case in many traditional hunter-gatherer cultures.

Self-Compassion Moment

I want to remind you again that I'm not judging any parent here, and I'm inviting you to be deeply compassionate with yourself. We're all affected by the culture we grow up in; we needed to believe certain beliefs to be safe, belong and be loved. However, as adults, we have the opportunity to question whether these beliefs truly resonate with us, and whether we want to pass down different beliefs and experiences to our children. I'm sending lots of love and compassion as you read what follows.

Cots and separation during the night

Cribs have been in use since the Roman days, however, they started to be used more in Europe from the 13th century.

In *The Aware Baby*, Aletha Solter says:

*"During the 13th century in Europe, the Catholic priests first began recommending that mothers stop sleeping with their infants..... the primary reason for this advice was probably the rise of patriarchy and the fear of too much feminine influence on infants (especially male infants)..... By the 14th and 15th centuries, the advice not to sleep with infants began to take effect, and cradles were commonplace items of furniture in most European homes with children..... **During the twentieth century, infants in technological societies became more separated from their mothers than ever before in the history of our species.**"* (pages 97-98) [emphasis mine].

She continues:

*"By 1950, very few babies in Western, industrialised nations slept with their mothers. **It is little wonder that parents began seeking advice for a whole new array of problems**... for the babies who would not go to sleep at night.... for toddlers who climbed out of their cribs and kept coming into their parents' bed, and for the young children who .... had nightmares and fears of the dark. **Many of these sleep-related problems could be the result of forcing babies to sleep alone.***" (page 98) [emphasis mine].

In addition to reducing the influence of mothers on babies and affecting the mother-baby bond, cots might have a cultural purpose in training babies to not depend on others so much, and instead to develop early independence. Early-independence paradigms teach parents that it's important for their baby to learn to 'self-settle'. Again, we can see the cultural effects at play.

*The **DDC** is based on disconnection (hence the 'Disconnected' Domination Culture) and it is common for parents to also experience disconnection. Many parents don't have – or expect – family and community support in child-rearing.[16]*

Disconnection and separation are needed for many of the structures of the *DDC* to operate.

Therefore, we could see the purpose of 'sleep training' being not just about 'training' sleep, but about training babies and children to expect to often do things alone, without support.

There are also other cultures that train babies in early independence, such as in certain colder climates. For example, in some Nordic countries, for the past 50 years, and possibly longer, babies have been left outside (now in prams or strollers, previously in specially made cradles) for daytime naps. Parents report that babies who sleep in a very cold environment whilst being wrapped in a lot of warm clothing sleep more deeply and for longer. We might wonder whether these practices have their roots in

---

16 In contrast, "The !Kung mother was almost never alone with a crying baby." In Hunter-Gatherer Childhoods. Hewlett, Barry S. (2017).

earlier traditions, when babies were swaddled and carried on sleds.

Ongoing swaddling

Ongoing swaddling for older babies – and cots for toddlers – *may* lead to feelings of powerlessness (in relation to not having freedom to move) and then to dissociation. Powerlessness and dissociation in infancy and childhood helps the *DDC* to continue, because children who feel powerless and who dissociate are more likely to be compliant as adults.

From a baby: It's funny, Mummy, because when you wrap me up tight, at first, I really want to move my arms and legs. I'm learning so much about what my body can do. Did you notice me reaching for my toy just now? My body moves so much and so often I wonder why it happens and whether I can make it do things. Am I powerful? Can I make things happen? When I smile at you, you smile back at me, so I know that I can make things happen sometimes! But other times I smile and you don't smile back, and I feel confused. Oh, you're wrapping me up now, and it's happening again. At first I want to move, I want to kick out and push. But I can't. It's too tight. I try again, but I'm pushing and kicking and nothing is happening. Hmm. I think it's one of those times when I'm not powerful. And this funny thing happens, Mummy, because I kind of stop trying. I kind of stop caring, even. The world changes and goes a bit more fuzzy. I stare out at you, but things are different. Maybe I don't even want to move after all. I stare into this different world. I am different, too. After a while, I fall asleep.

Suppression of feelings before sleep

In the *DDC* (as well as in other cultures) there are many ways in which children's painful feelings are suppressed before sleep. This leads to children learning to suppress their own emotions, which is necessary for the *DDC*. People trained to suppress painful feelings often buy more things to help them dissociate from those emotions, which supports the consumerist structure of this society.

Self-Compassion Moment

If you've used schedules, a cot, ongoing swaddling, and/or emotional suppression with your baby and you're tempted to pick up those guilt sticks, I invite you to put them down. I want to remind you that cultural conditioning is designed to make us believe certain things. The culture that most of us grew up in told us to think that schedules, cots, and emotional suppression were the 'accurate' way to respond to babies. Shame and guilt are part of DDC conditioning. Your unwillingness to hit yourself with the guilt or shame sticks is part of you freeing yourself from that conditioning.

Remember, we learn to internalise cultural beliefs by the time we are adults, so that we can pass those thoughts and practices on to the next generation. I invite you to be deeply compassionate with yourself. You needed to learn the beliefs of the culture you grew up in, in order to be safe, belong, or be loved. And now, if this Aware Parenting information resonates with you, I'm here to support you in increasingly feeling safe, having a sense of belonging, and being loved while believing these different thoughts and experimenting with these different practices.

This is why our own inner work is vital if we are to practice Aware Parenting. Because thinking and doing something different to what was done to us – and what is done by the majority of others around us – can help us connect with those original feelings we had as children, when we needed to fit in to our family and our culture to survive.

These sleep practices all work well if we're looking at the perspective of the continuation of the culture. They keep the *DDC* going by helping children fit in to that culture and pass it on to the next generation.

The practices do that through:

- schedules;
- isolation and early independence;
- lack of freedom of movement; and
- suppression of painful feelings.

However, if we look at optimal emotional, intellectual, and spiritual development, each of these practices can come at a cost for us as individual beings.

We:

- can become disconnected from our own intrinsic body clock;
- might disconnect from our innate needs for connection, support, and community;
- may not realise how strong, free, and powerful we are; and
- can learn to suppress our painful feelings, rather than express them in healing ways.

How sleep and children's wellbeing can be different with Aware Parenting

Aware Parenting is a very different approach, because we're aiming to meet the innate needs of a baby, child, or teen, so that they can thrive physically, emotionally, mentally, and spiritually within the culture they live in. We aim to support the intrinsic wisdom of their body, and deeply trust them, whether they're a six-week-old baby, or a sixteen year old teenager.

This is likely to mean that they grow up with different beliefs when compared with many other children growing up with *DDC* practices. As toddlers, they're likely to carry their dolls in slings, put them in beds all together, and 'listen' to their feelings. They are likely to be willing to cooperate more of the time, but they *won't* be compliant. They will be much more likely to listen in to themselves rather than just go along with what their peers think and do. They'll be freer to feel and express their feelings in healing ways. And they will be more likely to be able to sleep restfully, with less need to numb their painful feelings by dissociating.

CHAPTER SUMMARY

Sleep practices that keep the *DDC* going include:

- schedules;
- isolation and early independence;
- lack of freedom of movement; and
- suppression of painful feelings.

Each of these practices can come at a cost for us as individuals. We:

- can become disconnected from our own intrinsic body clock;
- might disconnect from our innate needs for connection, support and community;
- may not realise how strong, free, and powerful we are; and
- can learn to suppress our painful feelings, rather than express them in healing ways.

You are powerful, and what you think and believe has powerful effects on how you respond to your child/ren, including about their sleep.

4. *Classical Attachment Parenting* and sleep

Sleep practices and *Classical Attachment Parenting*[17]

Classical Attachment Parenting returned to industrialised countries of the West through the combination of two key occurrences:

1. Research into secure attachment, through the work of Bowlby, Ainsworth, and others in the 1950s and 60s.

2. With more easeful travel to remote countries, increasing influences from existing traditional cultures, particularly *in hot climates,* percolated over into the West in the 1960s and 70s.

Moving away from the cots, bottle-feeding, and prams that had become mainstream in many industrialised countries, some parents returned to original practices of co-sleeping, breast-feeding, and baby-carrying. In many industrialised cultures, these practices were judged and looked down upon as indicating inferiority or lower class status.

Remember the quote from Aletha Solter in *The Aware Baby* about how *each* culture has practices that support the continuation of that *particular* culture?

Classical Attachment Parenting aims to duplicate the practices that are common to many Indigenous cultures, with practices related to birthing, breast-feeding, co-sleeping, carrying, and prompt responsiveness to crying. Although all of these elements are beneficial for all babies in all cultures, *some* of the *specific ways* they are practiced *are not* most optimal for *all* babies and children in *all* cultures. Instead, the particular ways they are practiced reflect the needs of the babies and children – and the values of the adults – living in *those particular climates and cultures.*

---

17 A term created by me and taken up by Aletha Solter as an official Aware Parenting term to refer to the original attachment parenting paradigm, which was first described by William and Martha Sears. The Aware Parenting version of attachment parenting has several key differences from this original version.

For example, as Aletha Solter talks about in depth in *The Aware Baby*, very frequent breastfeeding in **extremely hot climates** is important for survival reasons, when there is a high risk of dehydration due to heat and diarrhoea. As well as providing plenty of fluids, frequent breastfeeding in hot climates reduces the expending of energy – and possible overheating – by suppressing crying. Being able to stop any crying through breastfeeding also reassures mothers that their baby doesn't have a serious health issue, which is vital information in traditional cultures that have high mortality rates.

One of the beliefs in *Classical Attachment Parenting* is that frequent feeding is the most helpful way to respond to *all* babies and children in *all* cultures, rather than recognising that this way of parenting is the most optimal adaptation for survival in a *specific* (hot) climate, within a *unique* culture.

Very frequent breastfeeding after early infancy both day and night is *not an intrinsic biological need*. It's a beautiful *adaptation* to a *specific* environment by a *particular* culture.

Self-Compassion Moment

If you've been practicing Classical Attachment Parenting up until now, and you're feeling angry or frustrated while you read this, I'm sending so much love to your feelings. I want to remind you that I'm not judging you, and I'm not trying to persuade you to believe what I do. Rather, I'm inviting you to see if this way of seeing things resonates with you. And I support you in believing what speaks to you, and doing what is a fit for you, including if that is different to what I talk about here.

If you have been practicing Classical Attachment Parenting and this is new information to you – and it resonates with you – and you're tempted to pick up the guilt or self-judgment stick, I invite you to put it down. Whatever you've done in the past, it is possible to change, as well as to support your children to heal from the effects of what you did and didn't do in the past.

If you're feeling sad that you didn't know this information earlier, I'm sending love to the sadness. I hear from so many parents who feel similarly, so you're not alone. So much compassion comes from me to you, however you're feeling when you're taking in this information.

Why breastfeeding practices in cold climates differ from those in hot climates

In Indigenous cultures in very *cold climates*, there are often very different patterns of breastfeeding, because babies don't need to be fed as often as they do in hot weather. This can then also affect how they are carried, and how much they are held close.

In *The Aware Baby*, Aletha Solter talks about *three* of the reasons why parenting practices in cold climates can differ from those in hot climates:

1. Babies don't need to be breastfed as frequently because the weather isn't hot, so they feed for longer at each feeding and receive more hind milk, which is higher in fat.

2. *"Because there is less of a need to nurse at frequent intervals in cold climates, mothers in the northern indigenous cultures are less likely to keep their babies close to their bodies. Instead, they place them in cradles or hammocks, and strap them to cradle boards, animals or sleds for transportation."* (*The Aware Baby,* page 77).

As I mentioned earlier in the book, this is replicated in some present-day far northern hemisphere European sleep practices, where babies are commonly left outside in prams in snowy weather for daytime naps. The cultural belief is that sleeping in cold air helps babies be healthier and stronger.

Again, I'm here to remind you that *each* culture has *different* practices. *Some* traditional cultures in very *cold* countries *did* still keep their babies close, such as carrying them on their backs, inside warm coats. Sometimes the babies were bare inside the coats, relying on the warmth of body contact. However, in other cultures, the babies might be swaddled for warmth before being placed inside the coat, or on a hard structured carrier or a sled.

In researching carrying in traditional cultures in cold climates, I found support for this understanding from 'The Baby Historian', Aradia Wyndham, who wrote[18]: *"Around the world, there seems to be two main approaches for transporting infants in cold climates: a **soft carrier** that shares body heat between child and caregiver... and a **hard carrier** that creates a micro-climate for the baby."*

Where wrapping and swaddling does occur in cold climates, that is different from how babies in very hot climates are carried, where the least amount of fabric is used for clothing or a carrier, to help with cooling. As a result, there is generally more skin-to-skin contact.

The *swaddling* piece is also vital in understanding the sleep picture we're building here, because swaddling can easily lead to dissociation, where babies stop crying when they have feelings to express to us.

3. Less frequent breastfeeding and lower fluid intake is beneficial for another reason in some very cold climates in pre-modern societies: there's less need to urinate. This is of obvious advantage when frequent undressing, offering opportunities to wee, or having wet clothing in cold weather might be uncomfortable or even dangerous for babies.

However, again, each culture has found ways to support babies with elimination in those very cold climates, such as by using moss inside carriers to wick away moisture, or having clothing that provides ease when offering the baby opportunities to eliminate.

In transposing the parenting practices from some hot-climate cultures, where *more* of babies' innate needs are met compared to in the *DDC*, *Classical Attachment Parenting* has assumed that *specific ways* those parenting practices are practiced are most optimal for *all* babies and children in *all* areas.

When in fact, *some* of those *specific* practices are most optimal in *specific* climates and are therefore *not* the most beneficial for *all* children.

---

18 https://thebabyhistorian.com/2018/11/14/the-inuit-amauti/

In addition, one tenet of *Classical Attachment Parenting* is that *all* crying indicates an unmet need. It doesn't recognise that *healing-feelings*[19] exist as well as *needs-feelings* and thus doesn't perceive the healing and relaxation-through-release processes.

Self-Compassion Moment

I'm sending love to you however you're feeling right now. If you're practicing Classical Attachment Parenting, and didn't experience that from your parents, I want to acknowledge all that you've already done to move away from how you were parented, and to change the beliefs that you grew up with. When we've already gone through this process of changing our parenting beliefs once, we can become very passionate about these new beliefs, especially if we've needed to fight for them, as is often the case with Classical Attachment Parenting in the DDC.

I want to emphasise that I really appreciate your passion for secure attachment and for meeting the attachment needs of your child/ren. I share that passion with you. I really enjoyed carrying my daughter and son and owned a smorgasbord of carriers to carry them in. I co-slept with both of my children for many, many years and absolutely loved it.

What I love about Aware Parenting is that we see attachment-style parenting as a wonderful cake, and healing from stress and trauma as the icing on the top of that cake.

If you do feel interested in shifting your beliefs from Classical Attachment Parenting to Aware Parenting, I'm here to support you with that. And if you aren't willing to, I deeply support your no!

As I already shared in the previous chapter, Aletha Solter reports in *The Aware Baby* that anthropologists have not observed much crying by babies in hot climates[20]. However, there are two situations when crying is observed, and both occur in children once they are past infancy.

---

19 This is a phrase I coined to differentiate them from needs-feelings. Needs-feelings indicate unmet needs. Healing-feelings are feelings which, when expressed with loving support, bring about healing. These are not official Aware Parenting terms.

20 However, with the Hazda of Northern Tanzania, parents frequently ignore crying babies, and mothers often stop mid-breastfeed, leading to crying. Blurton-Jones, in Hewlett, Barry S. (2017). Hunter-Gatherer Childhoods: Evolutionary, Developmental, and Cultural Perspectives.

1. Where babies are fed very frequently, when breastfeeding is stopped several years later, in some cultures, children often cry a lot, sometimes for weeks or months[21].

From an Aware Parenting perspective, we recognise that this is because the innate biological wisdom to heal from stress and trauma is not as important during infancy as survival is. Once past that most risky early stage, children do then use their innate healing and relaxation process through crying, thereby catching up on the *healing-crying* they didn't get to do as babies and younger children.

2. After a long in-arms phase, when babies grow into children, adults stop being willing to carry them, and make them walk themselves. In some cultures lots of crying was observed after this. In the Ache people of Eastern Paraguay, it was observed that children would "scream, cry, hit their parents, and try everything they can think of to get adults to continue carrying them[22]."

In those cultures, attachment needs and breastfeeding were prioritised during infancy and early childhood because they were most necessary for survival. Once survival was assured, then children could freely use their innate healing and relaxation process to release accumulated feelings and stress that had become pent-up in their bodies.

In the book *Voices of the First Day,* about Indigenous Australians, the author Robert Lawlor wrote about some traditional First Nations Australian communities. He reported that crying was stopped in babies but welcomed in children.

He said that babies and small children *"...are never allowed to cry for any length of time; the parents and the entire clan see that their discomforts are quickly soothed or alleviated."* (page 165).

However, when they are older *"...children are allowed to vent all their emotions in every form, from wailing lament to colossal tantrums."* (page 170).

---

21 "Weaning is an extremely unpleasant experience... with children screaming, hitting, and throwing tantrums for several weeks." (Observations of the Ache people in Eastern Paraguay, by Hill and Hurtardo (1996) in Hewlett, Barry, S. (2017).

22 Hill and Hurtardo (1996), in Hewlett, Barry S. (2017).

He went on to say, *"Perhaps because of the freedom to release emotions given them as children, when the occasion arises adults ... express their emotions with unrestrained intensity and then forget them. They do not harbour repressed feelings that can warp their relationships with their kin or with the metaphysical order."* (page 171).

We can see how this response to the natural healing function of crying at different ages is a precise fit with each particular culture and its climate.

Sometimes this pattern of differing responses to tears in babies and older children is replicated in modern societies, where parents often feel more comfortable with being with their crying child, compared to listening to their baby cry in their arms when all their needs are met.

However, without understanding Aware Parenting and what is required for the healing power of tears, a parent might not provide the most helpful support whilst children are expressing healing-feelings. For example, by encouraging the child to cry on their own, by leaving them alone if they tell us to "go away!" during a tantrum, or by interpreting the louder crying that happens when they come close as indicating that the child wants them to stay away, rather than that the closeness is helping them feel more safety to release.

From a child: I don't know what's happened, Mummy, but you won't breastfeed me any more. And you've stopped picking me up whenever I ask. I loved it when you fed me any time I asked, and carried me any time I wanted. I did sometimes feel a bit funny, though, as if I was a bit fuzzy and like I couldn't move. Like I had this hole inside me that would never be filled up. This is different. I feel so sad. All the tears of the world are coming out of me. I cry and cry and cry and cry. I haven't ever really cried before, so this is kind of strange for me. Crying is funny. There's all these tears and all this snot, and I want to stamp around and wave my arms everywhere. This is going on forever. Will I cry forever? You're there with me still, and you're listening. I can hold your legs. I cling on to you. I feel you. But I want to cry and cry some more. It goes on and on. It's like there were 10 rivers in me, and I've just cried a whole river.

But it's funny now, Mummy, because the river of tears has all gone. And I don't feel fuzzy, and I don't feel a hole inside me. Actually, as I hold my arms around your legs, with your hands on my back, I can actually feel you. I can feel me. I can feel us. This isn't like the fuzziness. I can really feel us. And I can feel some space inside me. It's not a big empty hole. It's like lots of lovely clear open space. And I look around me, and actually, everything looks a bit clearer. It's like the world is fresh and I can see it all. There are still nine rivers of tears inside me. But perhaps this crying thing isn't so terrible after all, as long as you're still here with me.

In Western, industrialised cultures, there is generally not huge concern about excessive heat nor cold, nor survival for babies and children.

And so, as Aletha Solter goes on to say in *The Aware Baby, "We are therefore free to focus on optimal psychological development right from the start."* (page 78).

Babies can go to sleep as a result of being fed, and can go back to sleep as a result of being fed frequently through the night. Just as they may often experience in *very hot* climates. They might be dissociating from painful feelings, but their bodies have this capacity so that they can sleep in very hot climates.

Babies also can go to sleep after being swaddled in a cot. Just as they may go to sleep in *some cold climates* wrapped in fur on a cradleboard or sled, while observing their family going about their day-to-day tasks. They might be dissociating from their painful feelings, but their bodies are able to sleep this way so they can sleep in cold climates.

With Aware Parenting, we can observe these different cultural practices, and choose responses which are most helpful for babies and children – in terms of both their intrinsic needs, and their innate wisdom for healing, *while* living in the climate, society, and era we live in. These practices also create the most relaxed and restorative sleep.

From a toddler in a traditional hot culture: *I am at home in my skin. Everywhere around me I look, and that is my home. The birds speak my name. My grandfather is in this rock. I belong here. My community is all around me. I have Mumma and Dadda, and all my aunties and grandmothers, uncles and grandfathers. They tell me that since I was born, I was carried everywhere. My siblings also carry me around a lot too. They are so strong. I sleep in their arms. Mumma feeds me often. So do my aunties. It is very hot here, and I get thirsty a lot. At night, we all sleep together on our bedding mat. There is often talking and singing. I love to hear my family. Mumma tells me that the time is coming where she and my aunties won't feed me any more, and that I am old enough now to not be carried, like my siblings. I think I will feel very sad. But I also want to be like them. Cousin stopped feeding and being carried and I saw him cry and cry and cry. But now he runs around like the bigger children and says he will one day carry his baby sister. Perhaps it will not be so terrible after all.*

From a toddler in a traditional cold culture: *I crawl out of bed. We are all cosy in there, Mama and Papa and brothers and sisters. After we eat, Mama will be carrying me on her back. Sister says that soon I will be too big to be carried, and I will walk like she does. Brother says that when I was a baby, I had no clothes on when Mama carried me on her back inside her big coat. I was cosy and warm next to her. Now I am bigger, I have clothes too. I still have mama milk when I'm inside Mama's coat, it's so warm inside there. I sleep sometimes in there too, but not so much now. My face gets so cold when we are outside, but I am used to that now as well. I watch Sister and Brother as they sew new clothing for us all. I am starting to learn too. I will soon be like them. Sister helps me and Mama get into Mama's coat. We are going out fishing now. I used to like sleeping when we were outside, so that I didn't feel the cold so much, but now I love watching. One time, Mama wrapped me tight in lots of furs and put me on our big sledge. We were moving camp, she told me. I was there for a long time, watching everyone doing lots of things. I didn't feel sad not being close to her. I didn't feel anything much. I felt kind of fuzzy and foggy. Usually I fall asleep when Mama is walking, but that time, I went to sleep simply watching, when the fuzziness and fogginess got so big that I fell asleep.*

CHAPTER SUMMARY

Classical Attachment Parenting aims to duplicate the practices of many Indigenous cultures, with practices related to birthing, breastfeeding, co-sleeping, carrying, and prompt responsiveness to crying. However, some of the specific ways those elements are practiced reflect the needs of the babies and children living in those particular climates and cultures, as well as the values of the adults.

Very frequent breastfeeding after early infancy both day and night is not an intrinsic biological need. It's a beautiful adaptation to a specific environment by a particular culture.

Breastfeeding practices in traditional cultures in cold climates can differ from those in hot climates. Understanding these differences can help us choose sleep practices that are most helpful for our unique baby or child's overall wellbeing in the specific society and era we live in now.

In some traditional hot cultures, children weren't prevented from crying once they reached early childhood. Once past that most risky early stage of infancy, children caught up on the *healing-crying* they didn't get to do as babies and younger children. Sometimes this pattern is replicated in modern societies, where parents generally feel more comfortable with their child crying compared to listening to their baby cry in their arms.

Babies can go to sleep as a result of being fed, and can fall back to sleep as a result of being fed frequently through the night, just as as they may often experience in *very hot* climates.

Babies can also go to sleep after being swaddled in a cot, just as they may go to sleep in some *cold climates* wrapped in fur on a cradleboard or sled, while observing their family going about their day-to-day tasks.

I'm here to support you to listen in deeply to yourself so that you really know which parenting beliefs you most resonate with.

5. Aware Parenting is the third way with sleep

Aware Parenting is the third way with sleep for babies and children

In industrialised countries, we are generally taught that we either need to choose between closeness with our baby or child, *or* restful sleep. (After reading the last chapter, you might almost see this as a choice between two different cultural practices.) The idea that *both* are possible can be a huge eye-opener for many parents.

I wonder if you're feeling surprised as you read this? Perhaps you can hardly believe that you might be able to support your baby or child to be securely attached *and* have more restful sleep? If so, I'm here to show you that it really is possible, and I'm going to be sharing stories from parents and Aware Parenting instructors with first-hand experience of this, so you can see that possibility for your family too.

After reading the past few chapters, you'll probably see *why* Aware Parenting is this third approach to sleep. It's primarily because of the first and third aspects of Aware Parenting: meeting their attachment needs, and supporting their innate ability to feel deeply relaxed by releasing stress and trauma.

I love this message from Carole, where she shares about her insights regarding this:

"I really always felt that you're either in the sleep-training camp or in the feed-to-sleep-until-they-grow-out-of-it camp (where I was). I can't believe there has been a third camp all along, built on absolute love and nurture."

Talking of camps, I invite deep compassion for all of us, whatever camp we're in – or have been in. Let's all set up camp together! In fact, that's so vital, if we're to move away from the DDC.

And I want to acknowledge that if you have an older child or teen, your focus is less likely to be on secure attachment. However, I will explain why connection and attachment is still relevant for this age range, and what *else* is important to consider for older children and teens in relation to trusting their innate body wisdom. The second aspect of Aware Parenting, non-punitive discipline – and finding the true causes of behaviours – becomes more relevant at these older ages. In addition, the natural outcome of secure attachment – self-connection and healthy independence (or interdependence) is also deeply relevant to sleep for older children and teens, as we'll talk more about later in the book.

If you are the parent of a teen, maybe you're wondering if it's possible for them to get enough sleep without you using coercion, threats, or punishments to get them to go to bed when you want them to. With Aware Parenting, we can support older children, tweens, and teens to be more likely to have the sleep that their body needs *without* using punishments, coercion, or harshness, by supporting and trusting their innate body wisdom and their desire to learn through their own life experiences.

Self-Compassion Moment

As always, I invite you to keep on listening to yourself and to how you feel in your body when you're reading, so you know what resonates with you and what doesn't. If you want to do things differently now with Aware Parenting, it's never too late, whatever you have done in your parenting up until now. This approach also helps children heal from past stress and trauma, including any that was caused by us. If you've left your baby alone to go to sleep, or you've used threats to get your child to stay in their bed, or you've punished your teen when they went to bed later than you, you can absolutely help them heal from those experiences with Aware Parenting.

Before diving in deeper, let's look again at some of the options given to parents of babies and young children in the other two paradigms.

In the *first way*, which I've termed '*DDC*' so far, but which could be called early-independence approaches, the belief is that babies and children need to learn to go to sleep alone, often through methods which are termed 'self-soothing', such as sucking their thumb or a dummy, or clutching onto a blanket or soft toy. There are many different forms of this approach, some of which include practices that are termed 'controlled crying' or 'cry-it-out'. Swaddling can be a part of this process, too.

Outcomes: babies and young children sleep separately and tend to not call out for connection in the night.

Benefits: parents get more sleep.

Disadvantages: during the night, neither the child's attachment needs nor the parent's bonding needs are met. Babies and young children are likely to be moving between states of dissociation and hyperarousal, which are not optimal for their physical and emotional wellbeing.

From an Aware Parenting perspective, the early independence paradigms do not recognise the intrinsic needs of babies and young children for closeness while falling asleep. Most also do not recognise the stress-release function of crying, and even those that do (for example, Brazelton), don't understand the baby's need to be held while crying for the crying to be healing.

Self-Compassion Moment

If you're tempted to pick up the guilt stick, I invite you to put it down. The phrase you could think instead might be, "I'm not willing to hit myself with the guilt stick right now. I am willing to be compassionate with myself." I'm sending you lots of love and I want to remind you of two things again. One: it's possible to learn new information without judging ourselves for not knowing it before. And two: if Aware Parenting resonates with you, it's never too late to change what you're doing, and to support healing from the past to happen. If you're feeling sad, I'm sending so much love to your sadness.

In the *second* way, the *Classical Attachment Parenting* perspective, the belief is that it is biologically normal for babies and young children to wake up several times at night for the first few years of their lives. Mothers are invited to co-sleep and breast-feed throughout the night, believing that they are simply meeting all of their child's needs if there is frequent night waking.

Outcomes: there may be frequent night-waking.

Benefits: a baby or child's attachment needs are met, and a mother's bonding needs are met.

Disadvantages: needs for relaxed, restful, and restorative sleep may be less fulfilled. Children also don't get to use their relaxation-through-release process and may show signs of stored tension both day and night.

From an Aware Parenting perspective, the **Classical Attachment Parenting** *approach understands the innate attachment needs of babies and children, but doesn't recognise their intrinsic relaxation-through-release process, hence the frequent night waking.*

Remember that Aware Parenting is a form of attachment-style parenting. The key differences from *Classical Attachment Parenting* include the recognition of the intrinsic relaxation-through-release process, and the differentiation between needs-feelings and healing-feelings, and thus between mild dissociation and true relaxation. These differences show us that children *can* co-sleep and breastfeed and not need to wake up several times at night for the first few years.

Later in the book, I'll explain why babies and young children tend to wake up more frequently at night if their parents are practicing **Classical Attachment Parenting** *compared to Aware Parenting. I'll also explain why those brought up with early independence sleep approaches appear to sleep for longer periods at night (notice the key word here, 'appear').*

Aware Parenting is the third way. It recognises the three ingredients needed for sound sleep, which include meeting both their intrinsic needs, and their innate relaxation-through-release process. It also offers a different set of practices, so that parents don't need to make a choice between restful sleep and secure attachment. It really is possible to meet both of these vitally important needs!

I've heard time and time again the relief that parents often feel when they first discover that it really is possible for them to have restful sleep *and* offer their baby or child closeness during the night. For example, Kate wrote to me and said:

"Thank you, Marion, for your sleep series on The Aware Parenting Podcast! *As a first-time Mum of a beautiful seven-month-old boy I stumbled upon some of your older episodes on my feed, then before I knew it, yesterday I was bingeing all your recent sleep episodes. It was so divinely timed: our little one slept a lovely stretch of five and a half hours for the first time since he was a four-month-old!*

He also didn't wake up soon after going to sleep, which he has been doing basically since birth, and the two times he woke up, he went back to sleep very quickly. We listened to his healing-feelings before bed, leant into playtime and didn't cut it short (as we would normally do) but followed his cues as to when he was satisfied and relaxed after playing, and we created a truly relaxing environment by not just 'doing' the bedtime routine (which just stressed us out when we moved through it), but actually enjoying it all with him.

Thank you so much for bringing Aware Parenting to my attention. Googling and trawling through Instagram, I was really thinking the only options were to sacrifice sleep for connection, or vice versa.

Our beautiful boy has never followed conventional age-appropriate 'wake windows' and trying to follow those types of rules to help him have lovely relaxed day naps and deep night sleep was leaving me stressed and feeling like a failure.

My core values (that tell me every human has inherent dignity in their diversity) were completely at odds with the pressure I felt from well-meaning family and friends who all subscribe to this mainstream way of viewing sleep as being 'one size fits all'.

Just under one week into this Aware Parenting approach to his sleep, and it finally feels like we are really giving our little boy exactly what he needs. We had been doing Classical Attachment Parenting *and really believed the lie that 'all crying = bad and should be avoided at all costs!'*

This new way, and third way of viewing sleep deeply resounds in my spirit. After years of therapy, I have learnt to not shy away from the 'hard' emotions and to not be afraid of releasing them. Raising our son this way feels empowering, dignified, and to be honest, very whole."

Self-Reflection Moment

How do you feel, having read about Kate's journey with sleep and Aware Parenting? Does anything particularly resonate with you and your experience? I'm sending loving compassion to any painful feelings you might be feeling.

Aware Parenting offers a different perspective on sleep for older children and teens

When it comes to older children and teens, the three camps may no longer be so clearly differentiated. However, yet again, Aware Parenting offers a compassionate, respectful, and effective approach.

It invites us as parents to trust our older children and teens, and to support them to stay connected with (or reconnect with) their innate body wisdom, as well as the natural process of them becoming increasingly independent. This is timely independence (or interdependence), as a result of secure attachment, rather than early independence, which is often promoted by the *DDC*.

In many hunter-gatherer cultures of the past as well as present-day Indigenous and non-Western cultures, children played freely in the evening, perhaps singing and dancing around a central fire, crawling into a lap if they still needed closeness when they were sleepy. Children often had free choice about when they went to sleep. This may have been influenced by what the community required, e.g. staying up at night to tend to animals. It may also have been affected by the time of year, with longer sleep in the winter and less in summer. We can see here again the cultural differences, where flexibility with sleep is important in cultures with wider seasonal fluctuations in temperature, very different to cultures near the equator.

This is in contrast to the *DDC*, where schedules for school and work dictate sleep requirements and often have very little to do with the seasons or other unique local influences. In addition, the *DDC* way of seeing the sleep of older children or teens is often that it's our role as their parents to choose when they go to sleep. Aware Parenting has a different way of seeing this. Instead, we aim to support them to listen to their bodies and trust them to learn through experience about when they need to go to sleep.

In many traditional cultures, children and teens are trusted to make their own decisions, such as about when to go to sleep, and are supported – and expected – to be helpful members of the society. For example, for the reindeer-herding Sámi Indigenous people of northern Norway, Sweden, Finland, and Russia, *"...the whole family adapts to whatever tasks need to be carried out, be that earmarking, travelling or other joint activities. Within that framework, children make their own choices. "They eat when they are hungry and go to bed whenever they are tired," says Tytti Valkeapää, a mother of six children ranging in age from 8 to 18, who lives in the northern Finnish village of Kuttanen ...... In the summer, during the bright Arctic nights, it is also normal for older children of 12 or so to go fishing with their friends at night, and only come home in the early morning hours."*[23]

Just as Aware Parenting with a baby or younger child supports secure attachment, Aware Parenting with toddlers, children, and teens is about nourishing the results of that – by trusting the unfolding of their own true independence, including with sleep.

Remembering that they are learning from us can be important here, so if we stay up late reading or on screens before bed, they will be learning those behaviours from us.

Trusting their innate body wisdom, whether we're the parent of a baby, child, or teen, is central to Aware Parenting. It's also about supporting secure attachment and the development of healthy and timely independence and competence.

---

23 https://www.bbc.com/future/article/20220105-the-arctic-parenting-style-that-fosters-resilience

That means keeping babies and children close when they require it, and supporting children and teens to be independent when they are ready for it.

In order to do both of those, we're invited to do two things:

1. *Question* our culturally conditioned *beliefs* and those we've acquired from other cultures.

2. *Listen lovingly* to our *feelings* from our own experiences of growing up *without* Aware Parenting (particularly from when we were the age our child is now).

Enquiring compassionately into our thoughts and feelings this way, we are more likely to be able to support our baby, child, or teen to stay deeply connected with both their intrinsic needs, and their innate body wisdom in relation to sleep.

Self-Reflection Moment

How are you feeling having read this?

Did anything resonate with you?

Did you have any 'aha!' moments?

Did you have any painful feelings or reactions?

I'm sending you love, whatever you're feeling and thinking.

CHAPTER SUMMARY

Aware Parenting is the third approach to sleep primarily because of its first and third aspects: helping babies and young children feel safe by meeting their attachment needs, and supporting their innate ability to feel deeply relaxed by releasing stress and trauma. However, the second element, non-punitive discipline, is relevant too, particularly once children leave infancy.

It also offers a different set of practices, so that parents don't need to make a choice between restful sleep and secure attachment.

Trusting their innate body wisdom, whether we're the parent of a baby, child, or teen, is central to Aware Parenting. It's also about supporting secure attachment and the development of healthy and timely independence and competence.

I'm sending love to your beautiful mind as you make your own sense of this information.

6. The three ingredients for relaxed and restful sleep

This chapter is perhaps the most central one in this book. You might want to return to it and re-read it several times.

I will explain in more detail what I have been referring to up until now as *intrinsic needs* (for closeness and safety) and *innate biological wisdom* (to release stress and trauma). You'll see that these are the second and third ingredients consecutively. These are both needed for the *relaxation* that is required for restful sleep.

Babies, children, and teens need to be *tired* and *relaxed* to sleep restfully.

Relaxation is created in two ways:

~ through a sense of **safety** (which comes from **closeness**, especially in the early years),

~ and by **releasing** any pent-up painful **feelings** that **naturally bubble to the surface to be expressed when they are tired.**

If children don't feel *safe*, they won't feel *relaxed*, and will need to *dissociate* to go to sleep.

If children have *accumulated painful feelings* bubbling to the surface when they are tired that aren't being released, they won't feel *relaxed*, and will need to *dissociate* to go to sleep.

If they *dissociate* to fall asleep, the sleep is not likely to be *restful.*

Thus, there are three ingredients required for restful sleep.

These are:

i. to feel tired;

ii. to feel connected (*closeness creating a sense of safety*); and

iii. to feel relaxed (*by releasing any healing-feelings present*).

As I go through each point in turn, I will invite you to see them from a different perspective compared to how you might have been perceiving them up until now.

In this chapter, I outline them in general ways. Then, in each of the following sections of the book – on babies, children, and teens – I will go into much more detail. There, I will illustrate what you can actually do at each of their ages with each of these ingredients to support them to sleep more restfully.

Self-Compassion Moment

I invite you to connect in with how you feel when you take in this information. I'm sending loving compassion to you and however you feel as you do. If you're hitting yourself with a guilt stick, I invite you to put that down. If you're feeling painful feelings, I invite you to reach out to a loving listener or do some journalling. My heart goes out to you.

---

i. To feel tired (sleepy)

This may seem obvious, but our bodies are so wise. If we are not tired, it is often very hard to go to sleep, whether we are a baby, child, teen, or adult.

Self-Reflection Moment

You might have experienced this if you've needed to get up super early for a trip or other event and you went to bed very early, way before you actually felt tired. Do you remember how difficult you found it to sleep? Perhaps you took a long time to drop off to sleep? How did you feel?

Babies, children and teens are just like us. This is why the following can all lead to challenges:

- giving babies sleep routines that aren't connected to their feelings of sleepiness;
- taking toddlers to bed at the same time each evening;
- telling children and teens to go to bed at the same time every night [24]

This is because we might be *working against* what their body is communicating to them.

Common signs of tiredness in babies include: red eyes and/or eyebrows, fluttering eyelids, blinking, rubbing eyes, pulling ears, losing coordination, jerky movements, yawning, eyelids drooping, or lying down.

Common signs of tiredness in children include: yawning, losing interest in activities, losing coordination and the ability to concentrate, and lying down.

Common signs of tiredness in teens include: yawning, losing the ability to concentrate, and lying down.

You might be wondering why I didn't include behaviours like crying, raging, or being super playful and rambunctious before bed as signs of tiredness for babies and children.

I'm going to skip to the third ingredient for a while, to explain why.

That's because, from an Aware Parenting perspective, those aren't signs of tiredness. Rather, they are indications of their innate relaxation process in operation when they are sleepy.

We are all born with this innate relaxation-through-release response to enable us to feel relaxed enough to go to sleep, and to sleep restfully and restoratively.

When we are a **baby**, that is crying in the loving arms of our parent.

---

24 In the section on teens, you'll discover why we don't actually recommend telling older children and teens when to go to sleep.

When we are a **toddler** or **child**, that can be through crying or raging with the loving support of a parent, or it can be through playing and laughing in particular ways that we call *attachment play*.

When we are an **older child** or **teen**, that might be sharing our feelings about our day, which can include talking, crying, laughing, and having fun with another person.

This is related to what I shared earlier on about pent-up feelings caused by stress and trauma, and how healing happens. Having this understanding about our innate relaxation process will lead to a very different perception of what's going on in the evenings. That clarity is likely to lead to actions different to those you might usually take.

Let's imagine six evening scenarios:

- a *baby* starts *crying* a lot (the so-called 'witching hour');
- a *toddler* starts *tantrumming* about something apparently small;
- a *three-year-old* is *asking* for one thing after the next, and is not happy with anything;
- a *five-year-old* starts getting rough and harsh with their sibling and then throws things;
- a *seven-year-old* wants to play *rambunctious* games while jumping on the bed; and
- an *older child or teen* starts *disagreeing* with everything we say.

If we're thinking that these are signs of tiredness, we will of course try to do everything we can to get them to go to sleep as soon as possible. We're likely to try to 'calm them down' through activities such as:

- rocking, jiggling, and shushing a baby;
- trying to placate a tantrumming toddler;
- saying yes to everything a child asks for;
- trying to get a child to be calm and gentle;
- telling a child to stop being rambunctious; or
- shutting down a teen's attempts at conversation.

If our child isn't going to bed or is taking a long time to go to sleep, and we believe that the behaviours in the evening scenarios list are simply signs of tiredness, we're likely to feel frustrated or powerless. This is likely to be exacerbated if we think thoughts such as, *"She's fighting sleep!"* or *"Why won't he just go to bed?"*

> ### Self-Reflection Moment
> *Have you ever had that 'fighting sleep' thought? It's a very common perception, and completely understandable if we believe that tiredness is the only ingredient required for sleep, and that agitation, aggression, playfulness, and crying are simply signs of tiredness.*

If we're feeling frustrated, it can be easy for us to slip into trying harder to get them to 'calm down'. This can lead to cycles of more frustration and powerlessness when, despite all our efforts, they're *still* not going to sleep. No wonder many parents find sleep one of the most challenging parts of parenting!

However, as you read more, you'll see that having a different understanding of what's going on leads to a very new possibility emerging.

I invite you to notice how differently you might feel and respond when you think about sleep in this Aware Parenting way.

We can change our perceptions of playing, rambunctiousness, agitation, aggression, reactivity, crying, and raging, so that rather than seeing them simply as signs of tiredness, we understand that they are indications that our child is trying to use their innate relaxation process when they are sleepy. *They are trying to release unexpressed painful feelings and tension from their bodies so they can sleep peacefully.*

How does that work?

When they're tired, they're *less* able to suppress their feelings.

I imagine you've found that for yourself too!

If we deeply trust our bodies, we can also trust that there is a reason for that.

In Aware Parenting, we see that it's because their bodies are trying to express pent-up feelings and release stress, so that they can feel more deeply *relaxed*, and can thus have more restorative sleep.

As I've already shared in this book several times (and will be repeating throughout!), this is one of the many things I love about Aware Parenting – the deep trust in our bodies and our innate wisdom.

Instead of seeing 'witching hour' as something 'wrong', we can *cooperate* with what our *baby* is inviting us to do and *listen* with deep presence to their healing-feelings while holding them in our loving arms.

Instead of trying to distract our *toddler* from their tantrum, we can stay close with them, keep them physically safe if necessary, and *listen* lovingly to those big emotions.

Instead of saying 'yes' to a million requests from our *three-year-old* which leave them still feeling agitated, we can offer them a *Loving Limit*[25] and listen to their painful feelings.

Rather than trying to talk our *child* into being calm and gentle, we can also offer them a *Loving Limit* and listen to the big feelings underlying their aggression.

Rather than trying to 'calm down' our rambunctious *seven-year-old*, we can *join in* with their play.

And rather than telling our *older child* or teen to stop arguing or to quieten down the talking, we can *listen* to what they want to share with us.

After our visit to the third ingredient, let's return to the first one.

In many other parenting paradigms, tiredness is perceived to be the only ingredient required for sleep. It's this belief that has led to such

---

25 I will explain more about *Loving Limits* later in the book!

a focus on tiredness and the invention of concepts and terms such as 'sleep windows' and 'sleep pressure' and being 'overtired.' (None of which are used or required in Aware Parenting).

As a result of believing that only tiredness is necessary for sleep, parents may believe that their baby isn't sleeping because they as the parent are not accurately understanding when their baby is tired, or that they are not taking the apt action at the exact time. As a result, parents can experience lots of painful self-judgment and stress, as you'll read in some moving stories shared in this book.

Night owls, early birds, and sleepiness

Another aspect to hold in mind with sleepiness is the existence of two chronotypes. These are genetic predispositions to either fall asleep and wake early (the early bird) or to go to sleep and wake late (the night owl). This is important information to take into account when looking for tiredness cues, since night owls are likely to feel tired *later* than early birds. Some researchers suggest that there is an even wider variety of chronotypes than just two.

So, tiredness is the first of the three ingredients for restful sleep. Let's turn to the second element, connection, and the relationship between closeness and children feeling a sense of safety.

ii. To feel connected (*closeness creating a sense of safety*)

We could say that at the most basic level, this second ingredient is actually the need to experience a sense of safety.

Children need to experience a sense of safety to feel relaxed.

If they don't feel relaxed, they will need to dissociate *in order to go to sleep.*

If they dissociate to fall asleep, the sleep is less likely to be restful.

Because the *main* way that babies and younger children feel safe is connection and closeness (and that need continues, albeit in a reduced form as they get older), I've used these as the title for the second element.

When children experience being safe, they can relax. If children don't feel safe and relaxed, they will need to dissociate in order to fall asleep, which is likely to lead to more restless sleep.

If they do feel safe and relaxed, they can fall asleep without dissociating, which leads to more restful sleep, with less likelihood of being woken by noise or movement.

If they don't feel safe and relaxed, their sleep is likely to be lighter, in case they need to wake up to try to fight or flee.

It makes complete sense, doesn't it, that for a baby or child to feel *relaxed* enough to sleep, they need to know that they are *safe*. To feel safe, they need to experience *closeness* and connection.

As they get *older* and *stronger*, they feel *safer*. As that happens, they are less likely to need closeness to feel relaxed enough to fall asleep without dissociating, and to be able to sleep restfully.

Children's bodies were adapted for hunter-gatherer times and continue to function in these ways.

In a challenging situation with a sabre-tooth tiger, a baby had little option to fight or flee and could only freeze. Toddlers and small children might have had some capacity to fight – but not with much strength, and to flee – but not very fast.

To feel the kind of embodied safety that is required for relaxed sleep[26], babies and young children need to feel a sense of

---

26 Later in the book, I"ll explain the difference between true relaxation and dissociation, which is relevant here.

connection – so that they intrinsically know that there are others close who are bigger and stronger, who care about them, and who will keep them safe whilst they are sleeping.

This innate and inbuilt survival system has great wisdom.

This body intelligence is matched by practices in many traditional cultures, as I've already shared about in earlier chapters. Even in Indigenous cultures in very cold countries, where in the *daytime*, babies might have at times been swaddled and attached to a solid wooden carrier or a sled, still able to see their family, *babies would not be isolated from others overnight*, for these safety reasons (as well as for warmth).

Co-sleeping is still practiced by the majority of families in many parts of the world, such as in Japan, Sweden, and Egypt. It's in English-speaking countries such as the UK, Australia, the US, and Canada where co-sleeping is practiced least.

If you do choose to co-sleep with your baby or child, please make sure you research how to do that safely.

Babies and young children will generally need to mildly dissociate[27] to be able to go to sleep alone in a cot in a separate room.

Using mild dissociation to help babies and children fall asleep is very common – across different cultures and climates, both in the present and the past.

---

27 Dissociation is one of two primary physiological reactions to real or perceived threats or trauma. (The other is hyperarousal.) During dissociation, the parasympathetic nervous system is dominant, and children are quiet, passive, compliant, inattentive, unresponsive, and numb.

> ### Self-Compassion Moment
> *I invite you to put down the guilt stick if you're tempted to pick it up right now. And if you're feeling frustrated or outraged reading this, I'm sending love to all of your feelings. I invite you to be deeply compassionate with yourself if you've left your baby to go to sleep in a cot in a different room. I invite you to listen in to whether you are willing to learn more about what I'm sharing about here. If you're feeling sadness or grief, my heart goes out to you. I hear you. I invite you to reach out to a friend or empathy buddy for some compassionate listening if you are feeling painful feelings.*

Children are so wise. Their bodies still hold the innate wisdom of their hunter-gatherer ancestors.

> In order to feel truly *relaxed* enough to be able to fall asleep and sleep restfully, babies and children need to know that they are *safe*, and for that, they need *closeness*. The younger they are, the more closeness they need.

> ### Self-Compassion Moment
> *Throughout this book, I will keep inviting you to drop the guilt and self-judgment sticks, and I'm doing that now if you have put your baby in a cot in a separate room. Remember, whatever you've done in the past, if this information resonates with you, you can support both secure attachment and healing to happen.*

I want to remind you that it's inbuilt in us that we imbibe the cultural conditioning we're surrounded by. From our own infancy, most of us have internalised the belief that babies have a nursery and sleep in a cot. We would have seen thousands of pictures of this in books, on TV programs (or *programming*), and movies. That simply becomes the norm, along with dummies and strollers. It's so understandable that many of us go on to use those with our own babies.

Discovering what many traditional cultures do, what our ancestors did, and what is still done in many countries today, can help us see our own cultural beliefs more clearly. As a result, we then have the *choice* to do what really resonates with us, rather than what we've been conditioned to believe is the 'right' way to do things.

As children get older, bigger, and stronger, they generally feel safer.

Physically, they are able to get out of bed and run towards connection and safety.

Cognitively, they understand that a parent is close by.

If we have offered them closeness before and during sleep, they will also have internalised that sense of closeness.

For all of these reasons, they will increasingly feel safe enough to fall asleep and stay asleep without having closeness.

Each child has their own unique journey and timing with this. This is partly because their experiences differ in terms of what kind of – and how much – stress and trauma they've experienced, including in relation to separation, and how many accumulated feelings are sitting in their bodies. We will go into this in the third ingredient.

Their unique journey will also be affected by their sensitivity levels.

Highly Sensitive Children[28] (who are picking up more information from their environment) will often need closeness to go to sleep for more years than children who aren't highly sensitive. They are also likely to want to co-sleep for longer. This makes sense from an evolutionary perspective. Their signalling system for safety is set higher, thus they receive more information that might potentially signal danger. So they need more connection and support to feel safe at night.

Each child's unique journey with closeness, safety, and sleep will also be affected by their environment, which includes the physical set-up

---

28 This term and concept is from the work of Elaine Aron.

of the home, and their parents' physical and emotional state. If we are stressed, scared, or dissociated, that will affect how safe they feel.

It is normal for all children to still prefer closeness at night, even once they are past early childhood.

Even for older children and teens, knowing that family members are close by is still likely to signal safety during the night for their hunter-gatherer bodies. Carrying over a general sense of connection from their day can also help them feel more relaxed, for the same reasons.

In many traditional cultures, it's common for older children, teens, and adults to sleep close together in groups at night. As a community, closeness would have been safer for everyone, whatever their age.

When needs for closeness, community, and safety are met, relaxation is possible.

Many adults in modern cultures enjoy bed sharing with a partner. Experiencing a sense of closeness during the night is such a normal and understandable need, whatever our age.

Again, we can see cultural differences at play here. In cultures where lots of physical closeness is common in adulthood, this will also be given to babies, children and teens. In the *DDC*, physical closeness and affection in adulthood are not as common, so we may have been trained as babies and children to not expect it as much.

Shaming children for needing closeness at night is a common *Disconnected Domination Culture* practice. (As is shaming parents if their child wants to be close with them while falling asleep and during sleep.) Hence the term, 'disconnected'.

There's a common perception in the *DDC* that all teens push away closeness from their parents. In Aware Parenting, this is not seen as a developmental stage, but rather, the result of cultural beliefs and painful feelings. Teens can develop increasing competence and timely independence *without* avoiding connection with their parents. With the practice of Aware Parenting, teens often continue to enjoy closeness and hugs with their parents.

I will be explaining the differing closeness needs that babies, children, and teens have in the relevant parts of the book, and what those needs invite you to do to help them sleep restfully.

In Aware Parenting, we understand that a sense of safety through closeness is *necessary*, but not *sufficient* for the true relaxation that is required for restful sleep. If a baby or child is tired and connected but they're not relaxed, it generally means that they have accumulated painful feelings that have bubbled to the surface to be expressed – but which haven't been released.

From a child: I'm feeling a bit sleepy, Mummy, I keep yawning and I just can't concentrate on what you're saying. It's funny, it's like you have some kind of a magnet, because I just want to be close to you. I wish we could cuddle up together. You're helping me brush my teeth because you say that I don't get in all the corners. I'm glad, because I don't even have the energy for brushing my own teeth now. We snuggle up together in bed, and I love being so warm and cosy with you. I'm like a kangaroo in your pouch. You tell me stories, and more stories, and I'm still yawning, but my legs are all wriggly. I wish I could go to sleep. Why aren't I going to sleep, Mummy? I really want to.

Instead of teaching babies and children to move into freeze – or mildly dissociate – from accumulated feelings to fall asleep, Aware Parenting invites parents to work with the innate wisdom of our children's bodies to release stress and feel deeply relaxed.

In the next section, I'll explain more about how that happens.

iii. To feel relaxed (*by releasing any healing-feelings present*)

The Aware Parenting understanding of true relaxation – and how it is different to mild dissociation (which I will explain more about soon) – is one of the key reasons why we look at sleep in a very different light compared to most other parenting paradigms.

Other approaches hold that as parents, we have two choices with the going-to-sleep process:

- To do things to our babies or children *while they are with us* to 'soothe' them to feel 'calm'.

- To teach them to 'self-soothe' *on their own* to help them feel 'calm'.

In Aware Parenting, we recognise that both of these tend to create forms of mild dissociation rather than deep relaxation.

> *Self-Compassion Moment*
>
> I invite you to drop any guilt sticks if you're tempted to pick them up here. As I'll talk more about soon, mild dissociation can feel pleasant. I'm not judging you if you help your baby or child to mildly dissociate before sleep. It's very common. I did it with my daughter when she was a baby, even though I knew about Aware Parenting (while I was still learning to understand it, and the nuances of it). I want to remind you that this isn't about judgment. It's about information, awareness and choice. Once you have this information, it's your choice about what you do as a result.

> In Aware Parenting, we have a deep trust that babies, children, and teens have innate healing and relaxation processes.

Rather than trying to do things to children to make them more superficially calm by 'soothing' them, or leaving them to 'self-soothe', when we *understand* these natural processes, we can *cooperate* with them, leading to a deeper sense of *relaxation*.

These innate healing and relaxation processes are:

- *crying* or *raging* with loving support;
- *laughter* and *play* with loving support; and
- *talking* with loving support.

We will go through each of these in more detail in the following chapters, because how this looks and how we can respond varies depending on whether we're with a baby, child, or teen.

For **babies**, crying in our loving arms when all their immediate needs are met is the main way that they express healing-feelings, release stress and tension from the day, and heal from past stressful events or traumas.

In Part 2, I'll talk about how you can help your baby feel connected and deeply relaxed.

I loved receiving this message from Gina about how her perception of herself and her baby's crying before sleep changed once she received this information. She said:

"Hi! I just wanted to say a big thank you for your post about babies' innate body wisdom and how they need to release energy via a big cry in our loving arms. I was having a hard time getting my baby to sleep. She kept on crying and crying in my arms, until she finally fell asleep. I was beating myself up, because surely I was doing something wrong if I (her mum) couldn't soothe her. And then I found your post, and it all made sense, and I don't feel guilty anymore."

Crying in arms when all their needs are met helps babies move *out* of the fight, flight, or freeze response, and into *deep relaxation.*

Later in the book, I'll explain the differences between mild dissociation and true relaxation. I'll also talk about how the things we are often taught to do to babies to 'calm them down' actually lead to a mild state of dissociation. That often results in:

- frequent night-waking;
- waking up crying;

- agitation during sleeping, and
- us walking on eggshells in case we make a noise and they wake up!

I absolutely adore Caitlin's description of the difference she experienced once she started practicing Aware Parenting with her four-month-old baby, Frankie. It clearly demonstrates what I'm talking about here:

"Aware Parenting has been simply life-changing for my family.

My son had never slept easily, sleeping on average 45 minute stints only after lots of bouncing on the yoga ball, loud music, singing and a dummy, or being fed to sleep via breastfeeding but then soon awakening. If I wanted him to nap longer, the house had to be silent, and the yoga ball nearby so I could start bouncing the moment he stirred.

We had initially tried to get him to sleep in a bassinet – my husband and I sleeping in shifts. We would bounce him to sleep then try to transfer him to the bassinet again and again, averaging about five hours each night of this routine, hoping this would be the night we would get it right. It was so disheartening to try so hard at something and then fail night after night.

We then began to survive nights by co-sleeping. He basically slept with my nipple in his mouth the whole night. This was causing me considerable hip pain from sleeping in a frozen position. Naps were short and always in the baby carrier. The pram or car seat I described as a battle ground – he screamed and screamed every time I put him in either.

I was adamantly against the idea of sleep training as it went against my every instinct to leave a baby alone to cry. But I couldn't understand why sleep was this difficult – I was devoting my life to attending to his needs 24/7. Well-meaning friends and family members described ways of getting him to sleep by crawling into the room and not looking at him, etc. It all sounded so ridiculous.

Also the idea of "sleep school" – we couldn't have evolved for sleep needing to be taught to infants at a school surely? It didn't make sense…

The moment I stumbled upon Aware Parenting, I knew this was the missing puzzle piece I had been searching for. I thought about how I felt in the postpartum period when I had cried in the arms of my husband, releasing all the emotions and stress I had been experiencing, and how much relief that had brought me. It made sense that Frankie also had emotions and feelings about this period of time too that he needed to express.

The first time I held Frankie in my loving arms and allowed him to cry (after first ensuring all his needs had been attended to) was profound – the results were instantaneous. He had a cry and then came out the other side bright and bubbly and ready to play.

My jaw dropped – I had spent months doing everything I could to suppress his crying – bouncing, singing, dummy, breastfeeding hourly, white noise, different temperatures/music and all I had needed to do was allow him to be heard.

Within a month he transformed into a baby sleeping 5-8 hours at night. We could even move him while he was sleeping to change his nappy and clothes and he kept on sleeping!! What a transformation!

He also happily went in the pram or car seat and allowed other family members to hold him. I also felt his concentration improved, he was able to spend more time independently playing and he was suddenly crawling at five months old. Life has become so much easier and more enjoyable.

I think of the trajectory we were on before Aware Parenting and the burnout we would have inevitably faced and I'm just so incredibly grateful to have found Aware Parenting."

Self-Compassion Moment

I'm sending so much love to however you feel when you read this. Perhaps you went through the bouncing, or all-night feeding, or your baby cried every time you went in the car, and you might be feeling painful feelings when you remember that time. If so, my heart goes out to you. Maybe you wish you had known this information earlier, when your little one was a baby. Or perhaps you are feeling excited and hopeful, if your baby isn't yet born, or your baby is fairly young, seeing that there is this potential for a really different experience with sleep. Or maybe you're feeling something else entirely. Whatever you're feeling, I welcome all your feelings. I invite you to share them with a loving listener.

For **children**, the main two ways that these natural relaxation processes work are through laughter/play and crying/raging with our loving support. As they get older, talking joins this list.

This can overturn two usual sleep maxims of trying to get children to calm down by stopping them from playing, and the fear that "it will all end in tears!"

We'll talk more about these in Part 3, and I'll show you how you can cooperate with their desire to play in the evening *without* playing for hours. I'll also explain how you can transform the fear of it all ending in tears into a deep welcoming of your child's big feelings.

For **teens**, talking while receiving loving listening becomes their primary form of expression that leads to relaxation. However, crying, expressing anger, and engaging in laughter and fun may also still be a part of this relaxation process at times, particularly after stressful or traumatic events.

In Part 4 (the teens section), I'll be inviting you to welcome those evening chats, and what you can do to maximise the likelihood that your teen will be willing to share their feelings with you.

You're probably getting a sense already of how holding these three things in mind means that not only are we seeing what is going on in the evenings in a very different light, we're going to respond to our baby, child, or teen in new ways too!

Trust in their innate wisdom

As you'll read many times in this book, one of the core elements of Aware Parenting is a deep *trust* in the *innate wisdom* of babies and children.

We recognise their innate drive for healing and wholeness, and the ways they are repeatedly trying to heal from daily stresses, as well as bigger traumas, such as birth or separation trauma. We also see their innate relaxation processes, the ones they try to use each evening, so they can feel relaxed enough to sleep restfully and restoratively.

It turns out that the healing mechanism and the relaxation response are one and the same. And that makes so much sense, doesn't it? When they release stress from their bodies, they feel more relaxed.

Deep *relaxation* is a *requirement* for *restful* sleep.

However, because our culture doesn't understand the innate healing and relaxation processes, most parents are taught to work against them.

With Aware Parenting, much of what we're doing is *freeing ourselves* from that cultural conditioning. The more we do so, the more we can trust children and cooperate with their natural wisdom. As a result, they can heal from stress and trauma, and they can sleep more *restfully* and *restoratively.*

Aware Parenting works with children's natural relaxation processes to support sleep

The simplicity of trusting their innate wisdom

Our bodies are amazingly *wise*. The ways that children heal from stress and trauma are the same ways that they feel relaxed enough to sleep; their bodies know how to release stress to have restful and restorative sleep.

The *DDC* often makes things very complex.

But if we return to our biological wisdom, things often become very simple.

If we *trust* the innate wisdom of babies and children, we can transform our understanding of what is commonly seen as 'wrong' and needing to be fixed, into something that *indicates intrinsic intelligence.*

We become detectives and researchers, willing to discern biological wisdom from cultural conditioning through clear observation.

What do many babies commonly do in the evenings?

Cry, or try to cry.

What do many toddlers and young children often do?

Be playful, or start crying or raging in response to something small.

What do older children often do?

Talk about their day.

What do teens and adults often want to do?

Also talk about their day!

If we are researchers, seeing the commonalities in all of these, we can see that these processes are their *inherent wisdom* at play, releasing the stresses of the day, or larger traumas from the past.

Each person at each age is *trying to heal*. Trying to move out of fight, flight, or freeze, to feel and express *healing-feelings*, so that those feelings, and the related stress and tension, can be released. Their amazing bodies are supported by this process to feel safe and relaxed, and thus sleep restfully and restoratively.

Sleep is so important for human health. Of course our bodies know exactly how to sleep most restoratively!

However:

For their crying to be healing, babies need to be *held* in our loving arms when all their needs are met.

Toddlers and small children need us to *join in* with their play, and listen lovingly to their tears and tantrums, for those to be healing.

Older children and teens need us to *really listen* to them talking with us for healing to happen.

They all *need our help* if they are to express and release stress and tension from their bodies. *The relaxation-through-release response requires our cooperation and support.*

They all need *our presence, our understanding* of what's really going on for them, and *our trust* in their innate wisdom.

That can require a lot from us.

If we don't know about this process, we might try to:

- *Stop* our baby from healing-crying by feeding them when they're not hungry. Jiggling, rocking, or bouncing them. Swaddling them. Or giving them a dummy;

- *'Calm down'* our toddler or child from playing, crying, or tantrumming before bed;

- *Distract, judge,* or *placate* our older child or teen in the evening, rather than really listen to them.

However, even if we *do* understand this process, we might find listening and playing *hard*, because we probably didn't receive it ourselves as children. This is why having our own feelings heard regularly as parents is a vital part of Aware Parenting.

Why do babies and children find it hard to go to sleep and stay asleep?

If we were to think in simple and clear ways, why would a baby or child find it hard to go to sleep and stay asleep?

Because they don't feel relaxed enough.

They need to feel relaxed to be able to fall asleep when they're tired and stay asleep during the night when they enter lighter sleep.

The *DDC* belief is that babies and children need to be 'calmed down' before going to sleep. Because the 'calming down' approaches don't take into account – and often work against –the natural relaxation-through-release process that happens when babies and children are sleepy, they often lead to a more *superficial* calm, rather than a *deep* relaxation.

Later on, I'll share why being able to understand the difference between superficial calm and deep relaxation is vital to sleep, and how we can learn to differentiate between the two in our children.

Sleep is a *barometer*. What happens with sleep tells us a lot about what is going on for our child, both physiologically and emotionally.

Babies, children, and teens have *incredible innate wisdom* in every area of life. Their bodies know exactly how to feel relaxed enough to sleep. But we're often taught information and practices that work against their intrinsic intelligence. This can lead to dissociation, rather than true relaxation.

We can work with their innate wisdom:

1. By offering closeness so they know they are safe to sleep[29].
2. By cooperating with their invitations to cry, rage, play, laugh, or talk with our loving support.

They can come out of fight, flight or freeze; heal from stress and trauma; express feelings such as overwhelm, powerlessness, fear, or sadness; and feel a deep and satisfying sense of relaxation.

This *deep relaxation* creates beautiful
restful and *restorative* sleep.

Not only does this process bring about sleep and secure attachment, but when we observe how powerful it is, we gain a deep *trust* in the innate biological wisdom of our children.

From an Aware Parenting perspective, sleep challenges at any age become *invitations* to support our children to feel more connected with themselves and us, freer from unhealed stress, and more deeply relaxed in their bodies.

These reframes can make a huge difference to both how we feel and what actions we take.

---

29 The older they are, the less likely it is that they will need closeness while going to sleep. However, for older children and teens, feeling a sense of connection in general will still help them feel more relaxed and sleep more restfully.

Alongside me offering you huge compassion if your baby or young child is taking a long time to go to sleep or is waking up frequently, or if you're having battles over sleep with your older child or teen, and your sleep is being affected, I will also be inviting you to see this as an opportunity for *profound connection and healing* for you both.

The three ingredients and how they are perceived in early-independence parenting, *Classical Attachment Parenting*, and Aware Parenting

Early-independence parenting

Early-independence parenting is generally based on the belief that only tiredness is required for restful sleep.

Needs for closeness and safety aren't generally recognised, so babies may need to learn to suppress those needs, as well as the feelings they feel when they don't have closeness and don't experience being safe.

The innate relaxation-through-release process is also not recognised. Instead, babies and children are taught to dissociate from those healing-feelings, such as through a dummy or clutching on to a soft toy or blanket, or they may start thumb-sucking.

Suppressing or dissociating from those uncomfortable feelings is called 'self-soothing' in early-independence parenting.

With the early-independence approach, babies and children will often still wake up at night. They will usually go back to whatever they were doing earlier on to suppress their feelings, without calling out to signal that they are awake and need connection. This is part of learning 'early independence', i.e. to be less likely to ask for help when they need it.

Because neither needs for closeness nor the relaxation process are recognised, all the *focus* is on *tiredness*. This is why complex calculations about 'sleep windows', 'sleep pressure' and babies being 'overtired' are seen as the causes of sleep challenges.

I have seen so many parents feeling really stressed when they believe that only tiredness is relevant to their baby's sleep, becoming desperate to work out complex 'sleep windows' and being concerned that their baby may be 'overtired'. Conversely, they tell me how relieved they are once they learn about Aware Parenting.

(Concepts such as 'sleep windows', 'overtired', and 'sleep pressure' don't exist in Aware Parenting – I'll share about why in Chapter 13.)

Self-Compassion Moment

I'm sending lots of compassion to whatever you're feeling right now, and so much love to you. I want to remind you that I'm not judging you, and I invite you to be unwilling to judge yourself. Remember that we are meant to believe what we are culturally conditioned to believe about babies and children and sleep, and most of these things are what we saw and experienced growing up. We needed to believe those things were the 'accurate' way to respond to children. Early independence is pushed as a core tenet of much of the industrialised world. It's common and understandable if you've been affected by these beliefs. If you've been stressed, trying to get your baby to sleep according to 'sleep windows', or you've been worried that your baby is 'overtired', my heart goes out to you. Aware Parenting offers a really different experience for both babies and parents.

Classical Attachment Parenting

Classical Attachment Parenting believes that both tiredness *and* closeness are required for restful sleep.

However, the relaxation-through-release process isn't recognised. Instead, it's perceived that babies and children need to be 'soothed' to sleep through breastfeeding, or with movement – through carrying them in a carrier, or jiggling and rocking them.

Aware Parenting sees this as interpreting a *healing-feeling* as a *needs-feeling* and creating mild dissociation.

From an Aware Parenting perspective, the reasons why babies and toddlers then wake up often at night is because they are trying to *express* the painful feelings that have been suppressed through the 'soothing' (i.e. the mild dissociation or suppression).

Self-Compassion Moment

If you've been practicing Classical Attachment Parenting and you're feeling angry, I'm sending love to your anger.

If you're tempted to pick up the guilt stick right now, I invite you to be unwilling to judge yourself.

If you're feeling sad that you didn't know this information before, I'm sending love to the sadness.

Practicing Classical Attachment Parenting means it's likely that you've already shed some DDC beliefs around attachment and closeness needs. I so acknowledge all that you've already done to change your beliefs. And I send love to all of your feelings.

Aware Parenting

As you've already seen, Aware Parenting recognises that three ingredients are required for restful sleep: sleepiness; closeness; and relaxation.

When I work with parents, they are often surprised when they move from *DDC* parenting or *Classical Attachment Parenting* and start practicing Aware Parenting. I hear phrases such as:

"My baby doesn't wake up when I transfer her."

"We don't need to tiptoe around him anymore when he's sleeping."

"My toddler no longer spends all night doing gymnastics in our co-sleeping bed."

"My four-year-old is so relaxed when she's sleeping now."

"I love feeling connected with my eight-year-old when we play silly games before bed."

"My teen and I have a new level of connection and trust together."

However, since parents practicing Aware Parenting are still learning (because we grew up in the *DDC*), we will probably only support a *percentage* of the relaxation process rather than 100% of it.

We may often breastfeed to sleep, or distract our child in other ways, so they might still be woken up by unexpressed feelings at times. If our older baby, child, or teen is still waking up frequently or showing other sleep challenges, we are being *invited to understand the nuances* of Aware Parenting even more deeply. I'll share more about how you can do that throughout this book.

> Babies and children *want to feel relaxed*
> enough to sleep restfully. They want to sleep
> as much as we want them to sleep!

Biologically, sleep is essential, so babies and children can obviously go to sleep *without* these three ingredients, often through mild dissociation. However, that sleep is generally not as restful, which is why they might wake up with the slightest noise or movement.

The less that these three ingredients are met, the *more* likely that a baby or child will:

- take longer to go to sleep;
- wake up more easily, e.g. with sound or movement;
- wake up more frequently; and/or
- wake up without feeling rested.

When we understand *how* they are inviting us to support their innate wisdom for relaxation, and we *join in* with that process, they can feel more deeply *relaxed* and can sleep *restfully* and restoratively.

CHAPTER SUMMARY

Babies, children, and teens need to be both *tired* and *relaxed* to sleep restfully.

Relaxation is created in *two* ways: through a sense of *safety* (which comes from *closeness*, especially in the early years), and by releasing any pent-up painful feelings that naturally bubble to the surface to be expressed when they are tired.

If children don't feel *safe*, they won't feel *relaxed*, and will need to *dissociate* to go to sleep. If children have *accumulated* painful feelings bubbling to the surface that haven't been released, they won't feel *relaxed*, and will need to *dissociate* to go to sleep.

If they dissociate to fall asleep, the sleep is not likely to be *restful*.

Thus, the three ingredients needed for restful and restorative sleep are:

i. to feel tired;

ii. to feel connected (*closeness creating safety*); and

iii. to feel relaxed (*by releasing any healing-feelings present*).

Rather than being *caused* by tiredness, behaviours such as crying, raging, being super playful and rambunctious before bed, or wanting to talk about their day are all signs of their innate relaxation-through-release process in operation *when they are sleepy*, because they're less able to suppress their feelings then. Being super rambunctious or agitated can also be a symptom of hyperarousal.

The main way that babies and younger children feel *safe* is *connection* and *closeness* (and that need continues, albeit in a reduced form as they get older). If they feel relaxed, they can fall asleep *without dissociating*, which leads to more *restful* sleep.

As children get older, bigger, and stronger, they feel safer. Physically, they are able to get out of bed and run towards connection and safety. Cognitively, they understand that a parent is close by. If we have offered them closeness before and during sleep, they will also have internalised that sense of closeness. For all of these reasons, they will increasingly feel safe enough to fall asleep and stay asleep without having closeness. Each child has their own unique journey and timing with this, depending on the stress and trauma they've experienced, their sensitivity levels, and their environment (which includes our physical and emotional state).

In Aware Parenting, we have a deep trust that babies, children, teens (and adults) all have innate healing and relaxation processes, and we aim to work with them. These are:

- *crying* or *raging* with loving support;
- *laughter* and *play* with loving support; and
- *talking* with loving support.

Our bodies are amazingly wise. The way that children heal from stress and trauma is the same way that they feel relaxed enough to sleep; their bodies know how to release stress so they can have restful and restorative sleep.

I'm here with you as you enquire into your thoughts and beliefs about sleep.

7. The physiology of stress and relaxation

The natural processes whereby babies and children feel deeply *relaxed* are the *same* methods by which they *heal* from *stress* and *trauma*. In this chapter, I explain more about:

- trauma;
- the fight, flight, or freeze response;
- the healing from trauma process;

and how all of these affect sleep.

In her book *Healing Your Traumatized Child*, Aletha Solter, PhD defines trauma in the following way:

*"...anything that causes physical or emotional pain or that threatens a child's wellbeing.... **Anything that a child interprets as threatening can be traumatic**, even when it does not pose a real danger."* (page 21). [emphasis mine].

If you haven't already read *Healing Your Traumatized Child*, I highly recommend reading it, even if you don't think that the concept of trauma is relevant to your child/ren. The book explains how children are affected by – and heal from – challenging experiences like medical trauma, as well as daily hurts. From an Aware Parenting perspective, *all* babies and children experience frequent mild stress and mini traumas, and many will experience larger trauma. For example, babies commonly experience birth trauma.

There are two key ways for babies and children to respond to threatening events which are stressful or traumatic:

- **fight/flight** (also known as *hyperarousal*); or
- **freeze** (which we refer to as *dissociation* in Aware Parenting, as do other paradigms).

The fight/flight response is mobilised when a child feels scared and experiences a threat.

They will either **fight** e.g. yelling, hitting, scratching, biting, or **flee** e.g. running away from something, or towards a parent.

Screaming, yelling, and vigorous movement are essential parts of the fight or flight response. This is part of the *innate wisdom* of our bodies to support survival.

I invite you to hold this in your mind when you think about a toddler having a tantrum before bed. They are releasing all that energy that was mobilised to fight or flee, and are returning to homeostasis.

When a baby or child experiences stress or trauma, their sympathetic nervous system is activated. This increases the heart rate so that blood flow can be diverted to their arms and legs so they can fight or flee, and away from the digestive system, which is of secondary importance at times of danger.

Experiences of stressful situations include:

- a *baby* awake and alone in a cot at night, without closeness and thus not experiencing safety;
- a *toddler* awake and alone in a cot at night, unable to flee to a parent if they feel scared;
- a *child* hearing a strange loud noise in the night and not knowing what it is; or
- a *teen* watching a scary movie late at night.

These can lead to *either* hyperarousal *or* dissociation, or a pattern of both, for example, a baby waking up scared and in hyperarousal, sucking their thumb to dissociate to go back to sleep again, waking up in hyperarousal again, and so on.

> ### Self-Compassion Moment
>
> *I'm sending so much love to any feelings you might be feeling right now. Your baby or child might have experienced these things. If so, I'm here to remind you that I'm not judging you and I invite you to be unwilling to judge yourself. If you're feeling sad, my heart goes out to your sadness. If you're feeling numb, I'm right here with you to remind you that it's so normal for us to dissociate when offered information such as this. If you're feeling scared, perhaps connecting in with your own experiences when you were younger, I'm also here to offer you lots of loving compassion. I invite you to do some journalling or reach out for some loving listening. And I'm here to offer you another reminder, that healing is possible, whatever age our child is, or we are. This is what Aware Parenting is holding so dearly, our innate wisdom for healing from stress or trauma.*

If a child goes into hyperarousal (fight or flight), the HPA (hypothalamic-pituitary-adrenal) system is set into motion. It increases the amount of sugar in the blood, thus giving immediate energy required to fight or to flee. Related to the HPA system is the well-known hormone cortisol, which is correlated with the levels of stress in the body.

However, if a baby, child, or teen *isn't able to fight or flee*, the next automatic survival strategy is *dissociation*. Babies are much more likely than children and teens to dissociate, because they have little capacity to fight or to flee.

With dissociation, the parasympathetic nervous system is involved, especially the vagus nerve, which reduces heart rate and blood pressure.

In *Healing Your Traumatized Child*, Aletha Solter says: *"Dissociation also involves high levels of endogenous opioids (endorphins), which **numb physical pain and reduce emotions of fear and anger, sometimes even producing narcotic-like euphoria.** Dopamine, which plays a role in addictive behaviors, is also involved in dissociation. The high levels of both endorphins and dopamine might help to explain why **dissociative states are both pleasurable and addictive.**"* (pages 25-26). [emphasis mine].

When *dissociated*, a baby, child, or teen becomes *very still and quiet*, and will *feel numb*.

I invite you to hold this in mind when you think about your child's sleep.

In our culture, we are taught *to see this stillness and quietness as a sign of* calmness.

> ### Self-Compassion Moment
> I'm sending love to any feelings you might be feeling as you read this.
> I invite you to pause if you need to, and to have your feelings heard,
> or do some journalling, if you feel called to.

Dissociation is *vital* for survival purposes. It saves energy which might be needed if fighting or fleeing becomes possible. The numbness reduces the experience of any physical or emotional pain.

A *spectrum* of dissociation exists, with *mild* dissociation on one side – such as with daydreaming, to *extreme* dissociation on the other end – which would include fainting.

If a baby or young child doesn't feel *safe* because they are alone before sleep and during the night, they will go into *hyperarousal*. In order to sleep while alone, they will need to *dissociate*.[30]

If a baby, child, or teen has pent-up healing-feelings from previous experiences of fight or flight that are bubbling up to be expressed before sleep, and *their emotions aren't welcomed*, they will need to *dissociate* in order to go to sleep[31].

---

30 This explains the second ingredient that I talked about in the last chapter.
31 This explains the third ingredient.

Dissociation at bedtime *temporarily overrides* the *hyperarousal* response, so that a child who is stressed can go to sleep. However, the calming effect is only *temporary*, and when it wears off, the child moves into hyperarousal again and wakes up.

This might mean that they are in a repeated cycle of hyperarousal and dissociation during the night.

A child who is in a state of hyperarousal before bed, e.g. fighting with their sibling, or fleeing by running around the house rambunctiously, might be seen as 'misbehaving' or 'hyperactive'. A child who is dissociated before sleep, e.g. thumb-sucking and gazing into space, or swaddled with a dummy in their mouth, might be seen as calm or relaxed.

Understanding that there is no such thing as misbehaviour, and being able to differentiate between dissociation and true relaxation, are two core keys to practicing Aware Parenting, particularly in relation to sleep.

From a child: Nanna, when I stay at your place for the night, sometimes I get a bit scared. My bed here is so different from my bed at home, and there are funny creaking and whooshing sounds in the night. You always tell me that I'm a good girl when I go to bed. I put my thumb in my mouth because it helps me not feel scared anymore. Then I can go to sleep. But last night, I could hear all these loud banging noises. I thought it was a monster coming up the stairs to get me. I needed to put my thumb in my mouth and cuddle Teddy, and even then I still felt a bit scared. Then I heard you cough and realised it was you all along. I know you tell me I'm a good girl because I'm quiet and I don't call out in the night, but I don't really like staying overnight at your house. I'm going to ask Mummy and Daddy if I can just come to your house for the daytime next time, Nanna. Mummy and Daddy don't call me a good girl and they always leave my bedroom door open at night. They leave a night light on for me and they tell me that I can come into their room anytime I want. If I feel scared and cry, they listen to my feelings. I hardly ever need to suck my thumb at home. And I don't need to hold on tight to Teddy.

In *Healing Your Traumatized Child*, Aletha Solter says: *"...a major trauma may not be necessary for chronic hyperarousal or dissociation to occur. **An accumulation of stress or unhealed mini-traumas can affect children's bodies in the same way as a single threatening event because their brain interprets a build-up of stress as a threat to their well-being**. Children can accumulate stress from daily overstimulation, anxiety, disappointments, frustrations, unmet needs, criticisms, punishment, their parents' stress, or unrealistic expectations by adults."* (page 31). [emphasis mine].

If babies or children don't get to regularly release stress and tension from their bodies using their innate healing processes of crying and raging, that stress *accumulates* over time. You can probably see how this plays out with sleep, such as when babies tend to start *waking up more* as they get older, or after busy days or stressful events.

It's this phenomenon which is often termed 'sleep regression' in other paradigms.

However much we aim to meet the needs of our baby or child, *all* babies and all children will experience stresses and mini-traumas, and many will experience bigger traumas.

This means that *all* babies and children will regularly need to release stress and tension before sleep.

How often? you might ask.

This book is the detailed answer to that question.

The *younger* the baby, the more likely it is that they need to do that before *every* sleep.

All babies will have *some stress to release* through expressing healing-feelings *every day* for *the first several months* (although *not necessarily before every* nap and sleep), gradually decreasing as they get older (if their healing-crying has been thoroughly welcomed at younger ages).

Personally, I think that the majority of babies growing up in the DDC *will have some healing-feelings to express pretty much every day for the first year, but that is not an official Aware Parenting perspective.*

Self-Compassion Moment

I'm sending love to your feelings, whatever they are, when you read this. I want to remind you that even though babies have lots of stress to release, this doesn't mean that you 'have to' listen to all or even any of those feelings (and 'have to' is another DDC phrase). Although they have healing-feelings to express before sleep, they also know how to mildly dissociate when there isn't the available listening space for them. In addition, we can catch up on listening to many of their healing-feelings if we start the process when they are older.

I'd also love to emphasise that any listening to their healing-feelings that we are able to do will make a difference to them and how relaxed they feel, even if that only happens occasionally, and if we generally distract them when we are stressed or stretched. Listening to their healing-feelings sometimes will still help them release stress from their bodies.

In toddlerhood, the quantity of healing-feelings they need to express is likely to reduce (unless they're still catching up on expressing healing-feelings that they didn't get to express during their first year), apart from when they're going through big developmental leaps or experiencing external stressors.

The *older* a child is, the *less* likely they will need to cry or tantrum before sleep, unless they've had a particularly stimulating or stressful day.

The classic tantrum after a birthday party, or extra crying in the evening during a house move, holiday, or parents' divorce are classic examples of the innately wise healing and relaxation process in operation – releasing stress, so that restful sleep can come.

Laughter and play also release stress and trauma, particularly fear and powerlessness. When a child sees their parents playing, it literally *signals safety,* since people wouldn't be playing if there was extreme danger.

Attachment play[32] and laughter become more and more common ways to release stress as babies become toddlers, but *they do not replace* crying and tantrums to release stress and trauma.

As children become older, talking also becomes a common way to release stresses of the day, although it's still a natural process for them to need to occasionally laugh and play, or cry and rage before sleep. This continues into the teenage years and adulthood.

After our beloved 10-year-old French Bulldog, Feather suddenly died one evening, my 22-year-old daughter and 17-year-old son both cried in my arms before going to sleep. I was so grateful to understand how important it was for them to express all their grief and shock through wailing, sobbing, and crying with loving support. It helped me remember all those times of listening to their tears when they were babies and children.

<blockquote>
Sleep is not a priority in the face of stress and perceived threat. There is a survival advantage to being awake and alert in the face of potential danger. This may be the reason why children cannot easily fall asleep when they are feeling stressed.
</blockquote>

However, children are innately able to release stress. As parents, this translates into trusting and supporting our children's tears, laughter, and body movements as they release accumulated stress from their bodies with our loving presence.

---

32 *Attachment play* is a core element of Aware Parenting.

After the stress is *resolved* and relaxation is *restored*, the body is then free to prioritise *rest*, growth, and *regeneration*, which occur during sleep.

Babies who experience birth trauma and medical interventions will have more stress and trauma to release from their bodies, which will then affect their sleep more. Nik, who is training to be an Aware Parenting instructor, shares about her journey with her son, who experienced a stressful birth and early separation, and later on, a medical procedure:

"After a traumatic birth resulting in an emergency C-section, our baby spent the first 48 hours separated from us in Neonatal care. We weren't even allowed to hold him. Bringing him home, breastfeeding became a challenge – he couldn't latch and had to be fed through a tiny tube for the first week. During that initial week, Blaze remained unusually quiet until we discovered he had grade three tongue and lip tie. Following the doctor's recommendation, we opted for a frenotomy to correct the tongue tie, hoping it would improve his latch. Shortly after the procedure, Blaze began crying incessantly. What started as a few hours in the evenings soon escalated to all day and night, for up to 12-14 hours a day.

Before giving birth we completed a course on newborn care, where they taught various techniques on how to settle a fussy crying infant. This included swaddling, bouncing, carrying, white noise, walking, and loud shushing combined with rather vigorous side-to-side swaying until the baby completely stops. I vividly remember a video demonstrating this technique that gave immediate results even with the fussiest baby. We tried all of these techniques but nothing seemed to 'soothe' him. I remember at some point my partner carrying and shushing him for four hours at night to the point that he lost his voice – yet Blaze's crying persisted.

Desperate for a solution, we consulted numerous experts, from chiropractors, osteopaths, craniosacral specialists, pediatricians, lactation consultants, and even energy healers, but to no avail. Most of the time when he cried I fed him, thinking he must be hungry since all of his other needs were met. He developed severe reflux and his body was always tense and wiggly. For eight long weeks, I felt utterly helpless, and physically and emotionally drained while recovering from a C-section. Then, the all-day crying ceased, but another challenge emerged – 'sleep refusal'. Getting him to nap became a monumental task, requiring swaddling, hours of bouncing, white noise, and a pacifier, only for him to wake up shortly after falling asleep. Seeking answers, I hired an attachment-focused holistic sleep consultant, who suggested Blaze might be highly sensitive. Therefore, he'd benefit from a lot of vestibular movement like bouncing and swinging, especially before sleep, but we were already doing that.

It wasn't until Blaze was six months old that my friend sent me an Aware Parenting podcast episode on sleep. Being a somatic coach and supporting adults with their emotions, the approach immediately resonated. I decided to give it a try. One afternoon, I listened to Blaze without relying on gadgets or bouncing, and something remarkable happened. When he woke up, he was a different baby – calm, serene, and engaged, playing with the same toy for 20 minutes. A sense of peace emanated from his gaze. Encouraged by this transformation, we embarked on our Aware Parenting journey, and the results were profound.

Working with an instructor, I learned to increase my capacity to listen and support Blaze in releasing his pent-up emotions. In one of the long listening sessions, I could feel him revisit his birth and process a lot of that trauma. He still cries before every sleep, yet our approach to it has radically shifted. Rather than working against him, we aim to support him in releasing his feelings. And the difference is palpable – Blaze is a bright, happy baby, captivating everyone he meets."

Self-Reflection Moment

How are you feeling, reading this? If you've experienced anything similar to what Nik went through, I'm sending you so much love and compassion. Supporting babies who have experienced significant trauma can be a huge journey. Receiving support from an Aware Parenting instructor can make a big difference in being able to help a baby in the healing process, as Nik's story illustrates.

From a child: There's a big tiger chasing me all around the house. I won't let him catch me, I won't! I'm bigger than him! I'm a lion! I'm the biggest lion in the world! I roar and I stomp and I jump over the sofa. He'll never catch me! I keep falling over, I don't know why. My sister Lynn is sitting on the beanbag. She always sucks her thumb when it gets close to bedtime. It's so boring, because then she never plays with me. I need to run even faster when I see her doing that, I don't know why. The more still she is, the more I need to move. I know Dad doesn't like it when I run around like this in the evenings. He always tells me to be more like Lynn, and to calm down. But I don't want to be like her. I don't really like how I feel though. I wish I could rest now. Perhaps I'll just run around the house again, a bit faster and louder this time. Maybe that will help me be able to sleep.

CHAPTER SUMMARY

The natural processes that babies and children use to feel deeply relaxed are the same methods whereby they heal from stress and trauma.

There are two key ways for babies, children, and teens to respond to threatening events which are stressful or traumatic:

- fight/flight (hyperarousal); or
- freeze (dissociation).

When dissociated, a baby, child, or teen becomes very still and quiet, and will feel numb.

If a baby or young child doesn't feel *safe* because they are alone before and during sleep, they will go into *hyperarousal*. In order to sleep while alone, they will need to *dissociate*. If a baby, child, or teen has pent-up healing-feelings from previous experiences of fight or flight that are bubbling up to be expressed before sleep, and *their emotions aren't welcomed*, they will need to *dissociate* in order to go to sleep.

Dissociation at bedtime temporarily overrides the hyperarousal response, so that a child who is stressed can go to sleep. However, the calming effect is only temporary, and when it wears off, the child moves into hyperarousal again and wakes up. This might mean that they are in a repeated cycle of hyperarousal and dissociation during the night.

A child who is in a state of hyperarousal before bed, e.g. fighting with their sibling, or fleeing by running around the house rambunctiously, might be seen as 'misbehaving' or 'hyperactive'. A child who is dissociated before sleep, e.g. thumb-sucking and gazing into space, might be seen as calm or relaxed. Understanding that there is no such thing as misbehaviour, and being able to differentiate between dissociation and true relaxation, are two core keys to practicing Aware Parenting, particularly in relation to sleep.

If babies or children don't get to regularly release stress and tension from their bodies using their innate healing processes of crying and raging, that stress *accumulates* over time. You can probably see how this plays out with sleep, such as when babies tend to start waking up more as they get older, or after busy days or stressful events. It's this phenomenon which is often termed 'sleep regression' in other paradigms.

All babies and children regularly need to release stress and tension before sleep if they are to sleep restfully. The younger they are, the more likely that they need to do that before each sleep. But even older children and teens will need to do this after stressful or traumatic experiences.

Sleep is not a priority in the face of stress and perceived threat. There is a survival advantage to being awake and alert in the face of potential danger. This may be the reason why children cannot easily fall asleep when they are feeling stressed.

Your child's body is so wise.
(And so is yours!)

8. Differentiating mild dissociation from true relaxation

What's the difference between true relaxation and mild dissociation, and why is being able to differentiate the two so important with children's sleep? I will answer both questions in this chapter. I'll also talk about how this information helps us understand what's really going on with children's sleep in different parenting paradigms.

This brings together all that we've talked about in the previous few chapters, including:

- The necessity of sleep, so there exist many ways for children to go to sleep.
- The two key elements and three ingredients for restful sleep.
- The physiology of stress and relaxation.

Self-Reflection Moment

I invite you to connect with your own memories of being deeply relaxed, and compare that to when you feel dissociated. Mild dissociation can feel pleasant.

You might remember your favourite way to mildly dissociate, e.g.[33]:

- *Eating chocolate while scrolling social media.*

- *Drinking alcohol.*

- *Reading a novel while eating chips.*

- *Twirling your hair.*

- *Watching a movie while eating cookies.*

- *Biting your nails.*

- *Watching one video after the next.*

---

33 Please note that we can do these things without necessarily dissociating. Almost anything can be done either with presence, or to dissociate. The difference is our presence, not the action itself, although certain actions can almost always lead to dissociation.

But it doesn't compare to the gorgeousness of feeling truly and deeply relaxed.

Perhaps you remember that from how you felt after:

- a powerfully releasing bodywork session where you cried;

- sobbing in the arms of a friend or partner;

- laughing 'hysterically' with a friend until your cheeks ached;

- watching a funny video where you laughed for half an hour straight and could feel all the tension in your solar plexus releasing;

- a deep and intimate conversation with your partner where you both expressed your honest feelings and experienced being deeply heard; or

- a day at the beach (perhaps before becoming a parent), alternating between swimming in the warm sea, dozing, and chatting with friends about your feelings and life.

What do you remember about being mildly dissociated?

What did you feel when you were deeply relaxed?

What differences do you notice between the two?

In most parenting paradigms, parents are taught to help their babies or children *mildly dissociate* in order to be calm enough to go to sleep.

Self-Compassion Moment

Remember to drop the guilt sticks! I'm sending love to you and compassion to whatever you're feeling as you read this, and I invite you to be deeply compassionate with yourself and your emotions.

Mild dissociation can be experienced as pleasant.

However, stronger dissociation is less likely to feel pleasant.

They might be dissociating from fear because they don't experience being *safe*. For babies and young children, this can be because they don't have closeness to go to sleep or while sleeping.

They might be dissociating from the accumulated painful *feelings* that are bubbling up to be released when they are tired.

Or they might be dissociating from *both* of these!

In contrast, Aware Parenting helps children feel relaxed for sleep in *two* ways: through offering them closeness when they need it to feel *safe*, and by *cooperating* with their innate biological wisdom to heal from stress and trauma, their relaxation-through-release response.

More relaxation = more restful sleep.

This also makes sense of many of the sleep issues parents experience, since mild dissociation is very different to true relaxation.

Firstly, the sleep is *lighter*, partly so they are more easily alerted to something that might indicate that they are not safe. Thus, they are more likely to wake up if they hear sound or experience movement.

Secondly, it tends to be *short-lasting*, since babies, children, and teens wake up when painful feelings bubble up again to be expressed. This can often happen when they move into lighter sleep.

Thus we might observe:

- babies waking up with the slightest sound or movement;
- frequent night waking for babies and toddlers;
- toddlers moving all around the bed while co-sleeping; and
- children and teens waking up tired and 'grumpy'.

Self-Compassion Moment

I invite you to drop any guilt sticks if you're tempted to pick them up. It's so common that we will do things to dissociate from our painful feelings. It's also so common that we will do things to our baby or child to distract them from their painful feelings too, and that our children and teens will have already learnt plenty of ways to mildly dissociate. If you're feeling concerned, thinking about the ways that your child has learnt to dissociate, I'm here to remind you that the innate capacity to heal from stress and trauma and to move out of dissociation always lies within our children, even if we haven't supported it up until now.

Dissociation is generally short-lasting, compared to true and deep relaxation.

Which means, if we encourage a baby or child to dissociate from their feelings of fear or loneliness because they are alone and don't feel safe, they will wake up again when there are light sounds or movement. They are communicating an unmet need for safety through closeness.

If we help them bypass the healing-feelings that naturally bubble up to be released when they are tired, those feelings are likely to emerge again once the mild dissociation wears off. They are trying to use their innate wisdom to release stress by expressing their feelings with our loving support.

It's also why, if they've had a stressful day, it's likely to take longer to bypass the healing-feelings. Once they are asleep, they're also more likely to wake up more often, to try to tell us about the overwhelm they experienced, and release the stress from their bodies.

So, with Aware Parenting, we are invited to help our baby or child to feel relaxed rather than dissociated, because they feel safe.

We're also invited to cooperate with their innate biological wisdom to express painful feelings when they are tired.

They can then move out of the fight or flight response and into deep relaxation if we support them to release emotions in the following ways:

- Through play and laughter.
- By crying in our arms or with our loving presence.
- By having a tantrum with our compassionate presence.
- By sharing their feelings with us through talking.

In this way they feel the kind of deep relaxation that indicates deep safety. Then they can have beautiful, restful, restorative sleep.

When a baby, child, or teen is sleepy, they need to feel safe in order to be relaxed enough to sleep.

It is also very hard for them to feel relaxed enough to go to sleep if they have accumulated stress and tension in their body.

Many other parenting paradigms encourage parents to help their babies dissociate from these accumulated feelings, either with or without our presence. These different forms of dissociation are commonly called *control patterns* in Aware Parenting, as they generally become repeated patterns that children use to mildly dissociate (or that we do to them to help them mildly dissociate).

Early independence parenting and dissociation

With early independence parenting paradigms, the encouragement of dissociation will be in forms that promote separation. Those paradigms tend to call this '*self-soothing*' or '*self-settling.*' (These terms are *not* used in Aware Parenting.)

This means that babies and young children are being taught to dissociate both from any feelings of loneliness, fear, or terror from being alone and not safe, and from any healing-feelings that are naturally bubbling up when they are tired.

This is through offering:

- a dummy;

- a soft toy or blanket to clutch onto;

- swaddling or preventing movement in other ways e.g. velcroed into a cot; or

- movement from a mechanical cot, or within a stroller (without eye contact).

Self-Compassion Moment

I'm sending love to any painful feelings you might be feeling when you read this. Again, it is so normal for our own innate healing wisdom to help us connect with emotions such as sadness, fear, or outrage when we take in information like this. We might connect with feelings from our own experiences from childhood, or from seeing babies and children, or our own baby or child. I'm also here to emphasise the putting down of any guilt or self-judgment sticks you might pick up. Having your own feelings heard by a loving and present listener is so vital if you are feeling upset. Are you willing for that listening and empathy?

From a child: *Dummy, where are you? Where's my dummy? I'm tired and I need it so I can go to sleep. I have lots and lots of them now. They are usually all over the place, but I can't find one anywhere. Sometimes I get scared if I can't find one anywhere, especially if it's all dark and night time. I so desperately need them. Oh! I've found one! I pop it in my mouth and start sucking. I lie down, and I find another one. I play with putting it in my belly button. Oh, that helps even more. I need my dummy to go to sleep. Sometimes my mouth feels a bit funny when I've been sucking it for a long time, but then the dummy takes away even those feelings. I'm sucking and sucking and I can feel myself drifting off to sleep.*

Classical Attachment Parenting and dissociation

In *Classical Attachment Parenting* style approaches, this encouragement of dissociation will be *with* the parent (using terms such as '*soothing*').

Here, a child has closeness, and the sense of safety that comes from that, so they will only need to dissociate from the healing-feelings that are naturally bubbling up to be expressed before sleep.

However, if we are stressed, scared, or dissociated, our presence might not signal safety, and so they might need to dissociate from the emotions they feel when they are with us.

> *Self-Compassion Moment*
> *I invite you to be really compassionate with yourself here. Even if we are stressed, it is more helpful for our baby or young child to be with us rather than alone when going to sleep. However, it is also an invitation for us to receive more loving listening for our feelings.*

Some examples of ways that we might help create dissociation are:

• feeding to sleep;
• singing;
• shushing;
• jiggling;
• bouncing;
• rocking; and
• movement while being carried in a baby carrier.

Babies and children learn from us. The ways we help them dissociate from their feelings often become the ways they continue to dissociate from their feelings, including before sleep.

Alternatively, thumb-sucking, nail-biting, and pinching skin are all ways that babies and children discover *themselves* to mildly dissociate from their feelings.

> ### Self-Compassion Moment
> *I invite you to be deeply compassionate with yourself here. I invite you to drop any guilt or self-judgment sticks if you've done any of these things to your baby. It's so understandable that we do things like this. We were taught to do these things. We probably experienced them ourselves. Whatever we did in the past, it's always possible to change the effects of those actions on our children. It's never too late!*

I would love to share Karenna's story of her journey with sleep and breastfeeding her daughter. It explains so clearly and beautifully what can happen when we inadvertently suppress our child's healing-feelings before sleep, and how we can then go on to listen to those accumulated feelings. This way, we can transform sleep while continuing with breastfeeding and co-sleeping. She wrote:

Although Tara's life began with lots of crying in arms and listening, a few huge life shifts when she was nine months old, plus a baby who seemed quite content most of the time meant that I 'forgot' about the healing value of crying and raging to release accumulated feelings. Unwittingly (and with lots of self-compassion), I now realise we had settled into a control pattern of excessive breastfeeding.

Fast forward to Tara at three years old and I was experiencing several wakeup feeds a night, a little one who wasn't eating much food in the day and a chronic constipation issue. At the time I didn't know how to connect the dots, although I had an inkling these challenges were somehow connected.

The lack of sleep was taking its toll as I realised I hadn't slept through the night for three years straight. I also noticed the wakeup feeds had an agitated flavour to them, and even after finishing her long feeds, Tara would be restless and wake up again and again. I knew what I needed for myself was to stop the night feeds and initially I thought this meant I'd need to stop breastfeeding altogether, which also didn't feel quite right.

I started to work with Marion for support around that and also to help me prepare for a weekend away – my first since giving birth. Marion helped me understand how the restless nights were directly connected with Tara's need to release accumulated feelings. Also, she helped me believe it really was possible to reduce breastfeeding to what I needed (and wanted), rather than give it up entirely. It seems so obvious now, but at the time I felt powerless to even imagine it was possible, let alone what it could look like.

I prepared Tara for stopping her night feeds with stories, attachment play *with her toys and talking it through. The first week was challenging, with lots of wake-ups in the middle of the night and her huge releases of rage (to the point where I needed to talk to my neighbours to let them know everything was okay!).*

There were also lots of big feelings in the day and some biting (Tara had never bitten me before) which I found very confronting and this really activated the younger parts of myself and my own unhealed feelings from childhood.

I came to realise these huge releases showed such innate wisdom – my little girl knew exactly what she needed to do to release all those feelings that not only built up during everyday challenges but also the ones that hadn't been released from the past. She was releasing two years of pent-up feelings, and my Loving Limits *around breastfeeding were supporting those releases.*

Thankfully, in a shorter time than I'd feared, the night wake ups and rages decreased and I was better able to be fully present with her releases in the day. Not only that, I came to deeply value her magnificent releases and was in awe of her full expression and power.

It was also deeply healing for me as I came to realise no one had ever held me in the way I was holding her, and the deep sadness I'd carried all this time because of that. There were times when tears would stream down both of our faces as I'd offer her my own loving presence while also meeting my own inner child's feelings.

At other times my heart would burst with joy, watching her in full expression and in complete confidence she was loved and safe in the full spectrum of her emotions. Within a short amount of time, her sleep improved (literally sleeping through the night!), her poos became regular, and she'd have periods throughout the day after her big releases when she'd be content to play and sing by herself. On the whole, she seemed so much more joyful and herself, which was very validating.

When we began the Loving Limit *around feeds during the night, I'd said to Tara that when the sun came up she could have mama milk. And I noticed that while at the beginning she'd wake up at her regular wakeup time, soon the wake-ups became earlier and earlier until she'd wake me quite roughly at the crack of dawn and demand a feed. Similar to when we were night feeding, these feeds had an urgency to them that was different to other feeds and I noticed that even within the reduced breastfeeding journey there were nuances of* control patterns *emerging again.*

This was another invitation to bring in a Loving Limit *around the early morning feeds and I chatted with Tara about my need for sleep and that I wanted to wake up a bit, brush my teeth and make a cup of tea before she had her morning feed. She wasn't very enthusiastic about this and the first few days had quite a few big dawn releases when I reminded her of the new routine.*

But after a week or so this settled and we were finally doing what I'd never thought was possible – only two feeds in the daytime and both of us sleeping through the night. Even better than that, I noticed I was becoming more and more finely tuned to Tara's feelings and her need to release. This empowered me to make space as best I could to listen and be present.

Each release also brought with it the chance to be with my own inner child, and it felt as if through being with Tara's feelings, I was also acknowledging and witnessing my own suppressed feelings as a child. This has been very healing on many levels, and I continue to be so thankful for Aware Parenting and my ongoing discoveries about parenting and myself."

Aware Parenting and true relaxation

Rather than trying to get a child to dissociate from the emotions that arise when they don't feel safe, or from the accumulated feelings in their body that naturally bubble up when they are tired, Aware Parenting works *with* both their innate need for *safety and* their natural processes to heal from stress and trauma, which are also their natural *relaxation* processes.

This leads to more *restful* sleep, especially if a child has been supported to *complete* the process of releasing a whole chunk of healing-feelings.

When babies, children, and teens are tired, they are less able to suppress their feelings, and will often try to use these natural relaxation processes, unless we have already taught them to dissociate, in which case they will try to do that thing instead.

However, with dissociation, all the stress remains in the body. The tension is still there. The feelings are still there.

If they are alone and are not old enough to experience safety while alone, they will easily wake up if there is sound or movement that indicates they might not be safe. They will then they call out for closeness and safety, unless they have already learnt to dissociate by themselves from feelings of fear, terror, or loneliness through behaviours such as sucking on their thumb or a dummy.

Self-Compassion Moment

I'm sending you so much love if you're feeling painful feelings as you read this. Imagining your baby, yourself as a baby, or other babies, feeling scared and lonely can help us connect with fear or sadness in ourselves. As always, I invite you to pause reading if you need to, and to reach out to someone to share your feelings with.

Whether or not they had closeness while falling asleep, If their healing-feelings were dissociated from before sleep, then when they move into lighter sleep, those feelings will often bubble up. This is when they will either try to cry (or play, or talk[34]) to release that tension, or will ask for whatever we've done to help them dissociate, if that's connected to our body – for example, breastfeeding. Or to dissociate themselves if their way is not related with our body – for example, clutching a stuffed toy.

This information helps us understand why, as babies get older, if we aren't listening to their *healing-feelings*, those accumulate and accumulate, meaning we need to do more to help them dissociate. The increased tension in their bodies wakes them up increasingly frequently.

As you've already discovered, the inbuilt healing processes are: crying and raging along with vigorous movement (while feeling safe); laughter and play; and talking (for older children and teens).

For pre-crawling babies to feel safe, they need to be held in arms whilst they are crying to release stress, and to have all their immediate needs met. Once they're *mobile*, they don't need to be held in our arms, but they do need us to be close, and to be held if they do want that.

If we don't understand these natural healing processes, we're likely to feel concerned when they're crying, thinking that they are communicating

---

34 Depending on whether we're referring to a baby, child, or teen.

an unmet need. We're likely to feel frustrated when they're playing, perhaps telling ourselves that they are deliberately staying awake.

Not understanding these natural processes – given that most of us never got to use them when we were babies, or children, or teens – means that as adults, we may think that the things we are doing to them when they are tired are just helping them feel calm, when they are actually making them dissociate from their healing-feelings.

However, the more we *understand* these natural healing and relaxation processes, and the more inner work we do so we can be *present* with these processes, the more we can cooperate with them.

Then we can *trust* that babies and children and teens not only have the fight, flight, or freeze response to help them be safe and survive, they also have healing processes to help them return to homeostasis, to *relaxation*, and to more *restful* sleep.

Babies

Actions that can help a *baby* feel *mildly dissociated* to go to sleep:

Sucking:

- Feeding
- Thumb-sucking
- Dummy/pacifier

Repetitive actions:

- Rubbing fingers together
- Playing with their hair or ours
- Twiddling with their skin or ours

Movement:

- Jiggling

- Bouncing
- Rocking

Preventing movement:

- Swaddling

Actions that help a baby feel *deeply relaxed* to go to sleep:

Holding them in our loving arms when all their needs are met, being present and still, and listening to the feelings that arise for them.

For most babies in the early months, before most sleeps, this will be through crying.

The crying is:

- *expressing* healing-feelings.
- *releasing* stress and trauma.
- *moving* them out of the fight, flight, or freeze response, and into homeostasis.
- *releasing* the sound that was mobilised to cry out for help when they were stressed.

The *kicking* of their legs and the flailing of their arms is them releasing the energy mobilised to fight or flee.

If we simply are present with them until they tell us the whole story, and release a chunk of feelings (such as about their birth, or how overwhelmed they felt that day), once they *complete* the healing process, they will move into a deep sense of relaxation.

How we can tell if a baby is *mildly dissociated* when going to sleep:

They may:

- show *tension* in their muscles, e.g., tensed up face, fists, or feet.
- *continue sucking* in their sleep.
- *wake up soon* after we place them down.
- *wake up* if there's any slight *noise*.
- need to be in one *particular* position, e.g. in the crook of our arm.

- *wake up* after one sleep *cycle*.
- *wake up crying (might be from unmet needs)*.

How we can tell if a *baby* is *deeply relaxed* when going to sleep:

They:

- are likely to show *relaxation* in their *muscles*, e.g. relaxed mouth, face, arms, and legs.
- are generally able to *stay asleep* when we *move* them.
- often *stay asleep* even if there's *noise*.
- tend to sleep until they've *had enough sleep* or they're actually hungry.
- don't need to be on top of their parent or in the crook of their arm to stay asleep;
- tend to *wake up happy*.

Children

Actions that may help a child feel *mildly dissociated* to go to sleep:

Sucking:

- Feeding
- Sucking on their clothes
- Thumb-sucking
- Dummy/pacifier

Repetitive actions:

- Rubbing fingers together
- Playing with their hair or ours
- Stroking or repetitive movements on their skin or clothes or ours
- Twiddling with or pinching their skin or ours

Distraction:

- Singing
- Reading books or being read to

- Audiobooks
- Using screens

Please note that singing, reading books together, and watching screens together can all lead to *connection or distraction*. Most actions can be used to bring about *presence or dissociation*, depending on the *intention and presence* with which they're used.

Actions that help a *child* feel *deeply relaxed* to go to sleep:

- *Cuddles* and *closeness* with us being *present* with them (especially if we feel relaxed).
- *Rambunctious play* and *laughter*, especially if they initiate it, and particularly if we're *joining in*.
- *Crying* and *raging* with our *loving support*.
- *Talking* to us, with us *lovingly listening*.

How we can tell if a *child* is *mildly dissociated* when going to sleep:

They may:

- show *tension* in their muscles, e.g., tensed up face, fists, or feet;
- sleep very *lightly*;
- need to be in one *particular* position, e.g. in the crook of our arm;
- *wake up* if there's any slight *noise*;
- have *nightmares* or *night terrors*; and/or
- *wake up crying*.

How we can tell if a *child* is *deeply relaxed* when going to sleep:

They:

- are likely to show *relaxation* in their muscles, e.g. relaxed mouth, face, arms, and legs;
- don't move around much, but don't need to be in one particular position;

- don't need to be on top of their parent or in the crook of their arm to stay asleep;
- often *stay asleep* even if there's noise;
- tend to sleep until they've *had enough sleep* and wake up rested; and/or
- tend to *wake up happy.*

Teens

Actions that may help a *teen* become *mildly dissociated* to go to sleep:

Sucking:

- Nail biting
- Smoking
- Vaping

Repetitive actions:

- Picking their skin/spots
- Eyebrow plucking
- Playing with their jewellery
- Playing with their hair

Distraction:

- Reading
- Using screens

Activities that help a *teen* feel *deeply relaxed* to go to sleep:

- *Physical contact (touch, hugs, cuddling, massages, rough and tumble play, wrestling).*
- *Talking* about their day and sharing their feelings.
- *Crying* with loving support.
- *Laughter.*

How we can tell if a *teen* is deeply relaxed when going to sleep:

They:

- are likely to show *relaxation* in their muscles, e.g. relaxed mouth, face, arms and legs;
- often *stay asleep* even if there's noise;
- tend to sleep until they've *had enough sleep* and wake up rested; and/or
- tend to *wake up happy.*

How to distinguish between an early bird or night owl, and accumulated feelings

Earlier on in the book I talked about night owls and early birds. The existence of these chronotypes support the sentinel hypothesis, which suggests that from an evolutionary perspective, humans have differing sleeping patterns. This is so that each individual could sleep according to their chronotype, yet the community as a whole would be more likely to be safe because there was always someone awake at any point during the night. Some researchers suggest that rather than two chronotypes, a variety of them might exist, for maximum likelihood of someone always being awake.

How do we tell the difference between a child who isn't going to sleep because they have accumulated feelings, and one who simply isn't yet tired, because they're a night owl? And what about between a child who is rested and wakes up early because they're an early bird and a child who wakes up early due to accumulated feelings that were suppressed before sleep?

If they are not going to sleep because they're a night owl, they will tend to be present and aware as the evening wears on, rather than agitated, upset, or trying to dissociate late at night.

If they wake up early because they're an early bird, they are likely to wake up happy, rested, present, and relaxed. Whereas, if they are woken by accumulated feelings bubbling up, they're likely to wake up upset, crying, agitated, tense, or trying desperately to do things (or to get us to do things) to suppress the feelings.

Of course, they might be a night owl or early bird *and* have accumulated feelings added to the mix! Understanding both their innate biological makeup and wisdom, and the effects of unexpressed painful feelings can really help us get clear about what's going on for them and what they really need.

As parents, we can start the day and finish the day with presence, or dissociation, and we have so much influence on whether our child experiences presence or dissociation on waking and falling asleep. This has a huge effect on not only our sleep, but our presence during the rest of our day.

From a baby: My world is so big and confusing. There's so much happening, and everything is new to me. I see shapes and noises and I don't understand what they are. There's movement and dark and light and it's all so much to take in. I'm learning so much every day, and I need your help. I need you to help me understand the world. And before I go to sleep, I need to let out all that newness, all the bigness. I want to let it all out. I'm so tired, but there's all this going on in me, and it needs to come out. Where are you? I search for you.

I call for you, and you come! You're here! I see myself reflected in your eyes! You pick me up and hold me, and I love how warm and safe I feel with you. I smile, and you smile back! I try to tell you about how big it all is, and you nod and smile. Yay! You're listening! I want to tell you more, because I am getting so tired and I want to sleep. I start to cry, and I want you to hear it all. But what's this? You start to rock and jiggle me. You sit on that big bouncy thing and we bounce and bounce. Oh I've forgotten what I wanted to tell you, after all. It's probably not that important, anyway.

CHAPTER SUMMARY

In most parenting paradigms, parents are taught to help their babies or children mildly dissociate to be calm enough to go to sleep. Mild dissociation can be experienced as pleasant. However, stronger dissociation is less likely to feel pleasant.

Children might be dissociating from fear because they don't experience being safe. For babies and young children, this may be because they don't have closeness to go to sleep or while sleeping. They might be dissociating from the accumulated painful feelings that are bubbling up to be released when they are tired. Or they might be dissociating from both of these!

Aware Parenting helps children feel relaxed before sleep in two ways: through offering them connection when they need it to feel safe, and by cooperating with their innate biological wisdom to heal from stress and trauma by expressing painful feelings when they are tired, which is their innate release and relaxation response. More relaxation = more restful sleep.

This also makes sense of many of the sleep issues parents experience, since mild dissociation is very different to true relaxation. Firstly, the sleep is lighter, partly so they can be more easily alerted to something that might indicate that they are not safe. Thus, they are more likely to wake up if they hear sound or experience movement. Secondly, it tends to be short-lasting, since babies, children, and teens wake up when painful feelings bubble up again to be expressed. This can often happen when they move into lighter sleep.

With early independence parenting paradigms, the encouragement of dissociation will be in forms that promote separation. Those paradigms tend to call this 'self-soothing' or 'self-settling.' (These terms are *not* used in Aware Parenting.) This means that babies and young children are being taught to dissociate both from any feelings of loneliness, fear, or terror from being alone and not safe, and from any healing-feelings that are naturally bubbling up when they are tired.

In *Classical Attachment Parenting* style approaches, this encouragement of dissociation will be *with* the parent (using terms such as '*soothing*'). Here, a child has closeness, and the safety that comes from that, so they will only need to dissociate from the healing-feelings that are naturally bubbling up to be expressed before sleep. However, if we are stressed, scared, or dissociated, our presence might not signal safety, and so they might need to dissociate from the emotions they feel when they are with us.

Babies and children learn from us. The ways we help them dissociate from their feelings often become the ways they continue to dissociate from their feelings, including before sleep.

Rather than trying to get a child to dissociate from the accumulated feelings in their body, Aware Parenting works with their innate need for safety and their natural processes to heal from stress and trauma, which are also their natural relaxation processes. This leads to more restful sleep, especially if a child has been supported to complete the whole process.

I'm so willing for you and your child/ren
to experience even more connected presence
as well as restful sleep.

9. Why understanding feelings is vital in supporting restful sleep

You've already read lots about feelings in this book, and yet, I'd love to talk a bit more about them here. In particular, I want to expound on why differentiating between *needs-feelings* and *healing-feelings* is so vital with sleep.

In this culture, feelings are not often clearly understood. If we don't know about Aware Parenting, we might easily feel confused, because:

- Stillness can be a sign of calmness, *or* dissociation.
- Smiling and laughter can express happiness, *or* can indicate the release of fear.
- Crying can communicate an unmet need, *or* be a way to heal from stress and trauma.

However, with Aware Parenting, we *know how to differentiate* between each of these in the list, so we can recognise the difference between:

- when a baby or child is crying because they have an *unmet need*, and when they are *healing*; and
- when a baby, child, or teen is quiet because they are *dissociated*, and when they are *relaxed*.

The differentiation is vital in supporting restful sleep, as you have already seen.

Feeling and expressing painful feelings in healing ways is inextricably linked to the level of deep *relaxation* that babies, children, and teens feel, and thus to the quality and quantity of their sleep.

Children who are trying to cry or tantrum to release pent-up painful feelings need our loving presence to help them know they're safe, so that they can move out of that fight, flight, or freeze response and resolve it.

However, for us to be able to be lovingly present, we need to:

- *understand* the biological function of crying and tantrums so that we can *welcome* them;

- be able to *trust* a child's innate body wisdom; and

- *feel comfortable* in our body when we're listening to those feelings.

However, in the *DDC*, there are (at least) hundreds of years where tantrums have been demonised (literally!). In the Middle Ages in Europe, people thought that a child who cried or raged was possessed.

Over the years, beliefs have become slightly more compassionate. The perception of a tantrumming child became that they were 'misbehaving'.

Nowadays, children who tantrum are often seen as having an 'immature nervous system' or it's believed that they need help to learn to 'regulate' their emotions. *(And, from an Aware Parenting perspective, we recognise that for some children, there can be physiological or other factors that lead to frequent tantrums. We observe, make sense of, and respond to each child as a unique individual.)*

All cultures have beliefs about children that have profound effects on the ways they are perceived and responded to. In Aware Parenting, we deeply value trusting children and their innate wisdom. As you know, we see crying and tantrums as ways that their wise bodies heal from stress and trauma, so they come out of fight, flight, or freeze, back into homeostasis. Particularly before sleep, when true relaxation is so beneficial.

However, children need physical and emotional safety for that to happen. They need to be truly releasing feelings and moving out of the fight or flight response, rather than still being in fight mode. For that, they need us to offer them our loving presence, and certain actions, so that they know they are truly *safe* to do what their wise bodies know exactly what to do. With that loving and powerful support, they can release stress and tension from their bodies, then feel deeply *relaxed*, so they can sleep *restfully* and restoratively.

In Aware Parenting, we differentiate between when a child is having a healing tantrum – where they are moving out of the fight or flight response into homeostasis – and when they are still in the fight response and are continuing to hit, bite, throw, or lash out.

If they're hitting, biting or throwing, it's our role as parents to help our child know that they are physically and emotionally safe, so they can move out of hyperarousal, and release the emotions and tension that were mobilised for them to be safe, so they can then feel truly relaxed. This will be through loud, angry crying and screaming accompanied by active body movements – but without attempts to hurt the other person.

How not understanding the difference between needs-feelings and healing-feelings leads to sleep challenges

In Aware Parenting, we recognise two different functions of crying: to express an immediate need, and to heal from stress or trauma. I think of these as two different kinds of feelings, and I call them needs-feelings and healing-feelings.

Needs-feelings indicate an unmet need. When the need is met, the result is relief, fulfilment, and presence.

Healing-feelings, when felt and expressed to a loving listener, lead to healing and deep relaxation.

If we think a baby or child is expressing a *needs-feeling* when they are actually expressing a *healing-feeling*, we may unknowingly be helping them dissociate from, or suppress, those feelings.

This has vital relevance to sleep, because babies and children often try to express *healing-feelings* to us when they're tired, so they can release stress and tension and sleep more peacefully.

However, if we think that they are expressing a *needs-feeling*, and we stop them expressing the *healing-feelings*, then the *healing-feelings* remain in their body. It's this that often leads to restless sleep and frequent night waking.

Soothing, self-soothing, emotional regulation, or mild dissociation?

These different interpretations – 'soothing', 'self-soothing', and 'emotional regulation' are based on different beliefs about the needs and feelings of babies and children.

Classical Attachment Parenting promotes '*soothing*'. In *Classical Attachment Parenting, all* crying is seen as indicating an unmet need.

In contrast, in Aware Parenting, we aim to differentiate between crying that communicates a need (which is a *needs-feeling*), and crying that is the expression of a *healing-feeling*. We recognise that mild dissociation can result if *healing-feelings* are interpreted as *needs-feelings*, and are responded to as if they were.

Early-independence parenting promotes '*self-soothing*'. In these approaches, crying is seen as something that children need to learn to stop themselves.

Why this is relevant to sleep

Interpreting *healing-feelings* as *needs-feelings* leads to suppression which may lead to restless sleep, because it bypasses the *healing-feelings*, which remain in the body. Those feelings will often bubble up, particularly during lighter sleep, or as the night wears on, leading to restless sleep and frequent night waking.

The relationship between feelings, sleep, and our responses and a child's daytime behaviour

We may see symptoms of accumulated feelings showing up in both daytime and nighttime behaviour. I wonder if you've noticed that? Perhaps you might even have experienced this yourself.

For example: A baby has a stressful birth, and the parents practice *Classical Attachment Parenting*, and don't realise that their baby has trauma to release. The mother breastfeeds a lot to suppress the painful feelings, including before sleep and throughout the night. When the baby is a toddler, they feed many times during the night and the mother either gets exhausted, frustrated, or wants to conceive another baby and her period hasn't returned, so she wants to stop feeding at night. Meanwhile, the toddler cries if cared for by anyone else apart from their mother, even though their dad and grandparents are attentive and present. The parents don't realise that this behaviour, as well as the feeding throughout the night, is directly related to their toddler's traumatic birth and the healing-feelings that have been suppressed for the past 18 months.

Or perhaps a couple have a young child and they say that he has 'never been a good sleeper'. In addition, he tends to hit other children, or push them over. They don't yet realise that the sleep challenges and aggression have the same cause: accumulated painful feelings.

Perhaps a couple are frustrated that their five-year-old has a tantrum before bed most nights: not realising that this is related to the separation he experienced after birth, and the feelings he's trying to express every morning before school, and every afternoon when he comes home.

Understanding the links between daytime and nighttime behaviour, and the causes of stress and trauma, can help us be willing to listen to more healing-feelings. We see that it helps them feel more relaxed both during the day and at night, which affects both their sleep and their behaviour.

From a child: *The sadness fairy comes to visit me every night when I'm in bed. I'm here with my Teddy, and Daddy left me and turned out the light. I lie awake, watching my night light shining out. I really wish Daddy wouldn't leave me alone. I get so scared. The night light makes all kinds of reflections and sometimes I think they're scary monsters. It's like I'm all alone in the world, and I can't go to sleep. I talk to the sadness fairy, and then I start to cry. My crying gets louder and louder, and Daddy comes back. On Daddy, you carry me back to your and Mummy's bed. You don't usually let me do that. But tonight, you put me in between you two and I keep on crying and crying. The sadness fairy is still with me. Somehow the crying feels different when I'm not on my own. I feel different when I'm not on my own. Oh, the crying is stopping.*

The sadness fairy is leaving. I guess you'll want me to go back to my own room now. Oh, you're letting me stay! I cuddle up in between you both. My body feels all funny and different, like it's all melty and floaty. I think I will fall asleep really quickly. Nighty night!

CHAPTER SUMMARY

In this culture, feelings are not often clearly understood.

With Aware Parenting, we aim to differentiate between *needs-feelings* and *healing-feelings*, and between dissociation and relaxation.

We see crying and tantrums as ways that children's wise bodies heal from stress and trauma, so they come out of fight, flight, or freeze, and back into homeostasis. Particularly before sleep, when true relaxation is so helpful.

In Aware Parenting, we differentiate between when a child is having a tantrum, which is them moving out of fight or flight into homeostasis, and when they are still in the fight response, and are hitting, biting, throwing, or lashing out.

If we think a baby or child is expressing a *needs-feeling* when they are actually expressing a *healing-feeling*, we may be unknowingly helping them dissociate from, or suppress, their feelings.

This has vital relevance to sleep, because babies and children often try to express *healing-feelings* to us when they're tired, so they can release stress and tension and sleep more peacefully. Suppressing their healing-feelings is likely to lead to restless sleep and frequent night waking.

I welcome all of your feelings, too.
Your feelings are beautiful gifts.

10. Changing our thoughts: our own de-conditioning process

I imagine you're already seeing how much our cultural conditioning about sleep affects:

- how *we perceive* sleep;
- how *we respond* to our children and their sleep; and
- how *they sleep*.

We could even say that many sleep challenges are actually caused by our own conditioning.

It's these thoughts and beliefs about children and why they're not sleeping that so often get in the way of trusting that our babies, children, and teens innately know how and when to sleep restfully and restoratively.

Our unexpressed feelings also have a huge effect, which is why I'll be inviting you to reflect on your thoughts here, and your feelings in the next chapter.

Self-Compassion Moment

I'm inviting you to be deeply compassionate with yourself as you contemplate all the ways you have been given information about sleep. It can take time for us to gradually get free from believing the things we thought were true. Changing our beliefs can be a painful process, as we let go of what we once believed in. This can also be hard, especially when those around us remind us of our old beliefs and try to persuade us to believe what they still do. Over time, we can more clearly see the effects that acting from those beliefs has had on our parenting and life.

Suze sent this to me:

"It took me a long time to realise what Aware Parenting was. I remember getting your emails and I resonated with what you were saying, but I just didn't put the pieces together. I didn't really get the whole bigger picture of it. Meanwhile, I went from having one daughter, to two, and the sleep challenges just got worse and worse. One day I listened to one of your podcast episodes and something just clicked in me and I really got it. That evening, I listened to both of my daughters' feelings for the first time, and they woke so much less. It all started to make more sense."

Trusting the innate body wisdom of children in relation to relaxation, sleep, and healing from stress and trauma is very different to what most of us are taught, growing up in *the Disconnected Domination Culture.*

I'm here to remind you to be unwilling to pick up any guilt sticks here. Growing up in the DDC, *we needed to believe in cots, dummies, and separation for sleep, in order to meet our needs for safety, belonging, and love. It's so normal and natural that we do that. Thinking differently from mainstream perspectives can be hard.*

In preparing for parenthood, you might have been told that you won't get any sleep for the first several years. Most of us are given information from friends, family, and advertisers that there are essential things that we need, and those generally include a cot, and a dummy. This conditioning is powerful. It's designed to affect us, and make us believe certain things, often that require us to buy lots. Most of us would have heard that children need to be 'put to sleep' at a certain time. Most of us will have seen shows with teens fighting with parents about bedtime.

The beliefs and practices that most of us were taught work against the innate relaxation-through-release response that babies and children have and can actually make them feel more tense and sleep less restfully. The lack of trust in teens can also work against their intrinsic body knowing.

Few of us received information and embodied wisdom from those around us to invite us to trust that we have innate and inherent wisdom in relation to sleep, from birth to adulthood.

In contrast, Aware Parenting invites us to see that babies, children, and teens do know how to feel relaxed enough to sleep peacefully. They have incredible innate body wisdom.

When we know *how* to trust and cooperate with those natural relaxation processes and we are *able* to do so, they can then sleep *restfully* and restoratively.

The more we free ourselves from the cultural conditioning that babies and children don't know how to feel relaxed enough to sleep, the more we can collaborate with – and regain trust in – that beautiful inbuilt wisdom.

I was so grateful to have this information early on in my parenting journey. It meant that in general, I didn't worry about my children's sleep. I just focussed on doing as much as I could to meet their needs and listen to their healing-feelings, knowing that the more of those I did, the more likely it was that their sleep would be restful.

The four main ways that our conditioning can get in the way of restful sleep

- Trying to get them to go to sleep when they're *not actually tired.*
- *Not supporting* their needs for *closeness* when they are young (which may get in the way of them feeling safe and thus relaxed enough to sleep).
- *Preventing* their *intrinsic relaxation-through-release process* (through distracting them from their *healing-feelings* in a myriad of ways).
- *Not trusting* our older children and teens and their capacity to be deeply connected with their bodies and what they need in terms of sleep; their process of becoming more independent in making their own decisions; and their own learning process (e.g. that if they stay up late at night, they'll find it hard to get up the next morning).

However, in our culture, we often think that the cause of sleep challenges in babies is *'overtiredness'*, and in children or teens is a *lack of information or willingness*. This perspective can occur if you are telling your child over and over again that, *"It's important that you get enough sleep,"* and you get louder and louder, thinking that they will cooperate once they have that information.

Emily shares what a difference changing her beliefs about sleep made:

"Knowing this and actively embracing all of it has made our parenting journey so far extremely smooth and enjoyable. We haven't struggled with any sleep deprivation and I find peace in knowing that we have been truly present with bub whenever she's needed us as opposed to wishing she would just sleep and stop fussing."

Getting free from the beliefs that we've been conditioned to hold can be a huge process. I wonder if you find it helpful to contemplate how long those beliefs might have been passed down from generation to generation, as well as through the media.

This isn't only to do with beliefs about sleep, it's also about trusting babies, children and teens in all areas of their lives. It's also related to recognising the beauty and wisdom of crying and raging, as well as laughter and play, and how central they are to truly relaxed sleep as well as presence, awareness, and cooperation during the daytime.

Most of us grew up learning that children aren't to be trusted. That instead, they need to be taught by adults to go to sleep. The phrases 'sleep schools' and 'sleep training' illustrate these concepts. In the *DDC*, teens are seen as rebellious and unhelpful beings who also have to be kept in line, including with 'bedtimes'. All of these beliefs can seep into us over time.

What about tantrums? You know that in Aware Parenting, we see them as part of a child's biological wisdom: a way for them to release stress and trauma from their bodies when they feel safe. It's how they move out of the fight, flight, or freeze response, release the tension from the mobilisation of their muscles, and move back into homeostasis, and thus the relaxation that is required for restful sleep. Yet, for hundreds of years, tantrums have been demonised. Some version of that was probably passed down in each of our own family lineages.

Self-Compassion Moment

Does thinking about the hundreds of years of cultural conditioning help you be more compassionate with yourself when you find yourself reverting back to beliefs you used to have about crying, tantrums, and sleep?

Cultural conditioning is hard to change. I celebrate your willingness to see sleep differently, as well as crying and raging, laughter and play, and human nature in general!

Self-Reflection Moment

I'm going to invite you to reflect on the beliefs you have about sleep, crying, and tantrums.

I invite you to simply respond with the first thoughts that come to mind as you read the following:

- Sleep as a parent is ...

- Babies sleep when ...

- If we want to get a baby to sleep, we need to ...

- Toddlers sleep when ...

- Everyone knows this about teenagers and sleep ...

- Fighting sleep is ...

- Tantrums are ...

- Babies cry to ...

- If a child laughs when we tell them to go to sleep, it means ...

And here are some questions for you:

- Do you believe that it's possible to have restful sleep as the parent of a toddler or young child?

- What do you notice yourself thinking most about sleep when you're reading this book?

- What do you think teenagers need in order to have enough sleep?

- When you read that teens can be trusted with sleep, what was your initial response?

Are you surprised by what showed up in response to these questions?

Are you willing for any of these beliefs to change?

As you read the book, I invite you to see if any of your beliefs about sleep (as well as about trusting children's innate wisdom, and crying and raging) change.

The more we choose thoughts that resonate with us and that are aligned with our values – rather than thinking things that have simply been passed on or down to us – the more we will feel deeply connected with ourselves. And the more self-connected we are, the more likely we are to be able to see our child more clearly and respond to them in ways that most meet their innate needs. That will also contribute to their levels of relaxation and thus their sleep.

I'll be inviting you to reflect more deeply on your conditioning as we move through each section of the book.

Katie shares about her experience of the powerful effects that changing our beliefs can have on the presence we are able to offer our children when they're not sleeping:

The information that Aware Parenting provides has made it so easy to let go of harsh thoughts about my toddler, because I see so clearly now that he wants to sleep just as much as I want him to! It's much easier for me to hold space if he wakes up in the night because I'm not caught up in judging him, and I can usually drop the self-judgement too. I'm automatically much more present in my body when I'm not having those harsh thoughts."

We are way more powerful
than we're led to believe.

Oshah tells her story about how she was affected by the *DDC* beliefs of others, and how she came back to her own values (and co-sleeping again) after she learnt about Aware Parenting. She says:

"From very early on, my son would wake every 20-40 minutes. I co-slept with him. When he was one year old, I was so exhausted and began thinking I couldn't keep going in this way. From what I was reading and conversations with other mothers, I began to think that being right next to him was causing him to wake up, and that maybe I needed to 'teach' him to sleep independently. I made the decision to move him into a cot to help us both get a better night's sleep. He was in the same room as me, and it still felt so painful to force this separation. Even though Classical Attachment Parenting *and co-sleeping felt so normal and natural to me, the* Disconnected Domination Culture *had infiltrated!* **Thinking that my baby just couldn't sleep with me, or that I was causing him to sleep terribly, was deeply painful.**

When I discovered Aware Parenting, I understood that he needed to express feelings so that his body could relax and sleep would come more easily. I started practising Aware Parenting principles when he was 20 months old, and after some time, began co-sleeping again. He started sleeping much longer stretches and it was such a relief to be close again without forcing separation multiple times a night. We still co-sleep (he is seven and a half years old) and the closeness we have is just so beautiful."

> ### Self-Compassion Moment
> If you made your baby sleep alone because you were persuaded to, or you did other things with your child and their sleep or crying because you were told to, I'm sending you so much love and compassion. I imagine you might feel some painful feelings, and if so, I invite you to express them and have them lovingly heard.

In the *DDC*, it's common for children to be shamed if they want closeness at night, and for parents to be shamed for co-sleeping, or for listening to their child's crying and tantrums. Shaming is so painful, so it's very understandable that we might be tempted to move back to *DDC* beliefs and practices to avoid being shamed.

Being aware of how shaming works can help you be less affected by it. For example, you might say, *"I'm not willing to hear the judgments of others about my choices,"* or, *"I'm not willing to be affected by the judgments of others."* Remembering that people are trained to judge in the *DDC* can help us be unwilling to take their judgments personally, because we remember that it's nothing personal and nothing to do with us. It simply shows us their *DDC* conditioning.

Another common cultural belief is that babies and children need to go to sleep in a bedroom after a 'bedtime' routine.

However, if we follow our child's lead, we may find that they fall asleep in other places. We might imagine this happening in hunter-gatherer cultures and present-time intact Indigenous cultures, with toddlers falling asleep during the evening, whenever and wherever they wanted, as a part of the family's and community's activities, such as after singing and dancing together.

I want to remind you this is about finding a way to follow your child's innate body wisdom, while *also* being willing for *your own needs to be met* in this time and this culture.

Often that requires experimentation and creativity!

I love this reflection from Marieke, after doing my *Sound Sleep and Secure Attachment with Aware Parenting Course* many years ago. It shows how changing sleep beliefs and practices can also help us get free from the beliefs that lead to guilt.

"The sleeping of my baby (14 months) goes so much better: he sleeps through the night. This means more energy for us, so finally the moment to pick up on my life... As for my five-year-old daughter... her hyperactivity during the day (which made her a handful kind of kid)... it is gone!!!! She doesn't need to twirl all the time, is less agitated. She really needed a lot of roughhousing. But now, she likes it, but the need is gone. And she says; 'Oh I love you,' (to all of us) a lot, which makes me think that her inner energies are flowing. It is such a joy to see my daughter much calmer and more grounded. We did a lot of Aware Parenting work with her the last two years, and this was really a last subtle 'intervention' which made such a difference.

As for me: my feelings of guilt keep eroding. I am such a happy mom at the moment! My energies are flowing freely too. I notice that I can choose for joy more often. And even patterns of feeling unworthy and unlovable are changing. And yesterday night something great happened: my 14 month old gave me a few hugs and a big smile, looked me in the eye communicating, I am totally fine, I love you, turned his head around and went to sleep!"

CHAPTER SUMMARY

Our conditioned thoughts and beliefs about children and why they're not sleeping can get in the way of trusting that our babies, children, and teens innately know how and when to sleep restfully and restoratively.

Growing up in the *DDC*, we needed to believe in cots, dummies, and separation, to meet our needs for safety, belonging, and love.

DDC sleep beliefs and practices are often kept in place through shaming from others as well as through the shame sticks that we internalised as a result. Being aware of how shaming works can help us be less affected by it.

I deeply celebrate your willingness to be open to changing your beliefs about sleep.

11. Being compassionately present with our own feelings

Compassion for ourselves when we find it hard to sleep can help us be compassionate with our child

Do you remember times when you felt very tired in the evening, but you were worrying about something, and you just couldn't get to sleep? Or perhaps you woke up in the middle of the night, feelings and thoughts churning, and despite being desperate to sleep, you were awake for hours?

Babies and children are so similar to us in this respect.

Even if they're really tired, if they've got big feelings bubbling, it's really hard for them to feel relaxed enough to fall asleep, and they will wake up easily and may find it hard to go back to sleep again.

When we see babies and children as beings with feelings that affect their sleep just like us, sleep challenges make so much sense.

As you know, with Aware Parenting, one of the ways we support our babies and children to feel relaxed enough to fall asleep and sleep as long as they need if they have feelings bubbling is to listen to those feelings.

If the pent up feelings are preventing them from sleeping, listening to those healing-feelings helps them be able to sleep restfully.

When we understand that babies and children have *healing-feelings* as well as *needs-feelings*, and we know how to listen to those feelings, we can support them to have restful and restorative sleep.

They also get the amazing benefits of having their feelings heard: i.e. they heal from stress and trauma, and feel more relaxed during the daytime too, not just at night.

Remembering our own similar experiences can help us with three things.

It can help us:

- Put ourselves in our child's shoes when they're taking a long time to go to sleep, or they keep waking up at night.
- Be deeply compassionate with them and how they feel at those times.
- Be less likely to tell ourselves unenjoyable things about why they're not sleeping, which might otherwise lead to us feeling powerless, resentful or angry.

Kaitlin shares her experience of this process:

"I first came across Aware Parenting when my daughter Aida was about five weeks old. I was scouring the internet for answers, wondering why she cried so much before sleep and what I could do to help her and myself. I felt like I was drowning in guilt, because I couldn't get her to be quiet and go to sleep calmly. I remember spending 45 minutes bouncing her on the exercise ball regularly to get her to sleep. Only to put her down and have her wake up 20 minutes later. I was exhausted, and I felt like I was missing something.

When I found Aletha Solter, Marion Rose, and Aware Parenting, it was like a light switched on in my brain. Before becoming pregnant with Aida, I had suffered with anxiety and was really struggling with sleep myself. After seeing a psychologist and discussing my feelings with her, my sleep improved. But I hadn't realised it was also true for my baby. She had so many scary and overwhelming things that would happen to her every day. Simple things like taking her for a walk outside and the neighbour's dog barking could be quite startling for her.

As she got older, I realised that she was a hyper-sensitive baby. She could get easily overstimulated. Even if I was just playing with her or reading her a book. She would get this franticness about her. I used to think she was hungry. But now I can see that she was just experiencing so many feelings. After applying crying in arms (after meeting all her needs of course), I found I could sit there and be with her and even though she was crying, I didn't feel guilt or that I wasn't being a good mother. I knew she was just telling me about her day.

She would do this at every nap and before bed at night. At times (when I was experiencing feelings myself) I really struggled to hear her cry. I realised it was because I wasn't having my own feelings heard. After getting support, I found it much easier to listen to her. Now she will often just lay in my arms and make some cooing and chatty noises. I talk quietly back to her and after five to ten minutes her eyes close and her palms open and her body relaxes. Before Aware Parenting, she used to sleep all tensed up.

It amazes me every time how attuned our babies are. They are so intelligent. We just need to support them. Obviously, she does cry sometimes still when she has had a big day. But I just hold her and give her space to tell me her feelings. I can't wait to continue this journey. I hope that she will become a brave, resilient, kind and empathetic young woman."

> ### Self-Compassion Moment
> How do you feel when you read about Kaitlin's experience? If you have had challenges with sleep yourself, my heart goes out to you. Having our own feelings heard by a loving listener can transform our own experiences of sleep.

How our own childhood experiences and feelings can affect our parenting regarding sleep

It's very common for our experiences with sleep when we were a baby, child, or teen to affect our own parenting. Often, our child's behaviour invites us to reflect on those experiences. We might then listen lovingly to the younger parts of us and how we felt, what we needed, and what conclusions we made based on the experiences we had.

For example, perhaps you always slept in a cot from when you were a newborn. That might lead you to feel uncomfortable doing that to your baby, or alternatively, you might feel discomfort imagining co-sleeping, because it's so unfamiliar to you. If you're feeling either of those, I'll be supporting you to connect in with your thoughts, needs, and feelings when you read Part 2 about babies.

Or maybe you were given a dummy to go to sleep as a baby or child and you really don't want to give one to your child before sleep, because you remember being shamed as a four-year-old for still needing your dummy to get to sleep. But now perhaps your toddler just won't go to sleep, and keeps crying every night before bed, and the dummy is the only way you can think of to help them fall asleep.

Perhaps you remember being made to go to bed at a certain time as a teen and not feeling tired, and lying in bed looking at the ceiling, pretending to be asleep if your parent came in to check on you. Perhaps you snuck a book and torch under the covers but were so tense because you were worried that they'd come in and find you and punish you. You might then feel worried when you see your teen always reading before bed.

The more we can tend lovingly to our younger parts[35] and to the feelings we experienced back then, and probably didn't ever have heard back then, the more we will be able to clearly see what is really going on for our child.

> When we become more aware of our own feelings, needs, and past experiences, we will be more able to respond from our adult self rather than from our younger parts and their painful unexpressed feelings. We can then more clearly see our child and what they are needing and feeling.

Many of us would have experienced being:

- left to sleep on our own in a cot as a baby;
- left alone to cry;
- breastfed or bottle fed to sleep;
- given a dummy to go to sleep, or sucked our thumb to sleep;

---

35 This concept is part of Aware Parenting, but the term 'younger parts' is from *The Marion Method*. In Aware Parenting, the term used is 'childhood memories'.

- distracted from our feelings before sleep in other ways;
- told to go to bed at a particular time, whether or not we were tired; or
- judged, threatened, or punished, so that we would go to bed when we were told to.

Self-Reflection Moment

I invite you to reflect on your experiences with sleep and feelings. But first, please check in with yourself about whether you're truly willing, and whether you have the emotional spaciousness to do so.

- Do you have any memories that jump out at you about your experiences of sleep as a baby, child, or teen?

- Is there anything that you remember enjoying about sleep and the going to sleep process when you were a child?

- How old were you when you first had the experience of choosing what time you went to sleep? Do you remember how you felt?

- Does your family tell stories about an aspect of your sleep when you were a baby, child, or teen?

- What feelings or memories have come up for you most in your reading of the book so far?

- Do you remember ever crying before you went to sleep?

- Do you ever cry nowadays?

- Do you cry alone or with support?

- What do you do if you want to cry in the evening?

- Do you dissociate before sleep? If so, what ways do you use?

- Do you ever wake up feeling agitated or upset in the middle of the night?

- If so, what do you do next?

- Do you receive enough empathy for your own painful feelings?

- If you are having challenges with sleep in your family at the moment, are they reminding you of something in your own childhood?

- If so, are you willing to share your feelings about this with a loving listener?

Louise shares about the difference having her own feelings heard meant in her ability to listen to her children's feelings, and the effect that had on their sleep:

"I heard about Aware Parenting when I was pregnant with my first son. I started reading The Aware Baby *when he was a few months old and although it really resonated with me, I wasn't able to listen to his feelings when he was so little. It was really painful for me to listen to him crying and I felt like I had to do something to 'help' him when he was so distressed. Singing, rocking and feeding him when he was upset or going to sleep felt very nurturing to me. We always did lots of* attachment play *before bed and throughout the day, with lots of connection, but Aspen would wake up frequently throughout the night (sometimes every hour, although I stopped counting) and I would breastfeed him back to sleep.*

When he was about 18 months I re-read The Aware Baby. *The information was a lot easier to integrate and put into practice with him being a bit older, it wasn't so painful for me to listen to his feelings. Once I learnt more and more about Aware Parenting, it became so much clearer to me how important it was for me to listen to his feelings. He started sleeping more peacefully, and through the night. I notice that when he has feelings, whilst sleeping he is restless, he wakes up early, and mouth breathes.*

With my youngest son we have been practicing Aware Parenting since birth. He is now 14 months old. I love seeing his body totally relaxed after having his feelings heard. He sleeps peacefully at night. I worry less about noise in the house because he sleeps more deeply. I'm also not so obsessed with sleep because I know that when he's tired, he will sleep. I have never sung, rocked, or fed him to sleep. Having my feelings heard by a Listening Partner has really helped me to listen to both my sons with deep presence. I am forever grateful to Aletha Solter for Aware Parenting and to Marion for being such a compassionate and knowledgeable mentor."

Laura, an Aware Parenting instructor who lives in Germany, shares her story with sleep:

"When I grew up, sleeping was like a sacred thing. One was not to be

woken up. With my understanding of it now, I can see how much in my family of origin it was a cherished strategy to deal with our feelings. Through my journey as a mother, my view of and relationship with sleep changed in so many ways. And I love it now more than ever.

The journey started in our beginning stages of becoming parents, where we experienced several miscarriages, medical interventions, and deep fears. Lots of unresolved trauma got stored in my body. During that phase I wasn't ready to feel those intense feelings. And so the birth of our firstborn daughter reflected so much of our former experiences. What followed was a time of gratitude for being with my baby on the one hand and lots of confusion, disconnection, and tension on the other hand. It mostly showed in the nights, as our girl was showing lots of restlessness and tension. The evening and nighttimes were the toughest times and I ended up the worst version of myself as a mother. For both of us, our deepest fears and pains were trying to be resolved during these times, but I felt powerless, overwhelmed, and terrified. I am deeply grateful my husband has been the fall back, whenever I was not able to be present anymore.

Learning about Aware Parenting when our firstborn was three months old, everything started to change. We listened to so many of her feelings and after a while I started my own healing journey. The nights got better and better. Our baby started to sleep longer stretches and deeper. Her body was more relaxed, less agitated... instead there would be those beautiful evenings she looked totally at ease when she fell asleep after a good cry in our arms.

I then saw the biggest leap when our younger daughter was born. Having healed so much of my painful experiences and practicing Aware Parenting from the start with her gave us such a different experience. Her birth was a reminder of her sister's birth at first and then became an intensely healing and empowering experience for me. I was able to listen to her feelings throughout the night during the first weeks, because I was so much more in balance and peace in my own body. And our girl slept such long stretches very early on, right beside me. It was a magical time that made me feel powerful beyond what I ever thought possible before.

Nowadays my own sleep is more relaxed and deeper so that the hours that I need to feel truly refreshed are less than before. I am less attached to it and I feel more recharged after sleeping. It's so much easier for me to get up in the morning and start the day powerfully. Although the nights often still show when there is tension going on in our family, the experience is so beautiful now, the four of us sleeping in our family bed and enjoying it together. Although we have been supporting the healing from early on for both of them, we nowadays still can see the difference in our older and younger daughter in the quality of their sleep. May the journey go on."

Being willing to receive support can be hard for many of us growing up in the DDC, where many of us were trained to not ask for help, support, and empathy.

Being willing to receive compassionate listening can, in itself, be deeply reparative. I highly recommend regularly having your feelings heard by an empathy buddy or Aware Parenting instructor if you choose to practice Aware Parenting. Receiving loving listening of our painful emotions is such a *vital* part of the process.

I'm here to offer these loving words to the younger parts of you:

I'm sending so much love to you, every time you were left alone to sleep before you were ready.

I'm here to listen to any sadness or loneliness you felt.

I welcome the parts of you who are scared.

I won't leave you alone, sweetheart.

I'm right here with you, and I'll stay with you as long as you need me.

All your feelings are welcome.

I'm here to listen.

I love you, however you feel.

You can cuddle up with me for as long as you need.

I will always be here.

CHAPTER SUMMARY

When we see babies and children as beings with feelings that affect their sleep just like us, sleep challenges make so much sense.

Remembering our own similar experiences can help us with three things.

They can help us:

- put ourselves in our child's shoes when they're taking a long time to go to sleep or they keep waking up at night;
- be deeply compassionate with them and how they feel at those times; and
- be less likely to tell ourselves unenjoyable things about why they're not sleeping, which might otherwise lead to us feeling powerless, resentful or angry.

It's very common for our experiences with sleep when we were a baby, child, or teen to affect our own parenting. The more we can attend lovingly to our younger parts and to the feelings we experienced back then, and probably didn't ever have heard back then, the more we will be able to see what is really going on for our child.

I highly recommend regularly having your feelings heard by an empathy buddy or Aware Parenting instructor if you choose to practice Aware Parenting. Receiving loving listening of our painful emotions is such a vital part of the process.

I'm sending so much love and compassion to you every time you were tired but couldn't go to sleep because of loneliness or pent-up painful feelings.

SECTION 1 SUMMARY

How are you feeling, having read this section?

This was the most theoretical section of the book, where we looked at a big picture of sleep, both in terms of human history, but also in terms of the ongoing relationship between biology and culture.

We looked at Aware Parenting and sleep, and related it to our hunter-gatherer origins, *Classical Attachment Parenting* (which has been deeply influenced by Indigenous cultures in very hot climates) and what we could call either early-independence parenting, or *DDC* parenting (and how that overlaps with what happened in some traditional cultures in very cold climates).

Understanding these big picture ideas can help us in our day to day practice of Aware Parenting, because it can help us have a context and container that actually builds emotional safety for us, which we can pass on to our child/ren.

If what you've read resonates with you, you will have a 'why', a sense of purpose, to why you are actually responding to your child and their sleep in the ways I will be talking about.

Having this 'why' can be so supportive, because practicing Aware Parenting can be really hard at times, especially when living in the *DDC*.

I'm so willing for your big picture understanding of sleep and Aware Parenting to help you in your parenting practice.

ABOUT THE NEXT SECTIONS

In the following chapters, I talk about babies, then children, and then teens. Then there is the final concluding chapter, all about trust and the longer term outcomes of practicing Aware Parenting.

I invite you to choose whichever are relevant to you.

In addition, if you have a child or teen, reading Part 2, about babies, might help you to see their sleep experiences as a baby in a different light.

If you have a baby or child, perhaps you may find yourself wanting to read parts 3 and 4, to prepare for what's to come.

I invite you to trust yourself in what you feel called to read, and in which order.

Self-Compassion Moment

And if at any time you notice yourself feeling guilty or ashamed, I invite you to drop those emotional sticks. You might say to yourself, "I'm not willing to feel guilty or ashamed about what I did or didn't do." Remember that if you are hitting yourself with those sticks, you will actually be less present with your child, because of the painful feelings those sticks create. You feeling guilt or shame will not help your child.

If you feel sad, outraged, or overwhelmed I invite you to pause and connect with some empathic support. Perhaps you might put your hand on your heart, or you might reach out to share with a friend. It's very normal and natural to have big feelings in relation to sleep, and I'm sending so much love to any feelings you do feel when reading the book.

Let's continue!

PART 2

Babies and Sleep

12. The three ingredients for restful sleep – and what you can do to help your baby sleep restfully

I'll remind you of the three ingredients required for restful sleep:

i. to feel tired (sleepy);

ii. to feel connected (*closeness creating a sense of safety*); and

iii. to feel relaxed (*by releasing any healing-feelings present*).

i. To feel tired (sleepy)

Common signs of tiredness in babies include: red eyes and/or eyebrows, fluttering eyelids, blinking, rubbing eyes, pulling ears, losing coordination and the ability to concentrate, jerky movements, yawning, eyelids drooping, and lying down.

Other paradigms perceive that 'fussing', back arching, and crying are signs that a baby is 'overtired'. If we think that our baby is 'overtired' and that 'overtiredness' is the cause of their crying, of course it's natural that we will do whatever we can to try to get our baby to go to sleep as soon as possible.

It's so common for parents to then feel frustrated, overwhelmed, powerless, or confused if their baby is just not going to sleep and they are interpreting the cause as overtiredness.

> *Self-Compassion Moment*
> I wonder if you've experienced that? If so, I'm sending you so much love and compassion.

However, when we perceive crying in the evening as a process whereby babies relax by healing from stress and trauma, we are going to feel and respond very differently.

Firstly, we will know that it is likely that nothing is wrong, and can trust that this is their intrinsic relaxation process at play. So we're likely to feel calmer.

Rather than trying to get the baby to go to sleep as quickly as possible, through trying to 'soothe' them or to get them to 'self-soothe', we can be lovingly present with our baby as they cry in our arms, until they naturally feel relaxed enough to fall asleep.

Soon, I'll share more about exactly how you can do that.

If babies are tired, connected, and already deeply relaxed, they will simply fall asleep in our loving arms. We won't need to do anything 'to' them to 'calm them down' or 'soothe' them to fall asleep. If a baby has experienced a relatively peaceful birth and time in utero, you might observe this easeful going-to-sleep process in the early days after their birth.

For these babies, in those first few days, you might simply hold them when they are tired, and they may fall asleep, without you jiggling, rocking, bouncing, or feeding them. This is because they have relatively few accumulated feelings in their bodies and thus can go to sleep without either expressing feelings or suppressing them. *They are already relaxed.*

However, for at least several months, the majority of babies *do* have feelings to express *every day,* and *generally* before *every time* they need to sleep. If we understand this, are able to listen to their healing-feelings,[36] and don't distract them from those emotions, they typically will cry before *every nap* and before falling asleep in the evening.

---

36 However, it's important to note that the top priority in the early weeks is making sure that breastfeeding and milk supply is established, so please take that into account here.

Self-Reflection Moment

How do you feel when you read this? Taking in information that babies have this many healing-feelings is huge for most of us. If you feel incredulous, overwhelmed, or confused, I'm sending you so much love.

I'm here to let you know that this doesn't mean that you 'have to' listen to their healing-feelings before every nap and sleep. Many parents choose to listen once a day in the evening, for example.

Self-Compassion Moment

If the information you're reading resonates, and you've distracted your baby from their healing- feelings, and you're picking up guilt sticks, I invite you to put down those sticks.

I wonder if you find it helpful to know that even though I learnt about Aware Parenting when I was pregnant with my daughter, and resonated with all of it, that up until when my daughter was three months old, I assumed that there was no reason for her to have any healing-feelings to express. This was because we had a calm birth, I was carrying her everywhere, co-sleeping, breastfeeding, and responding to her promptly. I hadn't realised that all *babies will have healing-feelings to express, however much we meet their needs.*

But by the time she was three months old, I was starting to see evidence that she had unexpressed painful feelings that were accumulating. Not to the extent that I noticed that it was affecting her sleep (although I wasn't counting or making note of when she woke up, so it could have been), but she was starting to be a bit agitated in her body, and she was beginning to avoid eye contact at times. I realised that feeding her all evening was me distracting her from crying to release those pent-up painful feelings.

It took me a long time to recognise how many healing-feelings babies commonly have. Observing my daughter, and then my son, and also working with lots of parents, helped me fully understand how normal it is for babies to have a lot of healing-feelings to express. I was so surprised. Almost all of the parents I've mentored have expressed surprise about how many healing-feelings their baby has, when given the full opportunity to express those feelings.

I'm here to remind you that tiredness is only one of the three ingredients for restful sleep, so if a baby is tired but they don't feel connected, and they don't feel relaxed, it may be hard for them to fall asleep.

Self-Reflection Moment

I invite you to reflect on your experiences with your baby's tiredness:

- In the early days after their birth, did you ever experience your baby falling asleep in your arms without you doing anything to them to fall asleep?
- Do you generally think that fussing or crying is an indication of tiredness?
- What signs have you been interpreting as tiredness cues?

What you can do:

Observation

You can observe your baby. When their tiredness cues indicate that they are sleepy, I invite you to move to the next step, which is offering them closeness and connection (if you're not already).

From a baby: I'm smiling, and I'm looking at my hand. I don't know that it's called a hand yet, but it's amazing. It moves, and the movements seem related to me, but I don't exactly know how. I've been concentrating a lot on it. You're here with me, and I look over at you, and you smile. I smile back, and then go back to this hand thingy.

Hmmm... but what is happening now? There's something happening to my mouth. I don't know what that's called yet either, but I feel this wave building and coming from nowhere, and my mouth opens and stretches wide. I look at my hand again, but it's wobblier, and I feel wobblier too.

My hand goes to my eye, and I'm rubbing it. This wave comes again, and I yawn. Everything seems a bit more fuzzy. I've felt this before, this wave of feeling. Like woozy waves. Here it comes again. I look over at you again, and although I don't yet understand the words, I see you nod, and sounds come out. You seem to know what's happening for me, and I smile again. You've got me. You know. You understand. You're here with me. I move towards you, like you're the centre of my universe. I want to be even closer with you now.

ii. To feel connected (*closeness creating a sense of safety*)

Babies need closeness to feel relaxed enough to sleep. If we think about our hunter-gatherer heritage, that makes sense, doesn't it?

Babies need closeness in order to feel safe enough to relax into sleep.

Babies are extremely vulnerable, particularly before they can crawl or walk. If something dangerous happens, their fight or flight response cannot achieve much, since they have very little strength to fight and no capacity to flee.

For a baby experiencing any kind of threat, such as being alone after calling out for help, their main option after some attempt to fight or flee is to freeze (dissociate). Dissociation is often mistaken for relaxation.

A baby needs to feel a sense of closeness to know that they are safe to fall asleep. However, when they *are* close with us, our emotional state affects whether they feel safe and also influences whether they will be able to feel relaxed enough to sleep.

As a baby learns to crawl and becomes a toddler, and then to walk, they have more capacity to fight and flee. However, if they are in a cot in a separate room, they also have little capacity to flee when they experience a threat or sense of danger, since they can't get out of the cot. The only options they have then are to call out for help or to dissociate.

Self-Compassion Moment

If you've been wanting to co-sleep with your baby, or you have co-slept with them, and you've been judged or shamed, or told that they will never sleep in their own bed or that you are "creating a rod for your own back", I'm sending you so much love. You might find it helpful to imagine that the people who said those things to you were once little babies wanting closeness at night, and who were later conditioned to believe what they are now telling you. (That's a powerful example of the difference between a baby's innate needs and a parent's culturally conditioned beliefs.)

If you have put your baby in a cot in another room, I'm also sending you so much compassion. If you are still doing that, I invite you to connect in with whether that is what you really want. If you do, is there anything you'd like to do to support them to feel more closeness and safety during the evening and at night?

If you didn't want to put your baby in a cot in a separate room, and you were persuaded to do it, I'm sending lots of love to all of your feelings. If you are hitting yourself with emotional sticks of guilt, I invite you to drop those sticks and to replace them with deep self-compassion.

The wonderful thing about Aware Parenting is that whatever we've done in the past, we can change what we do in the present. We can also support our baby to heal from stress and trauma, including from us, using their innate healing processes.

If you want to start co-sleeping, it's never too late to start. And if you want to help your baby heal from experiences of being left alone and feeling lonely, scared, or overwhelmed, with Aware Parenting, you can do that too.

What about babies who *do* go to sleep on their own in a cot? How does that happen, if closeness is necessary for restful sleep?

From an Aware Parenting perspective, if a baby is left to go to sleep alone, they may feel lonely or scared, but because sleep is necessary, even in the most challenging environments, they are born with the capacity to dissociate from painful feelings, including fear.

Babies can do this with a variety of methods, such as thumb-sucking or using a dummy, clutching on to a blanket or soft toy, or as a result of being swaddled (the lack of ability to move evoking the freeze response, i.e. dissociation).

When they move into lighter sleep, or if there is noise or movement, they are likely to wake up, back in hyperarousal again. They may then do whatever they do to help them to dissociate again in order to go back to sleep.

Self-Compassion Moment

If you've left your baby alone to go to sleep, I'm sending you a big hug right now. I want to remind you that I'm not judging you. And I'm inviting you to be unwilling to judge yourself. If you're noticing yourself picking up that guilt stick, you might say, "I'm not willing to hit myself with the guilt stick about this. I am willing to be compassionate with myself. I did what I thought was the most helpful thing at the time. I'm willing to support my baby with any healing from those experiences that they might need to do." You might connect with sadness instead, which I invite you to receive some loving listening for.

You might feel sad if you were left alone as a baby. You might feel grief imagining all the babies left alone to sleep. I'm sending so much loving compassion to any and all of your feelings, and I invite you to feel and express them with a loving and present listener.

What you can do:

I invite you to offer your baby your loving arms and hold them on your lap, or lie next to them, offering your presence, your love, and your care. Offering them eye contact, your loving gaze, and showing them that you are there with them.

From a baby: *I'm here, and you're over there, and I feel that tired wave thing happening again. I've had the yawn, and my hand just rubbed my eye. My world feels wobbly and out of focus. The worlds are moving. I want to be with you. I track you with my eyes, and I call out. Come! Come! I need you! You hear my cry, and you turn around, and smile, and* *you come over and pick me up. My world is pulled into your universe. I feel a rightness, that my world is all well, even with the wobbliness. I feel your arms around me. Your heart beats and I feel the rhythm. I love your familiar smell. I am at home. All is well with my world and the wobbles shift.*

A little story on waking up in the morning:

I created a little family ritual when my daughter was a baby. When she woke up next to me in bed in the morning, and once she was fully awake, I would sing gently to her, "Good morning, good morning! We'll dance the whole day through, good morning, good morning, to you, little picklepoo!" I loved shining the light of my adoration for her through the song, and I found that it helped me connect in with my love for her, and was a beautiful start to the day.

iii. To feel relaxed (*by releasing any healing-feelings present*)

What about if a baby is clearly showing tired signs and they do have closeness, for example, if you're holding them or lying next to them, but they're not going to sleep?

It's *this* situation which often leads parents to think that their baby is 'fighting sleep'.

From an Aware Parenting perspective, tiredness and closeness are necessary, but not sufficient, for sound sleep. True relaxation is also needed.

They might be safe because they have closeness, but if they have accumulated feelings that are bubbling up to be heard, they won't feel relaxed enough to sleep.

In order to understand what's going on with babies and sleep from an Aware Parenting perspective, it's essential to differentiate between true relaxation and dissociation (freeze). Mild dissociation is often inaccurately perceived as relaxation.

Self-Compassion Moment

If you're realising that you helped your baby move into dissociation to go to sleep, and you're tempted to pick up the guilt sticks, I invite you to put them down. Most babies are helped to go to sleep in this way! Punishing yourself won't help you or your parenting. It won't help your baby. Being deeply compassionate with yourself and with them will be the most helpful response here! You might like to choose a loving phrase for yourself, such as, "I'm not willing to judge myself here. I am willing to be compassionate with myself." If you feel sad, seeing things you didn't see before, I'm sending so much love to your sadness.

Self-Reflection Moment

I invite you to reflect on your experiences with your baby's relaxation:

- Have you noticed at times that your baby seems to be superficially calm?

- Does the calm seem to be temporary?

- Do they easily wake up if you move them or make a noise?

- Does this concept of differentiating dissociation from relaxation resonate with you?

As parents, we are taught to help our babies move into mild dissociation, away from their healing-feelings that naturally bubble up to be expressed when they are tired. However, if we do that, those feelings don't go away. They still reside in a baby's body.

The painful emotions that babies are dissociating from are real feelings that accumulate in a baby's body and over time, will probably affect their capacity for deeply restful sleep, as well as other aspects of their behaviour. In the daytime, they might show continued signs of mild dissociation – such as sucking their thumb or on a dummy, or they might move into hyperarousal and either bite or hit others (the fight response), or repeatedly crawl away (the flight response). Alternatively, they might keep trying to express the feelings, which can show up as ongoing low-grade 'fussing', or loud screaming or screeching, if they're not getting to actually cry or rage.

Self-Compassion Moment

If you taught your baby to 'self-soothe' or 'self-settle', and you're picking up the guilt stick right now, I invite you to put it down. You don't need to punish yourself for not knowing before what you know now. And if you want to change things, and help your baby or child feel more connected with – and express – their healing-feelings, it's never too late!

For babies to be able to go to sleep so they can sleep restfully and stay asleep until they've either had enough sleep or they're hungry, they need to feel a *deep* sense of relaxation.

Many other parenting paradigms suggest things to bring about calmness such as:

1. *Creating a relaxing sleep environment:*
   - *Dimmed light or darkness*
   - *White noise machine*
2. *Supporting presence:*
   - *Bathing*
   - *Massaging*
3. *Doing things to 'soothe' a baby to sleep:*
   - *Feeding*
   - *Rocking*
   - *Jiggling/bouncing*
   - *Shushing to sleep*
4. *Promoting 'self-soothing':*
   - *Putting the baby's own thumb in their mouth*
   - *Giving a dummy, blanket, or soft toy*
   - *Swaddling*

Aware Parenting supports the practices in the first two categories – creating a relaxing sleep environment (although we suggest not complete

217

darkness, so our baby can see us, especially if they need to cry with us, and you may find that you don't need a white noise machine because your baby won't be woken up by noise when they are deeply relaxed), and supporting them to be present in their bodies – seeing these as helpful for *some* babies. Bright lights, blue light, and EMF radiation *might* make it harder for babies to feel relaxed. A bath and/or a massage can offer physical calm and add to a sense of connection, especially if they are in the bath with you. A baby's tactile environment can also affect them – some babies will feel less relaxed if their pyjamas or bedding are made from polyester or are washed with chemical washing powder. Their digestion and the foods they've eaten (including secondhand via breastmilk) might also affect how relaxed they feel. Having a bath or shower or receiving a gentle massage might help with relaxation.

However, Aware Parenting has a different way of understanding the 'soothing' and 'self-soothing'. As you've already read, doing things to 'soothe' a baby to sleep and encouraging 'self-soothing' are seen as working against a baby's innate relaxation processes.

I want to remind you that I am not telling you what to do.

You might choose to continue doing whatever it is that you usually do to bring about sleep. Or you might do it sometimes, or most of the time. I invite you to always listen in to yourself and your willingness. I'm offering you a way of understanding what is going on so that you can then make a *true* choice about how you respond to your baby based on information that *deeply* resonates for you, which might be Aware Parenting, or it might not be.

From an Aware Parenting perspective, babies have an innate way to feel deeply relaxed, and when we understand this and trust this, we can choose to cooperate with this process.

However, that is often a lot for us in a culture where it's huge to even believe that babies have healing-feelings, or that they are affected by their birth. It's an even bigger step to actually listen to those feelings with our baby in our loving arms.

If our baby is tired and connected, and we are doing things to them to 'soothe' them, or to help them 'self-soothe', and they are still not falling asleep, this is where Aware Parenting's understanding of stress and trauma can be helpful.

Let's reflect on stress, trauma, and healing again, this time, with a focus on babies.

Stress and trauma and sleep

When a baby has accumulated feelings sitting in their body from experiences of overwhelm or frustration (which are common for all babies to experience every day), or from prenatal, birth, or postnatal trauma, those are real physiological sensations that prevent a baby from feeling deeply relaxed. The baby literally feels tense, agitated, or antsy.

When a baby experiences stress, they may move into the fight, flight, or freeze response.

Sources of stress might include:

- stress in utero if their mother was going through a difficult or stressful time;
- their birth experience (even if it was relatively calm for their mother);
- what happened immediately after birth, including separation or medical procedures;
- loud noises;
- going out in the car or public transport;
- the overwhelm of all the new things that they are experiencing each day; or
- a busy day with lots of visitors.

If the tension mobilised for fight or flight is not expressed, it sits in their body, waiting to be expressed and released. They may feel tense and agitated, so even if they are tired and connected, they're not in the relaxed physical state which is conducive to falling asleep. It's here that as parents in this culture, we are often taught to keep doing things to a baby to 'soothe' them – through feeding them or moving them (such a rocking, jiggling, bouncing, or putting them in a carrier, stroller, or even the car). Or we are told to help babies 'self-soothe' by giving them items such as dummies, a blanket or a soft toy, or to swaddle them.

Aware Parenting sees this process in a different light in two key ways. The *first* is that these things that we do to babies cause a particular kind of calm which is more akin to a state of dissociation than to one of embodied relaxation.

Instead of bringing resolution to the fight/flight response, these actions bypass the healing process, by temporarily calming the stress and numbing the feelings.

Second, if the environment is relatively calm and they don't have anything going on from other physiological causes, we can trust that *they know* how to feel relaxed enough to sleep. All that is needed is for us to be lovingly present, hold them in our arms, and let them know we're there and ready to listen to any healing-feelings they have to express to us.

With beautiful biological wisdom, a baby's healing process from stress and trauma is also their innate relaxation-through-release response. This process involves releasing the tension mobilised to fight or flee, by crying in loving arms while vigorously moving their arms and legs.

When babies feel tired, they are less able to suppress their feelings.

When they feel tired and connected, they can then naturally release any pent-up feelings from the day (or the past). When they cry in our loving arms when all their immediate needs are met, they can release the tension that otherwise makes it hard for them to go to sleep and that wakes them up when they are in light sleep.

Rather than babies fighting sleep, so often it is we who are fighting this natural relaxation-through-release response. Babies try to cry to heal from stress and trauma so that they can feel deeply relaxed in their bodies and sleep restoratively. Learning this, we may realise that we have been doing everything we can to prevent or short-circuit that process.

Self-Compassion Moment

As you read this, you might be feeling all kinds of feelings and be thinking all kinds of thoughts. You might be feeling incredulous, sad, angry, or some other emotion. However you're feeling and whatever you're thinking, I'm sending you lots of love. I'm here to remind you of my initial invitation at the beginning of this book. Are you willing to be open to changing some of your beliefs about sleep? Would you like to deeply listen to yourself so you can hear what resonates with you and what doesn't?

You may have been told that *all* crying indicates an immediate need, and thus that a crying baby is telling us that they have a need that we're not meeting. Or you may have learnt that crying doesn't mean anything and that babies need to learn to stop themselves from crying. Or that crying is just a baby 'exercising their lungs'.

Learning that crying can actually be profoundly healing, as long as the crying happens in loving arms when all immediate needs are met, can come as quite a shock to many people.

Remember that in Aware Parenting, we understand that there are two reasons for a baby's crying. The first is communication, and the second is healing. You may recall that I call these needs-feelings and healing-feelings.[37]

In Aware Parenting, we always want to make sure that **all** *of a baby's immediate needs are met before listening to their healing-feelings. This is vitally important.*

However, we also hold that *all* babies in Western industrialised countries will feel healing-feelings every day for the first several months (and personally, I believe that is often for much longer), however much we aim to meet their needs. This kind of crying, provided it is in our arms for pre-crawling babies, and with our loving presence and offer of closeness for mobile babies, brings about deep healing, as well as relaxation – which leads to restorative sleep.

---

37 These are not official Aware Parenting terms.

There's a big difference between the kind of calm that happens when we jiggle, rock, bounce, shush, feed to sleep, give a dummy or blanket or soft toy, or the baby sucks their thumb, and the type of relaxation that happens when a baby cries in our loving arms before sleep when all their needs are met.

The first kind of calm is temporary and superficial. This means that if we are doing something to the baby to 'make them' feel this kind of calmness, the relaxation doesn't last. This is why babies may wake up, such as when there's noise, or after one or more sleep cycles, or if we transfer them from one place to another.

I wonder if you've ever tried to move your sleeping baby, or tried to move away from them when they're newly asleep, only to find that they wake up?

From an Aware Parenting perspective, the temporary calm has worn off and the underlying feelings are waking them up, ready to be expressed.

We may then end up doing whatever it is we did to help them feel that initial state of apparent calm, over and over again with each wake up. This can be why babies start waking up more and more even though they are getting older and their stomachs are getting bigger, because more and more feelings are accumulating.

If our baby is doing something *un*related to our body (e.g. holding a soft toy) to feel a superficial calm enough to go to sleep, they will need to do that action again when they wake up to be able to go back to sleep. That's why a baby who sucks their thumb or on a dummy, or who clutches on to a soft toy or blanket will need to keep doing that again if they wake up.

In contrast, when a baby cries in our loving arms when they are tired and all their needs are met, and they complete the whole crying cycle, the quality of relaxation that they feel is much deeper and thus more long-lasting. This profoundly affects the quality and length of their sleep.

This is something we can clearly *observe*, *sense*, and *feel* as parents.

As a baby expresses their feelings in our loving arms, they literally become more relaxed. Their muscles relax and we can feel them increasingly melt into our loving arms. We will also be able to see this relaxation in other ways too. They will move around less in their sleep, their hands will be more relaxed, and they will have less tension showing on their face.

The less accumulated feelings they have in their body, the more they will be able to sleep until they have had enough sleep or until they are actually hungry.

I remember the first time that we listened to my daughter's healing-feelings. She finished the cycle of crying in my arms and there was a quality of presence that permeated the room. We gazed into each other's eyes as if we were connected for all eternity. She had been 'calm' before, but this was something completely different. I hear this so often from parents I work with, and they send me photos of their babies, exuding a quality of presence through their eyes and a deep relaxation clearly visible on their face and body.

How can we tell the difference between the more superficial type of calmness which is mild dissociation, and true relaxation?

There are two core differences which indicate embodied presence: *eye contact* and *muscle tension*.

Eye contact:

When a baby is dissociating from their feelings, they will often either avoid eye contact or might have a glazed look in their eyes.

A baby who is truly relaxed can gaze into our eyes for long periods and alertly engage with what they are doing.

Please note: whilst a baby is crying in arms to release stress and tension when all their needs are met, they will often have their eyes closed or will not be looking in our eyes. This is because they are deeply connected with themselves and it doesn't indicate dissociation. You may notice that from time to time they might pause the crying, look in your eyes, and then return to the crying again.

Muscle tension:

A baby who is suppressing or dissociating from feelings will tend to have tension in their muscles. You might experience that in the form of tight fists, stiffness, all-over body tightness, tension in their mouth whilst feeding, and not melting into hugs. Or they might seem calm, but you experience a sense of absence rather than presence in their body.

In comparison, a baby who is truly relaxed after completing a crying cycle, having expressed a whole chunk of feelings in our loving arms, will feel relaxed, with a quality of deep presence through their body.

They might sleep with their hands open. Some babies (particularly in warm climates) even sleep with their arms above their heads. When holding them, they will melt into our hug, and their facial features will look relaxed too.

Please note: whilst a baby is crying in arms to release stress and tension, vigorous movement is common. They might be arching their back, kicking their legs, and moving their arms about. This is part of releasing the physical tension accumulated from the fight or flight response.

Jess shares how Aware Parenting was life-changing for her:

"We started to look into Aware Parenting when I had hit the point of, "I can't do this anymore". I had been 'demand-feeding' and co-sleeping with my son for 20 months and he was still waking up four plus times a night. My first thought was to 'get him to night wean', though I wasn't sure how to go about that, nor did the idea of it feel very gentle.

We started working with Marion and our main focus was listening to feelings before bedtime (both with him and our five-year-old). Sometimes those feelings involved 10 minutes of intense raging, while at other times it involved up to an hour of sobbing. It became clear he had a lot of accumulated feelings that he had unknowingly been suppressing through breastfeeding.

As the weeks rolled by, we noticed two things happening in parallel; 1) while our son still needed to cry before bed, it was often less intense and a shorter duration, and 2) his night wake-ups diminished at an astonishing rate. Within a couple of weeks, he was only waking up once in the night and after a month or so, that wake-up was 5am. Even this was game-changing for me. I felt so much more rested and able to meet with life.

Then, after chatting to Marion, we explored what might have been happening for our son at 5am during his birth. He was able to connect to some painful feelings from that time in a few powerful releases, and since then, wakes up later at, 6am or 7am.

Gaining the sleep I need to be the parent I want to be has been absolutely game-changing.

Now when he goes to sleep, he lies down, gets into a very cute and cosy position and rests his little body until his eyes close and he drifts off. Never did I ever imagine he would go to sleep without "milkies". Never could I have envisaged him laying down of his own accord and gently drifting into a slumber. It is the sweetest thing and my mind is blown!

This is only one of the profound changes we have experienced with Aware Parenting. It has profoundly changed our lives."

From a baby: *It's happening again, that wave is coming. The waves come quick and fast. You're holding me in your arms and I know I am safe and I can let the wave come through me. I don't need to stop it. The force comes through me, and moves my body. My arms move everywhere, and my legs kick out. Big loud sounds come out of me, from the very centre of me, out into the space between us. They join us together. I close my eyes, at one with the wave. I am loud and I am big and I am wild. I open my mouth again, and more loud sounds come out. The crying, the noise, we are all here together.*

There's a pause, and I open my eyes. Straight away, your eyes and mine meet. We are here together too. We two are one with this. The wave is coming again. I close my eyes, and the movements and sounds wrap themselves around me. I am the wave. We are one. The wave is on the beach, and then it dives back again. There is quiet again. I open my eyes again. Yes, you're there. I see you and hear you. I close my eyes one more time; another wave is coming. I feel you holding me. You are my shore, always there. This wave is quieter. I move, but not as much. I cry, but it's quieter. The wave is gone.

I open my eyes, and this time, there is a fresh new day. Some gusts of wind come out of me, and then I sigh. And now, how different I feel. All the colours around me are bright. There's space in between things. I gaze into your eyes. We stay this way for so long. Ahh, and the waves have left my body, which melts into the sand of your shore. I melt into you. We two are one. I love you. I feel my eyelids closing now.

What this means in practical terms

Holding or lying next to your baby

There are lots of different options for how we can offer closeness and listening to our baby, while also listening to our own needs to feel comfortable.

We might:

- Hold our baby in our arms while sitting down.
- Sit in a chair and have them lying on their back along our legs, with their head at our knees. This way, we can offer them eye contact, perhaps with a pillow or one hand under their head (once they grow longer, a pillow along your legs, underneath their body might be necessary).[38]
- Lie down next to them with our arm around them, offering eye contact.

If you have a yes to doing this, I invite you to set up an environment of support for you so that you can then be their supportive space for crying in arms.

This might include having some big cushions behind you, and your feet up on a stool, or making sure that you're comfortable on your bed. I

---

38 There's a diagram at the end of the book showing this position.

invite you to take care of your immediate needs too, e.g. ensuring you are hydrated and have been to the toilet, to help yourself be as relaxed as you can be during the crying.

Then we can offer our baby our focused loving presence.

The more present and loving we feel, the more likely it is that they will feel that presence, which can create a sense of safety in their body which will help them express any big feelings and move towards restful sleep.

In this process, we are aiming for maximum connection. We are invited to be as present as we can be in our body, so that our touch or hold is full of loving presence that they can physically feel. We can gaze lovingly in their eyes if they are willing to make eye contact. We're communicating to them that we are fully there with them, that they are safe, that we love them, and that we are listening.

Our baby might move from 'fussing' to more intense crying. Our role is to stay calm and relaxed, physically supporting them whilst they do what they know how to do to release stress and tension. They can then gradually move into a state of calm relaxation.

If you don't feel resourced to listen to your baby's healing-feelings when they're tired, even though you feel confident that they're not hungry and that all their needs are met, one option is to wear noise-cancelling headphones. That way, you can protect yourself from more overwhelm, while your baby still has the opportunity to express their healing-feelings to you.

When you first begin this process, it's totally normal and natural to feel concerned or scared that your baby has an unmet need that you haven't met, such as hunger. If that's the case, you could simply let them know, *"I don't know if you're crying to let out feelings or crying to tell me you are hungry, so I'm going to feed you now."* Then I invite you to keep observing them whilst you're feeding them. If they're pulling on and off, or rejecting the breast or bottle, or sucking intermittently, or falling asleep straight away, it's likely that they weren't hungry after all and that they *did* have some feelings to express and release.[39]

Later in the book, we'll talk in more detail about the actual process of crying in arms before sleep.

How dads or the non-breastfeeding parent can help with sleep

Supporting a baby's natural relaxation response to go to sleep can be transformative for everyone in the family.

If the mother is breastfeeding and has a partner, or other family members who are willing to help, she doesn't need to be the one who always helps the baby to feel relaxed enough to sleep.

I often find that it's a way for everyone to get their needs met even more. The mum has a sense of support, knowing that she's not doing it all herself, the dad (or non-breastfeeding other parent) gets to experience the beauty of supporting their baby or toddler to express feelings, and the baby has the experience of more than one person welcoming all their feelings. This is likely to mean that they are expressing a higher percentage of feelings and thus feel more relaxed and present.

This was Katie's experience. She shares:

"Before discovering Aware Parenting, I had put my son, Solly, down for bed every night from birth to 16 months, because the only way we could get him to sleep was on the boob. It was so taxing on me, and my partner, Corey, felt frustrated because he couldn't help. After discovering Aware Parenting, we immediately changed up our bedtime routine, stopped breastfeeding to sleep, and Corey started doing most bedtimes. This immediately improved Solly's sleep, my mental health improved because I got so much more freedom, and Corey felt more empowered.

---

39 Please note that there can be other possibilities for some of these, such as a tongue tie, so if you're ever concerned, please contact your trusted health professional.

After a couple of weeks, Corey expressed to me that he felt so much more in love with Solly since he started putting him to bed. I used to gush all the time and say, "He's so beautiful," looking at Solly while he was sleeping, and Corey expressed that he finally understood the feeling behind those words and he started telling me to look at how beautiful Solly is! I have watched the connection between father and son blossom through this paradigm. Solly is so much more of a daddy's boy now and it makes my heart explode with joy and love!"

Self-Compassion Moment

I'm sending so much love to any feelings you might be feeling, having just read this. I invite you to reach out for some listening time if you need it. The idea that mothers can breastfeed their baby or toddler, but not need to be the one that supports their child/ren to go to sleep can be a huge paradigm shift.

From a baby: *I love being in your arms. This is my home. I am safe here. With you, I move through different worlds. And oh, I'm moving into a different land now. I can feel it coming. My mouth makes this movement – I think you call it a yawn. My eyes feel different, too. I still don't really know how to make my hands do what I want them to, but one of my hands moves to my eyes and kind of rubs it. The world feels different. Kind of slower, somehow. A rumble starts from inside me. My legs start to move. An energy comes from inside of me, and I make a sound. It needs to come out before I can go to sleep. I need to move through this world before I can go to the land of sleep.*

I look up at you, unsure. You used to start doing all kinds of busy things to me when I did this, but something has changed. You keep holding me, and you're still. Our eyes meet. You are the centre of my world. You nod. You're there. You say yes to this. Okay, I'm going to keep on going. The wave builds higher, and I can feel the storm in the centre of me. It bursts out, and my legs kick, and my arms move, and my mouth opens, and there it is, a cry.

I look at you again, checking. Are you still here? Is this welcome? Am I safe? Do you love me?

Our eyes meet again, and you nod again, and you say something. I don't understand words yet, but I know what you mean. It's a yes. You're there with me. What I'm doing is welcome. Okay. I feel a ramping up inside of me. I look away from you, all my attention focused on this storm building in me. With full force, I kick, I arch, I wave my arms, and I cry. These waves of storm come again and again. A crescendo, it's so big and loud. I feel hot and full and big. This storm is me and I am the storm. These waves are moving through me. I feel their energy and their power. Louder and louder, then an easing off.

I look again. You nod again. All is well. This is all welcome. I am welcome. I move in again. The wave builds again. Cry, move, arch, kick. You put your hands against my feet and I feel this satisfying force. I can feel this power, as I push with all my might against you, and my voice speaks the loudness of me.

Oh, this reminds me of when I was coming into the world. I feel it, I feel it all. More tears come. My voice is the loudest it's ever been. I'm telling you all about how it was for me. It was so big. I look again, to make sure you know what I'm telling you about. You nod again, and you say some things. I know you know. You understand me. You're listening to me. It's all coming out. I'm at the peak of the storm now. I'm hot. The waves are rolling through so quickly. I'm still pushing, and I can feel your warm and loving hands at my feet still. We meet there. We are in this together. You're here with me. One last yell.... ahhhhh, and I feel a change.

The energy has moved. I sigh, and I feel so much space and stillness around me. I look at you again. There's a quiet, as if we're here together forever and this presence is all there is. I'm here. I'm here with you. You're here. You're here with me. My body is as wide as the world, and relaxed as a lake. It's all clear, and it's all calm. I gaze into your eyes forever. Oh, that yawn thing is here again. I'm drifting off into sleep. My eyes are closing. I open them again for one more peek with you, until I move into my dreamy world. Nighty night.

Attachment play

Remember, that earlier in the book, I said that play and laughter are also a part of the innate relaxation response of babies and children?

In Aware Parenting, we call this *attachment play*[40]. This is often less relevant for younger babies, but as they get older, it can be an important part of the process of them becoming more relaxed. *Attachment play* can also help a baby feel a deep sense of connection. I imagine you've already naturally played games like peek-a-boo, or rough and tumble. This kind of play is so innate in us.

CHAPTER SUMMARY

There are three ingredients required for restful sleep:

i. to feel tired (sleepy);

ii. to feel connected (*closeness creating a sense of safety*); and

iii. to feel relaxed (*by releasing any healing-feelings present*).

Other paradigms think that 'fussing', back arching and crying are signs that a baby is 'overtired'. In Aware Parenting, we perceive crying in the evening as a process whereby babies relax by healing from stress and trauma. Rather than trying to get the baby to go to sleep as quickly as possible, through trying to 'soothe' them or to get them to 'self-soothe', we can be lovingly present with our baby as they cry in our arms, until they naturally feel relaxed enough to fall asleep.

Babies need to have closeness to feel relaxed enough to sleep. If a baby is alone, the two options they have are to be in hyperarousal (e.g. agitation), or to be in dissociation – which is often mistaken for relaxation.

From an Aware Parenting perspective, tiredness and closeness are necessary, but not sufficient, for sound sleep. True relaxation is also needed. As parents, we are taught to help our babies move into mild

---

40 *Attachment play* is another core element of Aware Parenting which I will be explaining more about later.

dissociation, away from their healing-feelings that naturally bubble up when they are tired. However, if we do that, those feelings don't go away. They still reside in a baby's body.

Doing things to 'soothe' a baby to sleep and encouraging 'self-soothing' work against a baby's innate relaxation processes. Rather than babies fighting sleep, so often it is we who are fighting this natural relaxation-through-release response. Babies try to cry to heal from stress and trauma so that they can feel deeply relaxed in their body and sleep restoratively.

In Aware Parenting, we understand that there are two reasons for a baby's crying: communication and healing. I call these needs-feelings and healing-feelings. In Aware Parenting, we always want to make sure that *all* of a baby's immediate needs are met before listening to their healing-feelings. This is vitally important.

However, we also hold that *all* babies in Western industrialised countries will feel healing-feelings every day for the first several months (and I believe that it is often for much longer), however much we aim to meet their needs.

When a baby cries in our loving arms when they are tired and all their needs are met, and they complete the whole crying cycle, the quality of relaxation that they feel is much deeper and thus more long-lasting than if we distract them from their healing-feelings. This profoundly affects the quality and length of their sleep. The less accumulated feelings they have in their body, the more they will be able to sleep until they have had enough sleep or until they are actually hungry.

There are two core ways we can differentiate between the more superficial type of calmness – which is mild dissociation – and true relaxation: *eye contact* and *muscle tension*.

If a mother is breastfeeding and has a partner, or other family members who are willing to help, she doesn't need to be the one who always helps the baby to feel relaxed enough to sleep. Everyone can then get their needs met even more.

I'm here with you as you take in all this information.
You're not on your own.

13. Translating mainstream sleep terminology into Aware Parenting

In Aware Parenting – as I imagine you have gathered by now – we have very different beliefs about sleep and what helps babies sleep compared to many other approaches.

My heart goes out to parents who have been taught about 'wake windows' and babies being 'overtired' and have found that these concepts bring tension and worry to their experience of parenting.

Time and time again, I've seen the relief parents feel when they learn about Aware Parenting, deeply resonate with it, and see how different their relationship with their baby and with sleep can be.

Nyssa shares her journey. I was moved to tears when I first read about what she'd been through:

"Before Aware Parenting, I had spent the first 11 months of my daughter's life stressed about her sleep. When she was born, I was gifted some guides for 'gentle sleep training' which I didn't realise incorporated controlled crying. After wrestling with appropriate 'wake windows' and the enormous stress of my baby getting 'overtired', I came across gentle baby sleep methods, which resonated with my desire to practice attachment-style parenting.

This was an improvement, and yet after an initial sense of relief I was once again consumed by timing 'wake windows', and the fear and anxiety of my baby getting 'overtired'. My mind was consumed daily by the fear and anxiety of not being able to get my baby to sleep, of having visitors (family and friends that I love) as they may disrupt our routine, and being so incredibly stressed about leaving the house because of how it might affect my daughter's ability to fall asleep at the 'right time'. I would allow my baby to nap in my lap, and went to painstaking efforts to ensure the bedroom had not one streak of light coming through. I would cancel health appointments for myself at the last minute if my baby was still asleep in my lap from the fear of waking her up and what that would mean for the next sleep time. I wouldn't go to the toilet or eat if my baby was napping in my lap out of fear of waking her up.

This constriction around her sleep was impacting my relationship with her dad, to the point that I asked him not to move around the house for the first half hour of her sleep. I was often irritated by the noise that he would make when she was asleep, incredibly stressed about it waking her up. I feared my baby crying and did anything and everything in my power to prevent her from crying. The were multiple naps where I stood in a pitch-black room, in the middle of summer in 40 degree heat, with my baby in the carrier, rocking and jiggling her so that she would have her required amount of daytime sleep. Some naps I did this for over an hour, my calves burning from the constant rocking and jiggling and bouncing. I would reassure myself that it was for her benefit and that her sleep was of the utmost importance.

Then, one day I was participating in an online parenting session about parental tiredness when the facilitator mentioned her appreciation for Aware Parenting. I made a mental note to check it out, and a couple of weeks later my journey began! My entire attitude towards my baby's sleep has been turned upside-down and inside-out. I am much less stressed about it, I leave the house more to see friends, take my baby to the local farmer's market, and my partner and I even went out for brunch with our baby! This was unheard of prior to coming across Aware Parenting. The way I perceive my baby's behaviour throughout the day (not just at nap and bedtime) has been revolutionised and I am so incredibly grateful. I feel more connected to her and I feel like I understand her better and am better able to trust my own instincts when it comes to being her mother and primary caregiver.

I have experienced significant trauma in the past 12 months (not related to my baby) and practicing Aware Parenting and having Marion's loving support has been the defining feature in my ability to start processing my grief. This parenting journey is not easy and I still have much work to do, but I am now able to access the joy and amazement at being a mother to this beautiful little girl and I will forever be grateful to Marion for welcoming me into the Aware Parenting family. I am now able to watch my daughter fall asleep in my arms again, her beautiful baby cheeks caressed by soft light, and then transfer her to the bed without her waking up. And if she does wake up, I don't stress about it anymore because I trust myself and my daughter to be able to manage whatever the day brings. Thank you, Marion."

Self-Compassion Moment

I wonder how you feel when you read this? I'm sending you so much love if you experienced something similar. If you have, I wonder if you've shared your feelings with a loving listener? It's so important for us to have our feelings heard as parents, especially if we've gone through stressful and painful experiences. Expressing our emotions and having them lovingly heard helps us to be able to listen to our baby's feelings, too.

Although practicing Aware Parenting can be challenging, particularly in terms of helping us connect with our own unexpressed childhood feelings, understanding sleep in this way can bring so much more ease, as well as rest!

Let's translate common sleep concepts into Aware Parenting understandings.

Self-Compassion Moment

Before we do, I'm here to remind you to put any guilt or self-judgment sticks down as you read this. This information is not designed to invite you to pick up the sticks. Rather, I'm sharing this so you can listen in deeply to yourself and continue to see whether the Aware Parenting lens resonates with you. If it doesn't, I want to remind you that you are so welcome to pause or stop and put this book down at any time you want to.

I'm also here to remind you about what I have said many times now, that questioning our cultural conditioning can lead to us feeling uncomfortable feelings. The terms I share below are very common if you search for information about babies and sleep. These ways of seeing sleep are still most dominant at this time in industrialised countries. If what you read about Aware Parenting is a fit for you, I invite you to be gentle with yourself while old beliefs are being replaced by different ways of seeing things.

Terminology that has an asterisk (*) next to it is NOT used in Aware Parenting.

Going to sleep

'Wake or sleep windows'*

Have you read about wake windows and felt overwhelmed, aiming to understand how much sleep your baby needs and when? Some parenting paradigms have the concept of wake windows at the core of their approaches. This is sometimes based on the belief that a parent needs to get a baby to sleep before they become 'overtired'. We perceive things very differently in Aware Parenting. We do hold the belief that the longer a baby has been awake, the more likely it is that they feel sleepy and experience a need for sleep. However, because we're not concerned about 'overtiredness', we don't need to try to help a baby sleep before they're even showing signs of tiredness. We can relax, observe our baby's cues, and trust them. When they're tired, they will let us know.

Once we observe their sleepiness, we can aim to be present in our body. Then we can hold them or lie next to them, and support them with their own natural relaxation process of crying in our loving arms[41].

---

41 Once they are mobile, they don't necessarily need to be held in our arms for the crying to be healing, as long as we are close with them and they can move to being in our arms if they want that.

We might hold an approximate idea in our head of how long our baby is generally awake for before they get tired. However, that doesn't need to be a rigid framework.

We also don't need to be concerned if they've been tired for a while and we haven't been able to be present with them and support those natural relaxation processes.

Yes, it may mean that they get too tired to complete the crying cycle and thus won't release the whole chunk of feelings that are sitting at the surface. This may affect how relaxed their sleep is that time around. However, they will keep giving us many more opportunities to listen to the rest of their feelings!

In summary then, we can trust our baby and our observations of them, and follow their cues, rather than needing to follow timetables from others.

Self-Reflection Moment

What do you think and how do you feel, when you imagine not having the concept of wake windows? Would you enjoy that?

Self-Compassion Moment

I'm sending you lots of loving compassion if you feel uncomfortable emotions reading this. Perhaps you put a lot of effort into following wake windows. However you feel right now, I welcome all your feelings.

Nixy shares the shift she made – from the stress she felt with the concepts of wake windows – to the relaxation she felt once she found Aware Parenting. She says:

"Thank you for your podcast, it has helped me to turn away from the sleep apps, wake windows and all the other things they tell you babies need to sleep. Every time I logged onto Instagram I was overloaded with sleep training advice and it was just so painful for me to do. It never felt right to let my baby cry on his own. The learning journey I went on

through crying in arms to sleep was quite profound with my first child. I started doing it when he was seven months old. From birth he slept amazingly, but at around four months, he started waking more frequently and I was feeding him back to sleep every two hours. I had heard stories of mums feeding like this until their babies were two years old. I thought, 'There has to be a better way'. I was searching for a podcast to gather other stories. I knew I didn't want to go down the sleep training route because it never sat well for me.

Once I found your Aware Parenting Podcast on sleep, I thought, 'This makes sense'. I could relax. When I searched online for anything about babies I would put '+aware parenting' in to find information. I made the decision to try crying in arms with my son. After 45 minutes of crying and raging, his body fully relaxed and he fell asleep. I cannot explain the feeling this gave me, it was absolutely beautiful. I continued this for the next few months and to my surprise, the cries before bed got shorter and shorter and some nights he would even laugh and chat to sleep. I think besides the benefits of sleeping longer stretches, you get to have that time for more connection.

My baby can come anywhere with me whilst I work and he will get the sleep he needs when he can. Now when I go out, if my baby is tired I can hold him and he will fall asleep in my arms anywhere. Then if I choose to, I can place him down somewhere. I was at a BBQ the other night, people talking and music going and he was tired, he had some crying to do, so I walked away and sat down with him and he had a bit of a cry and fell asleep in my arms. My friends were shocked.

I have learnt so much more about my baby. We were connected before but this has connected us more.

This is just a small example of how letting a baby cry in your arms before sleep gives you the ability to go out and do the things you need to do and not race home to a dark room, with white noise on. A little trust and patience, and the baby will sleep anywhere."

'Overtired'*

We do recommend observing a baby's tiredness cues and supporting them to go to sleep when they're tired – as we addressed in the previous chapter. However, in Aware Parenting, we don't perceive babies as being 'overtired', so we don't need to be concerned if they've been tired for a while.

Other paradigms believe that when a baby is arching their back, becoming rigid, making fists or crying strongly, that they are 'overtired'. If a parent believes that their baby is 'overtired' and that any crying caused by 'overtiredness' is uncomfortable or even painful, they will of course take lots of action to make their baby go to sleep as soon as possible. That might be through jiggling, rocking, bouncing, feeding, giving a dummy, and so on.

In Aware Parenting, when a baby is rigid in our arms or is arching their back, making fists and crying intensely, we don't perceive this as them being 'overtired'. Instead, we recognise this as a sign of their innate wisdom for healing. They are tired *and* have unexpressed feelings in their body that they are trying to express so they can feel relaxed enough to fall asleep.

As long as our baby's needs for connection are met (for a pre-mobile baby, this means being held, for a crawling baby, offering them closeness), and they have been recently fed, and all their other immediate needs are met, the back arching, vigorous movement, and crying are part of their natural relaxation-through-release process.

Rather than being signs that something is awry, these actions are the baby releasing stress from their body. We can trust that babies know how to feel relaxed, and in that moment, that is through crying in our loving arms (or with our loving support, for mobile babies) once all their immediate needs are met. The crying, back arching, and movements are all part of that innate relaxation process.

From an Aware Parenting perspective, all babies experience stresses. Tension remains in their body from those stresses until they release the feelings and heal from those past experiences.

To move out of the fight, flight, or freeze response, babies need to cry in our loving arms, while moving their arms and legs vigorously to release the tension that was stored to fight or flee. This crying and movement indicates that our baby is using their natural relaxation response, to release stress and tension from their bodies, so that they can feel relaxed enough to sleep.

This understanding leads to very different responses from us. When we see their tiredness cues, instead of rushing to 'get our baby to sleep', we can use that time to prepare ourselves so we can support their relaxation-through-release process. That might include finding a comfortable place to sit, getting ourselves a drink of water and going to the toilet or even having a quick snack (ideally, holding our baby all the while). Preparing ourselves in this way, we can then continue to hold our baby in our loving arms, feeling comfortable in our own body. Then, without jiggling, feeding, rocking, or distracting in other ways, we can simply be still and present, offer them eye contact, and offer phrases like, "*I'm here with you and I'm listening*". Then they can let out the feelings that were bubbling up to be expressed. We are trusting that our baby knows what to do, and recognising that they simply need our loving presence and arms to do that. Once they have expressed the chunk of feelings and completed the crying cycle, they will fall asleep. I'll share about that process in more detail soon!

'Overtired' = tired but not relaxed.

Note: we also don't use the term 'sleep pressure', which in other paradigms often combines both tiredness and a belief in 'overtiredness', i.e. it doesn't recognise the difference between tiredness, healing-feelings, and relaxation.

Self-Reflection Moment

How do you feel and what do you think when you read this?

Does it make sense to you?

Does it resonate with you?

Does it bring meaning to your past experiences?

'Sleep associations'*

In other paradigms, this term can indicate the belief that whatever a parent does to help their baby go to sleep, the baby will then expect that each time they wake up. Parents are often encouraged to 'break' those sleep associations.

In contrast, in Aware Parenting, we aim to differentiate between actions that help babies feel truly relaxed before sleep, and those which are helping them dissociate before sleep. For example, we recognise that closeness is an innate need for a baby to feel safe enough to relax into sleep. In contrast, feeding them 'to sleep' or rocking them are seen as actions that bypass healing-feelings, which then emerge again when the baby enters light sleep and wakes up. As parents, we might then repeat what we did the first time. The baby might then 'ask' to be fed if they're used to being fed to sleep.

But in Aware Parenting, that doesn't mean it's an association. Rather, we recognise that they have learnt to interpret the healing-feelings as hunger. Rather than 'breaking' a 'sleep association', in Aware Parenting, we can offer them closeness and listen to their healing-feelings so they can feel relaxed and sleep restfully.

Over time, the baby can re-learn to identify that those particular sensations in their body are feelings such as sadness, anger, frustration, or overwhelm, and can differentiate them from hunger or tiredness. This is a vital part of part of preventing what is commonly called 'emotional eating' in other paradigms.

'Contact naps'*

In some paradigms, parents are told either to offer (or not offer) what are called 'contact naps' – this is where a baby falls asleep with body contact and where closeness is maintained during the nap.

As a form of attachment-style parenting, in Aware Parenting we recommend that babies are held as much as possible, particularly before they can crawl, and especially when they are tired.

Remember the three ingredients for restful sleep? If a baby doesn't have closeness when they're going to sleep, they will need to do something to dissociate from the feelings that come from not getting that need met. From an Aware Parenting perspective, *all* babies need closeness to feel safe and truly relaxed enough to sleep.

However, the whole issue becomes a bit more complex if we have repeatedly distracted a baby from their healing-feelings while holding them, e.g. through breast-feeding or rocking them. This is because they will then mildly dissociate not only when we're doing that thing (such as breast-feeding to suppress feelings), but also simply when we are holding them when they have healing-feelings to express.

This means that babies can find it harder to express their feelings when we're holding them. It's why some babies will cry strongly with their dad (or non-breastfeeding parent), even though they are securely attached with him, and will stop crying as soon as they're in their mother's arms.

How can we tell whether the closeness with mum is meeting a true need for closeness before sleep, or whether being in her arms is helping them dissociate?

It's the same as how we can differentiate between whether a baby's needs are met or they dissociated in other situations – their muscle tension, presence, and eye contact. If, when the baby moves from dad's arms to mum's, she holds them and they melt into her arms with presence and are willing to make eye contact, that suggests she's meeting their needs for closeness. However, if they're tense, lacking presence in their body, and avoiding eye contact or staring, it's possible they are dissociating.

Aware Parenting is about meeting the needs of both babies and parents. Although babies need closeness to go to sleep without dissociating, from an Aware Parenting perspective, they often may not need to have closeness all throughout the nap to stay asleep (although that might usually be their preference, especially in the early weeks and months).

What's going on then, if a baby always wakes up if they are placed down somewhere?

It's commonly when breastfeeding has become a *control pattern,* or being held in a particular position has, and so when that position for dissociation is removed by placing the baby down, they wake up.

Alternatively, it might be that the baby hasn't completed a crying cycle, and being placed down helps them reconnect with the rest of the healing-feelings that haven't yet been expressed.

If you want to place your baby down somewhere after they have gone to sleep, I invite you to experiment with this process: Listen to their healing-feelings for as long as your baby needs, so that they complete the crying cycle. Then wait about 10-15 minutes after they fall asleep before placing them down. In general, your baby will then be able to stay asleep until they've had enough sleep. However, if they're catching up on expressing a lot of accumulated healing-feelings, this might not always 'work', because they still might have a lot of emotions in their body that make it hard for them to feel deeply relaxed.

'Wearing a baby down to sleep'*

Various parenting paradigms offer different types of movement to help babies feel calm enough to go to sleep. One of these is 'wearing a baby down to sleep' in a baby wrap, carrier or sling. From an Aware Parenting perspective, closeness is a core innate attachment need, and movement is a beautiful experience that many babies enjoy. However, when they are tired, their natural relaxation process is to release stress through crying in arms when all their immediate needs are met.

If we are moving around with a baby in a carrier, or rocking and jiggling them, the movement can create mild dissociation. This is often pleasant enough, but it can bypass healing-feelings.

This is why babies will often wake up if we stop moving them or take them out of the carrier, because those healing-feelings are still in their bodies, ready to arise again once we're not distracting them. Over time, if we repeatedly move them to help them feel calm enough to sleep, they will accumulate more and more feelings, and this will often require us to move them for a longer and longer time, or use more vigorous movement to have the same effect of bypassing the feelings that smaller movements used to have.

If a baby falls asleep in the carrier *sometimes*, they are likely to still have other opportunities to express their healing-feelings before sleep. However, if the baby is almost *always* falling asleep in the carrier, it may be that they are not getting much of an opportunity to express their healing-feelings, which may lead to symptoms of accumulation – such as avoiding eye contact, seeming less and less happy in the day, waking up as soon as the movement stops, and waking more frequently at night.

Self-Compassion Moment

I want to remind you that I'm not judging anyone here, and I invite you to refrain from judging yourself, if you've been tempted to pick up a guilt stick. Or you might be feeling other emotions. Whatever you're feeling right now, I'm sending you so much love and empathy. It's so natural for us to go through quite a process when we come across ways of thinking that are different to what we've known and believed. I invite you to be deeply compassionate with yourself in whatever you're going through.

'Self-settling' and 'self-soothing'*

This is when other parenting paradigms encourage parents to help their babies go to sleep *without* the presence of a parent. Babies might be given a dummy, blanket, or soft toy, or they might be encouraged to start sucking their thumb to fall asleep. When a baby wakes up on their own, they will eventually stop calling out and will go back to the same method to suppress their feelings again.

From an Aware Parenting perspective, these are all ways that babies dissociate from their emotions.

Those can be the needs-feelings of loneliness or fear because their needs for closeness and safety aren't met. The emotions can also include any healing-feelings that might have bubbled to the surface before sleep.

A baby who wakes up and doesn't call out for connection has given up on calling for help. This is the opposite of what we're wanting in terms of secure attachment. For a baby to be securely attached, they need to repeatedly experience that their needs are met and that their calls are responded to promptly in a sensitive and attuned way.

Self-Compassion Moment

If you've encouraged your baby to go to sleep in these ways, and you're tempted to hit yourself with the guilt stick right now, I invite you to put that guilt stick down. I also invite you to replace that with lots of loving compassion for yourself. I want to remind you that it's so understandable that you learnt to do these things to your baby. So many parenting paradigms teach this. It's the most common way to respond to babies in this culture. In addition, you may have been responded to like this when you were a baby. If you feel sad when you imagine your baby, other babies, or yourself as a baby being left alone to cry, I'm sending so much love to your sadness. You might feel called to share those feelings with an empathic listener.

The wonderful thing is that however old your baby or child is now, it's never too late to help them heal from any stress or trauma that they experienced. And whatever age they are, the same is true for responding promptly to them, and letting them know that whenever they need closeness at night, you'll give that to them. Change is possible at any age. Changing attachment status is possible at any age.

'Settling' and 'resettling'*

This is when babies wake up and parents do things to help them dissociate back to sleep again. This could be feeding, or it could be rocking them, turning up the white noise volume, patting them, or giving them a dummy.

From an Aware Parenting perspective, if a baby wakes up in the night, our role is to understand the true cause of the waking, and attend to that cause (at the time, or during the next few days or evenings, in the case of listening to feelings).

- If they're waking up because they're needing closeness, our role is to offer them closeness.

- If they are waking because they are hungry, our role is to feed them.

- If they're waking to wee or poo, it's our role to support them with that, either through offering a potty (if we're practicing Elimination Communication), or changing their nappy afterwards (if they would otherwise feel uncomfortable).

- If they're waking because of tension from accumulated healing-feelings, it's our role to listen to those feelings. That might mean listening at the time, during the night. But if we are too tired to do that, we might focus on listening to those feelings the next day and over the following few days.

Often, the cause of waking is because once they are in light sleep, babies' unexpressed feelings bubble up to the surface to be expressed.

If a baby is waking because they have healing-feelings to express, then rocking, patting, or giving a dummy is simply suppressing those feelings again.

If our baby is waking because of unexpressed feelings, one of the key things we can do is increase the amount and intensity of feelings we listen to our baby expressing before they go to sleep. The more feelings that a baby expresses during the day, and particularly before naps and sleep (when their natural relaxation process is often most primed to work), the less they will have feelings that wake them up at night.

This is particularly the case if they complete the whole release process, or crying cyle, which means that they finish crying themselves rather than us distracting them before the end of the feelings session.

Many of us don't want to be listening to healing-feelings in the middle of the night, and listening to feelings before bed means this will often not be necessary. However, if a parent does have the emotional spaciousness in themselves to listen to feelings in the night when their baby has feelings to express, they may choose to do that.

Self-Compassion Moment

I'm sending you lots of love as you read this. If you're feeling overwhelmed, frustrated, or any other feeling, I so understand. I welcome all of your feelings. I'm here to remind you not to 'should' yourself into listening to healing-feelings in the middle of the night, and to tend to your own needs as well as your baby's. Rather than coercing yourself to listen in the nighttime, you might choose to feed your baby back to sleep but then focus on listening to more feelings the next day.

Swaddling and sleep suits

Some parenting approaches promote swaddling for the first several months as a way to help babies sleep.

However, from an Aware Parenting perspective, we only recommend swaddling in the very early days.

This can help *some* babies with their transition into the world, since swaddling is similar to their experience in the womb. Swaddling can help *some* babies feel a sense of containment and can help prevent the startle reflex. However, those *same* needs can also be met by carrying a baby close in a sling or carrier or simply in our arms. In that way, they are *also* having other needs met – for closeness, for warmth, and for connection with our heartbeat, and our familiar smell.

As babies get a bit older, they will very soon need more agency and autonomy, by being able to move their arms and legs freely, which is also important for them in developing their motor skills.

If they are swaddled and aren't able to move their arms and legs, they may feel powerless and may dissociate. This is generally why swaddling can lead to sleep – via mild dissociation.

If they are crying in arms to release stress, they need to make active movements – such as with their arms and legs – while crying, to resolve and complete the healing process.

In Aware Parenting, we're aiming to meet as many of our baby's needs as we can – for:

- closeness;
- security and safety;
- touch; and
- gentle pressure,

which can all be met by holding them. Carrying them in a carrier can make it easier for us to do other things, such as attending to an older sibling, too. We're also aiming to meet their needs for agency, through them being able to choose to move their arms and legs. And our intention is also to support them to heal from stress or trauma through crying in our loving arms, where they need to make vigorous movements as part of moving out of fight, flight, or freeze.

The more we are able to meet the majority of those needs, the more they will feel deeply relaxed in their body and will be able to sleep more restoratively and for longer periods.

So why can swaddling seem to help a baby go to sleep?

It's possible that it may help them feel a sense of containment and safety.

However, it's more likely that it's helping them move into a state of mild dissociation. It may lead them to feel powerless, which is why they freeze.

In contrast, with Aware Parenting, we want them to feel powerful.

Self-Compassion Moment

If you've done this with your baby and you're picking up guilt sticks, I invite you to put those sticks down. I'm here to to remind you that you were doing what you thought was most helpful at the time, and that you can always support your baby or child to feel powerful and release past stress and trauma, however old they are now. Your willingness to feel and express any feelings of sadness that you didn't have this information back then will help you create more of an emotionally safe space for your baby to express their healing-feelings to you.

Feeding a baby to sleep

Some parenting approaches advocate feeding a baby to sleep as a way to help them feel calm enough to go to sleep. In Aware Parenting, we invite parents to see if they're willing to respond most aptly to what a baby needs. If a baby is hungry, the most helpful thing is to feed them.

However, if they are trying to cry in our arms to release stress so they can feel relaxed enough to sleep restfully, then it's most beneficial for them if we lovingly listen to those feelings.

Remember at the beginning of the book, where I said that I wasn't going to judge you, and I wasn't going to tell you that you 'should' do certain things and that you 'shouldn't' do other things. That still stands here! I won't tell you that you 'shouldn't' feed your baby 'to sleep'.

What I love to do is give you this information, so you can:

1. *See* if it resonates with you.
2. *Decide* what you are going to choose to do.
3. *Observe* your baby and how they are affected by the actions you take.

I'd also love to share about why it can be more beneficial for a baby if we listen to their healing-feelings before sleep rather than to feed them 'to sleep'.

Expressing their uncomfortable emotions when they're tired is their innate wisdom in operation. It's how they feel most relaxed in order to sleep. Their healing-feelings are most accessible to be felt and expressed when they're tired.

If we feed them at this time instead, it **may** *have the following consequences.*

They *might*:

- not access their healing-feelings at the easiest time, so it might become harder for them to connect with and express those feelings both when they're sleepy and other times of the day;
- start to interpret that their sensations of tiredness to mean they are hungry, so they might not know how to read their own tiredness signals as they get older;
- develop a breast or bottle feeding *control pattern*, which means they might start asking for milk when they have painful feelings to express;
- not have the opportunity to heal from daily stresses and larger traumas;
- accumulate more and more healing-feelings, meaning that they feel more agitated in their bodies, take longer to go to sleep, and wake up more easily;
- find it harder and harder to express their painful feelings to us;
- learn to believe that we do not welcome their healing-feelings and aren't willing to listen;
- want to eat or drink when they're tired or have painful feelings to express as children or adults.

You might love breastfeeding to sleep. You might love the closeness, the quiet, the connection, and the ease.

I so support you doing whatever you have a 'yes' for.

I'm so willing for you and your baby to both get your needs met.

Emma sent me this, about her journey with breastfeeding to sleep:

"When I first came to you Marion, for mentoring, I had known about Aware Parenting for about six months, having come from what you call Classical Attachment Parenting. I was feeding Max, who was about 19 months old at that time, both for his nap and before sleep. I remember really not wanting to stop doing that, because I really enjoyed that time that he and I had together. At the time I thought it was really peaceful and connected. I remember feeling so mad when I first heard on the podcast that I might be suppressing his feelings. I turned that episode off the first time!

But then, the feeding to sleep got longer and longer and I stopped enjoying it as much. He was so wriggly and grumpy. It stopped being relaxing for me and I actually started to resent breastfeeding. Over the next few months, he started waking up more and more, and then he started hitting other children at daycare. By then, I realised that I really did want to listen to his emotions before sleep. But at that point, it was really difficult for him to do that. I guess it was because I had suppressed his feelings so often before sleep that he thought I didn't want to listen. Getting close to me would mean that he would just stop crying. He'd play with my hair and zone out and wouldn't cry with me. He started waking up more and more, and was still hitting. It was such a hard time for both of us.

It was then that I started asking his dad to help him express his feelings before bed. When we were doing just the attachment parenting, it always had to be me to take him to bed, because I was always breastfeeding him to sleep. But, nowadays, it's generally his Dad who helps him go to sleep. They do some rough and tumble together, and Max has a cry too, most evenings. His Dad was really unsure with the crying at first, but now he's more used to it, even if he's reluctant to listen. However, I'm really sad, because Max will hardly ever express his emotions to me at all.

When I look back on that time when I always breastfed him to sleep and I reacted to Aware Parenting, I wish I'd got some support earlier on to see why I had those big emotions. I know now that it was because my Mum only breastfed me for eight weeks and so when I thought about not

251

feeding Max to sleep, I felt my own sadness. But of course his experience was completely different to mine. I wish I'd known that I could have carried on enjoying breastfeeding, and also listened to Max's feelings, by avoiding feeding him to sleep.

Nowadays, when I tell other mums about Aware Parenting, I always share my experience, because I know how painful it is that Max won't tell me his emotions now. I really want other mums to have a different experience to me. I want to let them know that they can still enjoy breastfeeding and listen to their baby's feelings before bed. I really want to start working with you again, because he's not crying with me hardly ever. It's hard for me to be with the feelings that it brings up for me. I feel it's possible that this can change, but it's so hard for me at the moment. I'm learning to put down those guilt sticks, though!"

Each of us who practices Aware Parenting is on a spectrum as to the extent to which we aim to practice all the elements of Aware Parenting. Many parents who practice Aware Parenting will sometimes, or always, feed their baby to sleep.

The key in Aware Parenting is understanding that this is probably distracting the baby from their healing-feelings and that those feelings might mean that they wake up more frequently, or sleep less peacefully.

Again, I invite you to remember that **I'm not telling you what to think, and I'm not judging you**. I profoundly care about you listening in to yourself and connecting with what deeply resonates with you. **I'm not willing to tell you what to do, or that you 'should' do anything**. That would be coercion, and it wouldn't help anyone, least of all your baby.

I invite you to listen in to yourself, and to do what most resonates with you.

I invite you to do what you're willing to do, and not to coerce yourself to parent in certain ways because of the information I, or anyone else, gives you. I invite you to remember the triangle of research, which is to listen in to your own intuition and needs as well as observing your baby, and making sense of what you see.

You are powerful and wise, and it is your choice how you respond as a parent.

Self-Compassion Moment

This is one of the places where self-compassion is most needed, as well as having our feelings heard. Feeding to sleep is one of the most common parenting practices, and most mothers will have done this at least some of the time, if not all of the time.

If you're picking up the guilt stick, I invite you to put it down.

If you're feeling frustrated or outraged, I welcome your feelings.

If you're feeling numb and dissociated, I'm sending you lots of compassionate warmth.

If you're feeling sad, I'm sending love to the sadness.

It's so natural for this topic to help us to connect with lots of painful feelings. If you have an empathy buddy or friend with whom you can share feelings, or if you're working with an Aware Parenting instructor, I invite you to share your emotions with them.

'Cluster feeds'*

This is a term used in other paradigms to describe when a baby feeds very frequently or continuously, often in the evening.

From an Aware Parenting perspective, when a baby is feeding very frequently, it can often be a sign that they have healing-feelings to express to us.

From this viewpoint, they are trying to cry with us, and we keep suppressing those emotions through feeding them. Soon after we stop feeding them, they may start being agitated or crying again.

If we assume that they are hungry, we will of course keep feeding them. However, if we trust that babies know how to feel relaxed, we can do the following: After giving them a full feed, as much as they want (and from both breasts if breastfeeding), if they start fussing or crying soon after, when we are confident that they are not hungry, we can hold them in our loving arms, without feeding, jiggling or rocking them, and listen to those healing-feelings instead.

Babies will often seem to want lots of feeding when they are going through a developmental leap.

From an Aware Parenting perspective, that's often because babies have more feelings of frustration to express to us at these times. Similarly, if they're experiencing big events such as moving house, or we've been on a trip, babies will generally have more healing-feelings to express to us.

I'd love to share about my own experience with this. Back in 2002, the term 'cluster feeding' wasn't used – or if it did exist, it wasn't a commonly used phrase and I'd never heard of it. For the first three months of my daughter's life, despite deeply resonating with Aware Parenting, I assumed that she didn't have any healing-feelings to express. I also loved breastfeeding her. I really enjoyed the experience of it, and I also loved it because I had not been breastfed at all as a baby, and I was so happy to be giving her this experience that I hadn't had.

At the time, I made no connection between breastfeeding her most of the evening, every evening, and my assumption that she had no healing-feelings to express.

Really deeply understanding the nuances of Aware Parenting is such a huge process. I just thought that I already 'got' it. If I could go back in a time machine, I would have regular sessions with Aletha Solter, so that I could understand Aware Parenting more deeply, more quickly. It would have made a huge difference to how things unfolded for me and my daughter.

I also didn't make the connection between me feeding her very frequently all evening and my daughter often vomiting up milk. If I had reached out for mainstream support with her vomiting, I imagine she would have received a diagnosis. I had bought about 50 bibs, because of the amount of vomiting she was doing!

The vomiting disappeared once we started listening to her healing-feelings in the evenings at three months. It had indeed been caused by me often feeding her when she had healing-feelings to express.

At that three month mark, I had begun to observe that she did actually have healing-feelings to express that I hadn't been seeing – because I started to observe the effects of accumulated feelings. She was starting to be a bit agitated and to avoid eye contact. I was willing to feed her all evening, and wash 50 bibs, but I began to realise that the feeding all evening was a signal that I wasn't reading her cues accurately.

I realised that feeding her all evening was distracting her from her healing-feelings.

The first time her dad and I listened to her healing-feelings, she was three months old. It was the evening, and I'd already been feeding her lots, and she had only just recently fed. Her dad and I took turns holding her, and she cried for somewhere between 30 and 45 minutes. When she completed the crying cycle, an exquisite sense of peace and presence filled the whole room. She gazed into my eyes. Her dad and I said that she exuded a kind of spiritual presence. It was very clear that, although she had been pretty 'calm' most of the time (no doubt she was dissociated quite often, because of all the feeding I was doing!) that this was a whole different quality of relaxation. She was deeply present.

That is the big difference between true relaxation and freeze. True relaxation is pure presence. Dissociation is very different.

However, even after that experience, I was worried. All my fears from my own infancy bubbled up. I was grateful to have one friend who was practicing Aware Parenting, and I phoned her that evening and told her all my worries, and had a cry with her. From that day onwards, my daughter's dad and I listened to her healing-feelings pretty much every evening before sleep. We would often take turns eating dinner in the same room. I still remember those times, 22 years ago now, as if they were yesterday. They became deeply precious and connecting experiences.

'Dream feeds'*

In some parenting paradigms, a 'dream feed' is where a parent feeds a sleeping or drowsy baby just before going to sleep themselves.

Because Aware Parenting is a form of attachment-style parenting, we aim to respond in an attuned way to a baby's needs, which in general means feeding them when they are hungry. However, Aware Parenting is also about finding ways for everyone to get their needs met. If feeding your baby when they are asleep and not hungry helps you have the sleep that you really need, you might choose to do that.

In general, though, we are aiming to find ways for *both* baby and parent to get their needs met. When focusing on tiredness, closeness, and true relaxation, parents are more likely to get more sleep, and so they may then prioritise listening to their baby's cues, and feeding them when they are hungry.

Reading books

Many parenting paradigms recommend reading to babies before sleep. Like many activities, reading can be done to bring about more presence and connection, or can create dissociation and disconnection. In Aware Parenting, our aim is responding aptly to what they really need. Very young babies are more likely to enjoy our presence and eye contact than us reading them a book. Reading can be a lovely activity as babies grow older, and can bring deep connection and fun. However, if they are trying to cry in arms to release healing-feelings, our most apt and helpful response is to listen, not read to them.

Rocking, swinging, and bouncing to sleep

These are ways that are very commonly used to get babies to feel more calm so they can go to sleep. However, this is generally bypassing healing-feelings which still sit in their bodies, which may cause waking up later on.

These motions tend to create a kind of dissociation which can be quite pleasurable, although not so pleasant if the movement is very vigorous.

Over time, as a baby's feelings accumulate, this might mean rocking, swinging, or bouncing for longer and longer periods or with more intensity, because there are more feelings to be suppressed.

When we frequently use movement to get a baby to go to sleep, they are likely to then internalise this and then move around when they are upset. This can lead to a toddler being hyperactive before bed when they have healing-feelings bubbling.

Jenna shares:

"We were always rocking Heli to sleep. We had one of those baby hammocks, so we either put her in there while we were eating dinner, swinging her all the time, or my husband would hold her and bounce her while sitting on the fit ball. Sometimes we'd just rock her in our arms, or walk up and down the corridor between our bedroom and kitchen. We enjoyed it when she was little, but as she got older, we were needing to rock her for longer and longer to get her to go to sleep, and we were both pretty over it. By the time she was 18 months, we had a hyperactive little girl. She wouldn't sit still, even to eat. We were often following her around to try to get her to do things. She was just always on the move, even when she was eating.

Her dad and I were at our wits' end, because we were also feeling so exhausted, being around her energy all the time. When I came across the control patterns *episode on* The Aware Parenting Podcast, *suddenly everything clicked into place. I realised that all that movement we'd been doing became what she did herself when she needed to express her feelings. We made changes from that night on, and it made a big difference. However, movement is still her default when she's upset. I'm learning to not hit myself with the guilt sticks, but I do wish we had learnt about Aware Parenting earlier. It would have made such a huge difference. We were exhausted with all the rocking and all her hyperactivity, but kept going with it because we thought it was what she needed. We would have loved more peace and stillness!"*

Putting baby in a carseat or stroller

Movement while in the car or pram or stroller to get a baby to go to sleep is a similar form of distraction to rocking, only in this case, it happens away from a parent's body, so a baby might also be needing to dissociate from feelings of loneliness or fear. The movement is bypassing the feelings. However, those feelings still remain in a baby's body, which may mean that they might wake up soon after the movement stops.

Shushing

This is another way to distract a baby from their feelings. As with all of these approaches, we might put ourselves in our child's shoes and imagine how this might be for them, trying to share their feelings with us and we keep on shushing them.

White noise

This is also often used as a way to help babies go to sleep. From an Aware Parenting perspective, you might want to use it to block noise if your home is really noisy. However, what I've experienced – and have heard from many parents – is that if a baby gets to regularly express their healing-feelings to us, they are generally so deeply relaxed that they can sleep even if there's quite a bit of noise around.

Sucking

Sucking is a powerful way to create a mild form of dissociation, which can be pleasant, but which bypasses painful feelings that remain in a baby's body.

This is why breast and bottle feeding, thumb-sucking, and using a dummy can produce a temporary calming effect without true relaxation.

Raja said:

"We actually taught Zen to suck his thumb. My mother-in-law suggested it would be a good way to help him to go to sleep, so we encouraged him to do it. We were so pleased when he learnt to suck his thumb before going to sleep. We thought it was making him more independent. But then he started sucking it more and more often, until it seemed as though he was doing it most of the day. His eyes would look kind of glazed and I started to feel worried about it. I did some searching and found Marion's article on thumb-sucking, and Aware Parenting resonated with me straight away.

I couldn't believe that I hadn't realised what was going on. It's been quite a journey to help him return to being able to express his feelings before bed, but we're seeing a much happier and more present boy now, although he does still suck his thumb sometimes, especially on more stressful days or times when I've got a lot going on. Nowadays it's more like a barometer for me, an invitation to factor in some slowing down days for us all, so we can be more present with him and do more play and listening to feelings sessions."

Self-Reflection Moment

If you're feeling uncomfortable feedings as you read, I so understand. I'm sending you lots of love and compassion. I also want to keep reminding you to connect in with whether these ways of understanding babies and their needs and feelings resonate with you and to remind you that this is information, rather than judgments.

'Comforter' / 'transitional object'*

A blanket or soft toy ('comforter') used to be called a 'transitional object' and was seen as a way for a baby to transfer their attachment from their mother to an object. From an Aware Parenting perspective, they are another way that babies can learn to dissociate from their painful feelings.

Lullabies

Do you ever sing lullabies to your child? Are you wondering whether they suppress healing-feelings? The answer is: it depends! For some babies, singing lullabies can bring about a sense of emotional warmth and connection. For babies who are crying, our singing them a lullaby is likely to suppress their feelings. However, for yet other babies, a lullaby can help them connect with their healing-feelings and facilitate healing-crying. One mother I've mentored shared that singing touching songs sometimes helped her daughter move into crying. Yet, for other children, lullabies might actually help wake them up more.

If you do choose to sing lullabies to your child, I recommend avoiding language that includes suppressing feelings e.g. "Hush now baby, don't you cry".

When I was pregnant with my daughter, her dad and would sing a particular song to her, which we also sang to her after she was born. In the song, the usual words were: "Hush now baby, don't you cry". Instead, we sang, "You can cry as much as you want to with us." Because I'm passionate about the power of language, I changed the words of most songs (and books too!).

If you do choose to sing a lullaby, from an Aware Parenting perspective, we would recommend *not* doing it with the intention of trying to calm a baby down.

Instead, I recommend that you do it with the aim of connecting with your baby, and sharing love and the joy of music with them.

You mght want to wait until your child has cried, raged, played, laughed, or talked enough to be relaxed before sleep. Then, if you want to sing a lullaby, they are already relaxed and can enjoy it from that state.

Waking up

Waking up after they've fallen asleep and we place them down

From an Aware Parenting perspective, if we're holding our tired baby and they fall asleep and we wait for about 10-15 minutes for them to fall into a deeper sleep, and then we place them down somewhere and they wake up, this often tells us that there are still feelings sitting close to the surface that are waking them up.

Generally, the reason why babies wake up so easily when they are placed down somewhere – or moved whilst they are asleep – is because they're not in a deep enough state of relaxation, because of accumulated feelings.

This can also often happen if they have done some crying in arms before sleep but didn't fully complete the crying session with us, either because we stopped them before they were finished (in subtle or not so subtle ways), or because they were too tired to complete the crying cycle.

'Catnapping'*

This is when babies wake up after very short naps. From an Aware Parenting perspective, it's generally because either they are needing closeness, or they have feelings sitting close to the surface that are making it hard for them to stay relaxed enough to continue sleeping.

Waking up after one sleep cycle

This is the same Aware Parenting response as for catnapping, and similarly is often caused either by a need for closeness, or by accumulated unexpressed healing-feelings.

Waking up more and more frequently as the night goes on

This is very common when babies have healing-feelings that they are trying to express and we keep distracting them from those feelings. Those uncomfortable emotions are sitting at the surface and become harder and harder to suppress. They are bubbling up to be heard.

Feeding them straight after they wake up

Babies don't necessarily wake up because they're hungry, especially after waking from a nap (rather than after a night's sleep).

With Aware Parenting, as we observe our baby, we can become more and more competent at reading their cues and responding aptly to them. This includes not necessarily feeding a baby as soon as they've woken up. We can offer our loving presence, and discern, by taking in other information, whether or not they are actually hungry.

For the first several months when my daughter was a baby, whenever she woke up, I would always feed her. I didn't think to observe what she was actually needing and feeling in that moment. However, with my son, I would only feed him when I discerned he was hungry. I worked that out through a lot of detailed observation so that I really understood what he was needing and feeling.

Waking up crying

If a baby wakes up crying, it could be that they are uncomfortable or are needing closeness, it could mean that they are hungry, or it could mean that they have healing-feelings to express to us. Again, the more we understand our baby and their cues, the more we will know which one of these it is.

From an Aware Parenting perspective, a common cause can be because unexpressed painful feelings have woken them up, ready to be expressed. However, it is very important that we work out what they are really needing by observing them closely.

'Sleep regressions'*

From an Aware Parenting perspective, if a baby starts waking up more often, it may be because they have more accumulated feelings (although of course I invite you to always check whether there could be other things affecting their ability to be relaxed, such as teething, illness, diet, temperature, etc.). If a baby isn't getting to express their healing-feelings, or a percentage of those feelings, more emotions accumulate as time goes on.

In addition, when babies are going through new developmental stages, it's also very common for them to frequently feel frustrated. Therefore, they have more emotions to express to us so they can be relaxed enough to go to sleep and stay asleep until they've either had enough sleep or are actually hungry.

'Sleep regressions' = more accumulated feelings. This can coincide with developmental leaps that other paradigms sometimes call 'wonder weeks'. In Aware Parenting, we don't use the term 'wonder weeks', for the same reasons.

Sleeping through the night

You'll notice in this book that I won't talk about ages of sleeping through the night, nor about how much sleep babies need at each age.

Instead, I invite you to observe your baby closely, so you really understand their unique needs and timings in relation to sleep.

The more we respond to our baby's tiredness cues, meet their needs for closeness, and listen to their healing-feelings in our loving arms, the easier it will be for them to have enough restful and restorative sleep.

If they aren't getting enough restful sleep, it's often an invitation for us to receive more support and more information so we can listen to more of their uncomfortable emotions and support them to complete the crying cycle when they're in it.

I believe that each baby is unique and that you will receive the most helpful information about your baby and their needs and feelings from observing them – not by trying to fit into a timeline suggested by someone else.

CHAPTER SUMMARY

Many of the concepts that exist in other parenting paradigms *are not* a part of Aware Parenting, such as: wake or sleep windows, overtired, sleep associations, contact naps, wearing a baby down to sleep, self-settling, self-soothing, settling, resettling, cluster feeds, dream feeds, transitional objects/comforters, catnapping, and sleep regressions.

Instead, Aware Parenting invites us to return to the three ingredients for restful sleep to see what a baby is needing in the moment: *to feel tired*, *to feel connected,* and *to feel relaxed.*

I'm here to support you to really listen in to yourself so that you know what resonates with you and what doesn't.

14. Observing, trusting, and cooperating with babies' relaxation processes

The more that you understand the theory of Aware Parenting and sleep, the more you will know what to look for in your baby, and the more you'll understand what they are communicating to you.

Observing our babies in this way can help us feel more deeply connected with them. I've heard this from so many parents over the years.

We need to be present with our baby to be able to observe them and be attuned to them. Babies really feel our deep presence.

Each baby is unique.

If we look at individual differences in terms of the three ingredients required for restful sleep, each baby will have a unique experience in terms of each of these.

Babies differ physiologically. For example, Highly Sensitive Babies[42] might get tired more quickly and easily after a certain amount of stimulation. They're also likely to need to cry for longer and/or more intensely to release the stress from those experiences than other babies might need to.

With Aware Parenting, we can observe each individual baby to understand when they are tired, how safe they feel, and when they have healing-feelings to express. Rather than thinking about complex sleep windows, we can observe when they are tired, and then offer them our loving presence so that they feel connected and safe, and free to express any healing-feelings that are ready to be expressed.

---

42 Who are more affected by what they experience, as described by Elaine Aron.

Each baby is also unique in terms of the amount of stress and trauma they experience, such as in the following situations:

- *in utero* (such as if their mother was stressed or depressed);
- *during birth* (e.g. Caesarean, ventouse, forceps, very long, or very short births);
- *after birth* (such as being separated or having medical procedures).

In the early weeks and months, babies are highly susceptible to overstimulation and overwhelm. They will also experience more stress if their parents are stressed, and if there are lots of loud noises and stimulating environments.

The more stress a baby has experienced, the more often they will have gone into fight, flight, or freeze (hyperarousal or dissociation). This means they will hold increased levels of stress in their body, and they will need to cry in arms more loudly and for longer to release that tension.

This is why babies who have experienced birth trauma may take longer to go to sleep and might wake up more often – because they have more accumulated painful feelings.

The beauty is that with Aware Parenting, we can support each unique baby, with their individual physiology and specific experiences, using their innate process to heal from any pre or perinatal stress or trauma.

With Aware Parenting, each parent becomes their own parenting authority. Once we understand the principles and practices, we know what to look for and what it means, so we can respond to each individual baby as the unique being that they are.

Observing babies – what can we look for?

How can we tell if a baby is tired and connected but is not feeling relaxed enough to sleep? We can discern that this is likely to be the case if:

- we have *ensured* that our baby's *needs are met*; and
- they have clearly shown *tiredness cues*; and
- we are *holding* them in our arms *without rocking or jiggling*; and
- we are simply *being still* and *offering them our loving presence*; and
- they *aren't falling asleep*; and
- **they are starting to cry.**

This tells us that they are not yet feeling relaxed enough to sleep and are using their natural relaxation process to expel tension.

From a baby: *My eyelids are starting to feel heavy, Mummy, and I yawn. I look up at you, and I see you smile at me. I smile back. I love being in your arms, Mummy. I feel so cosy. I yawn again, and I see you looking at me. You're here. You understand. I know that you're here to help me sleep. I love going off to sleep when I'm tired, Mummy. But first, the storm is coming. Small waves at first. I wriggle and move. I stretch, and I cry. I can feel you with me. I can feel the love in your arms. The waves get bigger now, and the clouds come overhead. My crying is bigger and louder. I open my mouth wide. I kick and kick, and my feet meet your hands. I feel so powerful when I do that, when all this sound and power comes through me and out of me. My arms wave around too.*

The wave quietens a bit. I look up at you again. I see you saying words to me. They float to me like soft pink waves. I feel them in my heart. I cry again. A bigger cry this time, more movement. I kick and push, and you meet me again. A big wail comes out of me. Waaaahhhh!

Ahhh, it's gone. I feel softer and meltier now, as if I'm sinking right in to your body. So soft and lovely. I could go to sleep now, but there's still more here. I look up at you again, and you gaze into my eyes. You're still here. I want to let out more. I cry again. The waves are really big this time. I'm loud, I'm big, I'm strong. Waaaaaaaaaaaaaaaahhhh! There are so many waves flowing through my body. I cry and I cry. Oh that was so satisfying, Mummy. The sound tapers off. I'm melting into you even more, as if we were one again. I sigh. I could go to sleep now.

But what's this? You change position, and you talk with me again. There's a place in me I couldn't feel until now. Oh I want to tell you this bit, Mummy! I cry again. I kick, I wail, my arms flail. This bit is important too. Thank you for reminding me of it!

Oh, now it's all gone! I look in your eyes again and now I can see all the love. We are a raindrop on a rose together. There's such stillness in my body and all around us. There are love beams of light in between our eyes. My body is melting so much and I love it. My eyes flutter closed. I open them once more, and a little smile comes. They close again. Nighty night, Mummy.

CHAPTER SUMMARY

Observing our babies in this way can help us feel even more deeply connected with them. We need to be present with our baby to be able to observe them and be attuned to them. Babies really feel our deep presence.

Each baby is unique, and babies differ physiologically. For example, Highly Sensitive Babies might get tired more easily and quickly after a certain amount of stimulation. They're also likely to need to cry for longer or more intensely to release the stress from those experiences than other babies might need to.

Each baby is also unique in terms of the amount of stress and trauma they experience. In the early weeks and months, babies are highly susceptible to overstimulation and overwhelm.

The more stress a baby has experienced, the more stress and tension they will have in their body, and they will need to cry in arms more loudly and for longer in order to to release that tension. This is why babies who have experienced birth trauma may take longer to go to sleep and wake up more often – because they have more accumulated painful feelings.

With Aware Parenting, we can support each unique baby, with their individual physiology and specific experiences, using their innate process to heal from any pre or perinatal stress or trauma.

I invite you to be your own
parenting authority.

15. The actual process of crying in arms before sleep

Self-Reflection Moment

If you've just read the last chapter, I wonder if you felt any painful feelings when you received the invitation to listen to your baby's crying when they are tired? Perhaps you felt scared or stressed when you imagined listening to your baby crying in arms? Maybe you felt uncertain or unsure? Or perhaps you resonate with the information, but feel curious how it would be when you imagine listening to your baby crying in your arms without jiggling them or doing other things to stop the crying. I welcome all of your feelings.

This seemingly simple action is actually a huge thing to do. Most of us haven't ever experienced crying in arms ourselves, and probably have never seen anyone else practice it.

If what you've read so far resonates with you, I invite you to experiment. You are the one who is there, holding, listening in to, and observing your baby.

With the crying in arms approach, we are offering our baby our loving presence and stillness. This can be very unfamiliar, since most of us are used to rocking or jiggling a crying baby or moving them in other ways, such as in a hammock or pram. Being still and present while holding them is a very different experience.

We can offer this calm space in our arms when we are confident that they don't have any unmet needs.

For example, they've been recently fed, have a fresh nappy (or we've offered them a wee or poo if we're doing Elimination Communication), and we're holding them.[43]

There are so many different ways of supporting crying in arms. You might:

- Hold them *similar to a feeding position.*
- *Lie next to them,* with your arm wrapped around them.
- *Sit with your feet up on a stool or chair,* with your baby lying on their back along your legs, with their head at your knees.[44] You could put a pillow or your hand under their head, or a pillow underneath their whole body if their torso is longer than your thighs.

You might start off by holding one of your baby's hands gently with your hand. However, it's important that babies have the opportunity to move vigorously when they are crying in arms, because this is how they release the energy accumulated for the fight or flight response.

You might offer them loving words, such as, "*I'm here and I'm listening, sweetheart,*" and you might keep offering eye contact and being present with them.

If you've already observed their tired signs and you're offering them closeness, I invite you to trust that if they can feel your loving presence and they have healing-feelings to tell you, they will do so.

If they're not already crying, they might start off with what is often called 'fussing'. If you simply stay present, offering your warmth and loving presence, their crying will generally become louder and more intense. They are likely to move their arms and legs vigorously and may arch their back. The movements of their arms and legs are releasing the tension from the fight or flight response. The sound they make is part of that release too, since the sound would have been an important part of the fight or flight response, to call out for help.

---

43 Once a baby is mobile, they do not need to be held to experience emotional safety to cry, as long as we are close and can offer to hold them if they want that.

44 See the diagram at the end of the book.

271

Back arching may indicate that they are revisiting their birth and are healing from that experience – through making the movements and expressing the feelings they felt while being born.

If they were born vaginally, they probably needed to do a lot to move through the birth canal. They might arch their back and make other movements while crying in arms. They might twist or spiral, as they did during the birthing process. These movements are how they complete the healing processes. You might even notice them getting into positions that you know they were in whilst in utero or during birth.

Vigorous kicking is a typical movement while crying, especially if there was a long birthing process.

The baby might be revisiting the birth experience, trying to push their way out of the womb. The kicking helps to release tension from their legs.

Some babies at some times might only have a few minutes of crying to express, and the crying may then naturally taper off and finish. Other babies at other times might have big, long, and loud crying sessions, particularly if they have experienced more stress or trauma.

This can also happen if you started Aware Parenting later and they are catching up on expressing pent-up painful feelings that have accumulated from the times they didn't get to let the emotions out.

Once they've finished expressing a full chunk of feelings, and have completed the crying cycle, they are likely to fall asleep.

About 10 to 15 minutes after they've fallen asleep, if you want to place them down somewhere, you are likely to find that you can do that without them waking up. However, if they do wake up, they are probably telling you that they didn't finish expressing that chunk of feelings.

Natalie wrote to our free Aware Parenting Facebook group asking for help. She said:

"I recently came across Aware Parenting as I'm looking for something to help with sleep. I've been having constant wake-ups with my daughter for 15 months now, since birth. I'm so exhausted and depleted and feel

like I'm losing my mind. I've listened to some Aware Parenting podcast episodes about sleep but can't get any clarity about what listening to feelings looks like at night. I do it with my four year old son in the day but how do I do it with a 15 month old who constantly just wants to nurse and will scream and cry if she doesn't? Do I just let her cry while sitting there? I'm not sure what the process looks like but I'm ready to try it because I can't take much more of this sleep deprivation."

A few days later, after receiving responses from the Team about what she could do, she wrote again, sharing about the effects of listening to her daughter's healing-feelings:

"Just wanted to share some amazing news. My daughter woke up about 30 minutes after I put her down to sleep at night and instead of nursing her I told her 'I'm here and I'm listening' and she just started crying and cried for about 10 minutes. I held the space for her and she then rested her head on me and fell asleep immediately. It's so crazy to think this is what she needed all along, my little angel. I'm hoping this release makes a difference in her sleep tonight, and if not, I'm confident to listen some more."

From a baby: *You used to stop me from crying, but now you listen to my feelings. I can sense your feelings and I know that sometimes you are all tense when I am crying with you, Daddy. I feel a bit unsure when I sense that in you. I know that you really want me to go to sleep. When I'm crying with you and I get more sleepy, you go all quiet and still. But I haven't finished yet, Daddy. I've only told you the first half of the story. It was such a busy day today, and I felt so overwhelmed. There was the ride in the car, and then we went to that place with all the new things. I don't know what it was or what was going on. I've told you that bit, but there's so much more to share. But when you go all still and quiet and you want me to sleep, it's hard for me to tell you more. I start to drift off, but I do really want to tell you about all the things that happened today.*

I will have a little rest....... what's this? I wake up. I can see you walking away. I cry out. Come back! I hadn't finished! I want to tell you more!

You come back. I'm so glad! You pick me up. Are you willing to listen this time, or do you want me to just go to sleep? You close your eyes for a moment and sigh. You open them again, and I see you. You look me in the eyes and I see you. You say some words to me, and you nod. You DO want me to tell you all about it! Oh yay, Daddy! So, I will tell you the rest of the story with my tears. I open my mouth and shout it out. I cry. I wail. My legs kick and my arms move all around. That was such a big day, Daddy. I felt so much. It was so big. It was so much. I cry some more and then a bit more, and I feel you with me. You really care. I tell you everything. Ahh, that was the whole story. That was my day. I feel so relieved. I open my eyes for another moment, and you smile at me. You see me. You hear me. I can sleep now. I feel sleep come to me. Lovely, lovely, sleep.

Rebecca shares about the huge difference that Aware Parenting made for her daughter Amy's behaviour and sleep, and the big insights she also had about her own childhood. She says:

Amy is now five months old. We free birthed at home with just myself, my partner, and our doula present. We were very specific about not having any medical interventions, and after a nine-hour excruciating but simple labour, she was born into our arms. Amy is absolutely perfect and we called her the angel baby because she was so easy and sweet. The one medical complication that we did encounter was that she had jaundice on day five of her life and we were told to go to A&E. Being petrified first-time parents, we rushed there, and Amy was immediately put into an incubator with a tube down her nose and a needle in the back of her hand. Having worked so hard to birth her outside of the medical system, I was devastated (being anaemic after her birth, exhausted, and very emotional played a part in this!). Nevertheless, things got better after that. I have been exclusively breastfeeding. Amy and I co-sleep on a huge mattress on the floor, and she never goes into a pram – always in a sling on our bodies. I didn't know about attachment parenting in the beginning – I did what felt 'right' to me – but it seems I was pretty by-the-book.

She was smiling and starting to laugh, and we prided ourselves on her never crying. My parents told me over and over again that babies only cry for three reasons: hungry, dirty nappy, or wind. If she ever got fussy, we would check those things, and then bounce her, sing to her, or give her boobie – before she got to the point of crying. We had a range of techniques. At some point she was always fussy when we sat down with her – but we assumed that she was just inquisitive and wanted to be on the move all of the time. So that's what we did! We never sat down.

At around three months she started doing something so strange during the night while half asleep – she had full blown temper tantrums. She was kicking her legs and shouting out, her face was screwed up in anger. I couldn't reconcile this ball of fury with my sweet daytime baby! Of course, I comforted her and gave her boobie to get her out of it and she soon calmed down. But still, it didn't feel right to me, I sensed that there must be a root to this behaviour. This probably happened a dozen times.

Between months three to four she started to fuss regularly during the night. She sleeps a long time – from 6pm-6am – but she fusses and wants the boobie throughout the night. It got to the point where she was crying out, looking for boobie nine times during the night.

In all honesty I would have kept doing that if it made her happy! I have plenty of stamina and can do whatever is necessary.

However, two things were confusing me: a) all research said that babies' stomachs should be getting bigger and they should need to feed less often, not more! and b) she wasn't happy.

During the day I noticed the following in her. She was:

- *making **less eye contact**;*
- *more and **more fussy**;*
- ***fighting me** when I tried to put clothes on her;*
- *(apparently) **refusing to be held** to our chest (she would cry) – she would only stop crying if she was held facing outwards (I now see that she wasn't refusing to be held, but was trying to express her feelings to me);*
- *increasingly **fighting me when trying to put her to sleep** – even though she was clearly exhausted she would physically fight me for 45 minutes or so before bed (I now see that in a different light with Aware Parenting);*
- *having a very **tense body**, especially while breastfeeding.*

I was increasingly afraid to go out with her because I didn't know when she would start fussing, and that I'd need to be able to find a place to breastfeed to placate her. One morning I had probably gotten two hours of sleep and I tried to feed her and dress her to go to a playgroup (which I was already afraid of in anticipation). She made no eye contact with me, she was tense and agitated while feeding, and then lashed out so I couldn't dress her.

I broke down to my partner and told him that I couldn't do it anymore, and that it made no sense – how could I do everything 'right', cater to her every need, and her still be fussy, angry and frustrated?! My confidence was in pieces, and I'm a very sensitive person so it really hurt me that I wasn't getting this 'right' for my baby.

Fortuitously the universe had my back – I had talked to my doula about Elimination Communication (EC), and she had an ex-client, Maru Rojas, who was an EC instructor. We had a call booked with Maru the next day. I was bedraggled and exhausted and trying to keep Amy happy while my partner did most of the talking. In passing I asked Maru about the sleep issues I was having with feeding, and she told me, "Ah that's a totally different call – that's suppressed feelings coming up – I will send you a podcast to listen to". As it happens, she is an Aware Parenting instructor. We listened to your podcast and were hooked from the first minute. I signed up to your course that afternoon and we did our first crying in arms that night.

That first cry probably lasted around an hour until she fell asleep. I also cried. To me it felt like being crucified; it was incredibly painful and emotional. My mind was filled with doubts even though the theory made perfect sense. That night, Amy woke up to feed four times (instead of nine). I couldn't believe it. In the morning she made eye contact with us and was happy and smiley. She sat on our laps for around 30 minutes while we ate breakfast – unheard of! I had usually needed to eat while standing and bouncing around. She now allows us to hold her to our chest (i.e. she doesn't cry when we do that), she doesn't fuss when we dress her, and she's relaxed and calm while feeding.

Her cries are almost always before naps/nighttime sleeps, and for a few weeks they were long and painful cries. Now they rarely last longer than 15 minutes. Often she falls asleep after having a big cry but sometimes she stops, is totally calm, and just drifts off. Sometimes she doesn't cry at all and she just sits in my arms, getting increasingly sleepy until she nods off. This is entirely different to the 45-minute routine we had gotten into when I was trying to get her to sleep before Aware Parenting!

Doing this work with Amy has also had a very profound effect on me. I saw that I had been breastfeeding Amy to placate her because I was afraid of her crying – and in doing so had been repetitively suppressing her emotions. It was a painful realisation. I also started to connect the dots from what my parents had mentioned about their parenting style when I was a baby, and from what I can remember of them in childhood. I realise now that their 'babies only cry for three reasons' mentality led them to assume I was always hungry – and I know that they were feeding me baby rice at one month old. I suddenly saw very clearly the 'placating through feeding' cycle. I know that as a toddler, when I got too old to feed every time I was upset and was moved to a three meal per day model, I started to have huge tantrums. My parents have always told me the narrative that I was a 'naughty' child. So, they smacked me. Now I look back and see a little girl who just wanted to express herself and was given a control *pattern only to have it taken away and be met with violence instead. I've been ever so sad about that – and in between doing your course, making my adjustments to parenting Amy, and getting to grips with her crying in arms, I've had a cry here and there with my partner.*

Crucially, I can see many ways that the parenting paradigm I grew up in has had a tangible effect on me. One example is in my eating habits. When the feeding control *pattern was taken away from me (and we were too poor to ever have snacks at home), my grandmother's house had a sweetie cupboard that I was allowed to take from at any time. She filled it with chocolates and sweets just for me. It was a low cupboard – at child height, and I didn't even have to ask. So, when I was there I would revert to my original* control *pattern of eating – and I would eat and eat until I was ill, especially in the knowledge that at home we had none.*

This pattern of stuffing myself with sweets has been a consistent theme in my life. As an athlete who works in the fitness industry, it's embarrassing and has always been very shameful for me – but the shame has never been enough to stop me from overeating. I've had gut heath issues that have plagued me as an adult because of it. I could never understand why – as a person who is very disciplined in most areas of life (I am vegetarian, don't drink alcohol, and have never smoked or taken drugs) could be so inept when it came to food.

Doing your course put everything into perspective and I could see the connections so clearly. It's been really sad for me. I also became very fearful that I'd already repeated the cycle and contributed to Amy having some eating disorder in later life!! But I've worked through much of my fears as well as my sadness for myself as a child, and the positive changes we have seen in Amy have given me a confidence that didn't exist before. It's given me a blueprint for how I want to parent – where I was almost afraid to be with her before, I'm happy and confident in any situation with her because I know what's going on and what she needs. I feel so much more capable as a mother, as well as very connected to her. I think that feeling confident and capable as a first-time mother, at five months postpartum, and with a very happy baby to show for it – is some kind of miracle! It has changed the trajectory of both our lives – as well as breaking the maternal generational patterns in my family. Again, I want to thank you from the bottom of my heart."

Self-Reflection Moment

How do you feel when you read this? I'm sending love to all of your feelings. I wonder if you resonate with any of Rebecca's story, such as doing all the things recommended to support your baby, but seeing them increasingly unhappy and agitated, and waking up more and more frequently at night as time goes on. Or perhaps you've been having aha moments about your own control patterns and how your healing-feelings were responded to as a child. If so, my heart goes out to you. I invite you to reach out for some loving listening if you need that.

Just as Rebecca shared, it's really common for Aware Parenting to open all kinds of realisations for us about how we learnt to respond to our feelings in our family of origin. It often opens channels for feeling and expressing our unexpressed painful feelings. It's part of the Aware Parenting journey that so many of our own unexpressed painful emotions will show up as part of this. That's why having regular listening support from an empathy buddy or Aware Parenting instructor is so vital!

We may start off on the path of Aware Parenting because we're wanting more sleep, and then discover that we've been invited on a huge journey of healing and transformation!

CHAPTER SUMMARY

With the crying in arms approach, we are offering our baby our loving presence and stillness. This can be very unfamiliar, since most of us are used to rocking or jiggling a crying baby or moving them in other ways. We can offer this calm space in our arms when we are confident that they don't have any unmet needs.

You might offer them loving words, such as, "*I'm here and I'm listening, sweetheart,*" and you might keep offering them eye contact and simply be present with them.

If they're not already crying, they might start off with 'fussing', and if you simply stay present, offering your warmth and loving presence, their crying will generally become louder and more intense. They are likely to move their arms and legs vigorously and may arch their back. The movements of their arms and legs are releasing the tension from the fight or flight response, and the sound they make is part of that. Back arching may indicate that they are revisiting their birth and are healing from that experience.

Some babies at some times might only have a few minutes of crying to express and the crying may then naturally taper off and finish. Other babies at other times might have big, long, and loud crying sessions, particularly if they have experienced more stress or trauma. This is more likely if you started Aware Parenting later and they are catching up on expressing pent-up painful feelings that have accumulated from the times they didn't get to let the emotions out.

Once they've finished expressing a full chunk of feelings, and have completed the crying cycle, they are likely to fall asleep. About 10 to 15 minutes after they've fallen asleep, if you want to place them down somewhere, you are likely to find that you can do that without them waking up. However, if they do wake up, they might be telling you that they didn't finish expressing that chunk of feelings.

I'm sending you so much love and I invite you to keep on listening in to yourself and your baby, and to go at your own pace with all of this.

16. Releasing stress before sleep at different ages

The practice of Aware Parenting changes as babies move through different stages and ages.

Newborn to three months

If you're breastfeeding, I invite you to focus on building and maintaining your milk supply as the top priority.

However, if you:

- are already a confident breastfeeder;
- are familiar with Aware Parenting;
- have an older child with whom you practiced Aware Parenting; or
- see that your baby clearly has some feelings to express from their birth (particularly if it's affecting their feeding or sleep) –

then you might want to start listening to *healing-feelings* right from the beginning.

You could hold your baby as much as possible and trust that when they are tired, they will cry in your arms and will then fall asleep. Or you could offer them a particular opportunity to cry in your arms soon after feeding them, so you're confident that they're not hungry.

After about three weeks of age, if you offer both breasts at each feed and support your baby to feed for as long as they want, they will fill their stomach. This means you will then be less likely to feed them when they need to cry, and it will help them sleep for longer stretches at night.

But as always, please observe your baby and what they are communicating to you, and trust yourself and your observations. Each baby is unique.

Katie shares about her experience of practicing Aware Parenting with her second child right from the beginning:

"We've been listening to our newborn's feelings since the moment after he was born. He's just over a week old now and his sleep is so much longer and more restful than it was for my older son with whom we only practised Classical Attachment Parenting. *My older son was on the boob 'cluster feeding' constantly and waking frequently. My newborn will sleep restfully for 2-3 hours at a time during the day (and much longer at night although I don't check the time), he regularly and comfortably goes three-and-a-half hours between feeds, and he has often has hour-long periods of calm alertness when he is awake.*

We listened to many hours of feelings on his first couple of days that I felt intuitively were him healing from his birth (a very calm home-birth). I was surprised to see how many feelings he had about his birth and it was such a gift to support him and listen to his experience of that!

We did a Lotus birth with him and on his fourth day we listened to over four hours of feelings and he dramatically kicked off his cord during a release in the late afternoon. I sensed that this day he was truly landing and choosing to let go of his placenta. Since then he has generally had about an hour or two of feelings over the span of the day. We prefer to try to listen as feelings arise during the day rather than one big session in the evening.

We don't tiptoe around when either the baby or my toddler are sleeping. The baby crying does not wake my toddler in the evenings, even though the baby can get quite loud at times! And my toddler's rambunctious play during the day doesn't wake the baby. Aware Parenting makes newborn life so much easier, because we understand him so much more and can read his cues so much more clearly."

At this age range, if you regularly offer your baby an opportunity to express their healing-feelings, they may cry in frequent bursts with pauses in between throughout the day. They're likely to have some healing-feelings to express before every sleep, if we give them the opportunity to express those emotions.

Some parents will choose to listen to healing-feelings throughout the day, such as before every nap, or simply when the feelings arise. However, others choose to listen to their baby's healing-feelings just once or twice a day, perhaps in the evening, in which case those will be longer chunks of crying in arms.

Cross-cultural research has found that babies around the world tend to have a peak in crying at around 6-8 weeks. From an Aware Parenting perspective, we might hypothesise that they are crying to heal from birth stress or trauma as well as daily overstimulation and developmental frustration, because these are common experiences for babies, wherever they live.

Three to nine months

Now, babies may need to cry less frequently than they did when they were younger (if they were supported to express their healing-feelings in the first three months) but more intensely and for longer periods each time. However, this really depends on the frequency of when we offer them our loving presence to cry in our arms and on how many accumulated feelings they already have.

It's still typical for babies to need to cry in our loving arms before most naps and sleeps (as part of their innate relaxation-through-release process) – if they are not prevented from doing so.

Depending on the amount of stimulation and stress in the day, and how many feelings have already accumulated, you might find that sometimes they only cry for a few minutes. At other times (and for some babies in particular), they might have much longer crying sessions, which could be for longer than an hour. Some babies may have several hours of crying to express every day in the first weeks and months.

In this age rage, there is generally more of a sense of a beginning, middle, and end to a crying session. You're likely to see clearly when they've completed a crying cycle and have released a whole chunk of feelings. You'll probably be able to clearly observe that they feel much more relaxed at the end of a cry than they did at the beginning. Their muscles will be more relaxed and they are likely to be willing to make more eye contact afterwards, or to fall straight off to sleep.

During the cry, the crying may reach a crescendo of intensity, and then become quieter, and you might think that this means that they have finished the cry. You might find yourself not moving and being really quiet, because you're wanting them to drift off to sleep.

However, this lull in crying can sometimes happen when they are just having a pause and actually have more healing-feelings to express. In which case, if we don't realise this and encourage them to go off to sleep and quietly place them down somewhere, they are likely to wake up again, ready to express more healing-feelings to us.

The more experience we have, the more we will understand when the crying is just tapering off for a pause and there are some more healing-feelings to come. In that case, we might change the position we're holding them in, offering some loving words and our eye contact, *"I'm still here and listening. Do you have more feelings to share with me?"* You might find that the crying intensifies again, because they feel your love and presence and the emotional safety that creates. When they've finished crying in your arms, they might then drift off to sleep, or they might gaze into your eyes. You might even be surprised to see that sometimes they don't seem to be tired after all. You could simply keep holding them and connecting with them, to see what happens next and what they indicate to you that they need.

Nine months onwards (depending on when they become mobile)

When babies begin to crawl, they no longer always need to be held in arms while crying, so our response changes from the crying in arms approach to what I call '*the crying dance*' (please note that this is not an official Aware Parenting term).

They still need closeness with us for the crying to be healing, but because they can choose to come and be in our arms if they need to, they don't necessarily need to be in our arms to feel enough connection for the crying to be healing and relaxing.

Because they can now move towards us or away from us, they become an active participant in finding the level of connection they need for the *balance of attention*[45], so that the crying is indeed healing for them.

The shift between crying in arms to *the crying dance* requires a significant change in our practice of Aware Parenting. Parents often find this phase challenging, particularly in knowing how to respect a toddler's needs for agency and autonomy, while also supporting them to express their healing-feelings. Extra support and guidance from an Aware Parenting instructor can be really helpful at this time, especially if you're feeling unsure.

At this age range, a baby might move around a lot while they are crying to heal. They might move away from us to feel the *balance of attention*. Or, they might need our loving presence to while they are moving around, through us crawling along next to them, or walking beside them. Each baby is unique and their experiences (and ours) will be different in terms of exactly how much closeness they need for the healing crying to happen. That may also change between each crying session.

---

45 A state in which a child feels physically and emotionally safe while revisiting past stress or trauma. *The balance of attention* is necessary for both emotional release and healing to occur (through crying, play, laughter, etc.).

In general, as babies move towards the end of their first year, they will tend to need to cry less to release stress. This is in part because they experience less overwhelm and overstimulation, since they've become accustomed to many daily experiences. Those who have expressed a large percentage of their healing-feelings up until this point will also have less to catch up on. However, each baby is unique in terms of their past and present experiences, sensitivity levels, and amount of accumulated feelings, so some may need to cry less a long time before this, and some will need to continue to cry every day for a long while more.

Some babies may no longer need to cry before every nap and sleep, and as they get even older, they will increasingly not need to cry every day, unless there is a new source of stress or trauma in their life. Again, each baby is unique in this respect.

However, if there are healing-feelings sitting in their bodies, those are often likely to bubble up at the end of the day. This is still their innate wisdom to release stress, so they can sleep more restfully.

The later in their life that you started listening to their healing-feelings, the more accumulated feelings they will have to express, and this catching up process can often take some time, i.e. months or even years.

With our daughter, we started to listen to her healing-feelings when she was three months old. We listened every night before she went to sleep. At the time, I thought we were listening to close to 100% of her feelings, but by the time she was 18 months old, I realised that it was much more likely to be about 50%. So, I believe that she was catching up on expressing healing-feelings for the next year and a half. As a result, she would generally cry before going to sleep every night until she was three years old. If we'd listened to closer to 100% from the start, that would have probably looked very different. I'm sharing this story to remind you that whatever we do at earlier ages, we will have the opportunity to catch up on listening to feelings before sleep.

As always, observing your baby and their behaviour will clearly tell you whether they have a build-up of feelings that they're wanting to express to you.

As babies get older, *attachment play*[46] tends to become a more significant part of their relaxation process.

You can trust them and follow their lead with this.

Peek-a-boo type games, blowing raspberries (with no tickling) and chasing games where they chase you can all bring laughter, and are all part of this additional form of the relaxation-through-release process.

From a toddler: *I'm so tired, Daddy, I can feel it in my bones. My edges are all fuzzy and crawling is much harder. The waves are rising inside me, and I can see a storm in the distance. I'm crawling around the bedroom – there are so many interesting things to look at! You join in and crawl along beside me and I feel my world tilt, and the storm is here.*

Tears come, and crying comes, and I move from the side of the storm to the centre. I'm crying and crying, and you're here with me, Daddy. You used to hold me when I cried as a baby, but now I can move, everything is different, and we are dancing around together, me the storm and you the calm land. My storm meets you and I feel your welcome. The storm gets louder. I cry and rage, and lean against you. I feel your land, as I move around. My legs need to push against you, so my storm moves me in place, and as my legs push, the storm gets really, really loud. It's all coming out! Stormy me rolls and pushes and rains and cries, and you are here, my steady land.

Ahh, the storm is quietening again. I wonder if it's finishing? I look at you, wondering. You smile, and I see the love in your eyes. That love is a lightning spark, reigniting the storm, and I cry so loudly again. All the water in the world is leaving me. Tension runs out of me like the rain we saw running out of the drainpipe the other day. I push with my legs, and

---

46 *Attachment play* is another core element of Aware Parenting. There are nine types of *attachment play*, which we will explore later in the book.

more loud noises come out of me. My feet and your hands stay together and I love that.

Ahh, what's this? The storm is easing now. The rain lessens, the thunder quietens. Will there be another one? I look at you, and you smile, and nod. I see into the deepest places in me and I am seen. No, this storm really is finishing. I can feel the lightness of light and I feel soft and heavy. I snuggle in with you, and some sighs come out of me. You hold me in your big warm arms and I am held by the whole world. I am the breeze in the trees. I am as soft as our puppy. I'm falling asleep with you, Daddy. I love you.

Toddlers

Toddlers and sleep in general

As babies become toddlers, *attachment play* increasingly joins crying as a way to release tension and become relaxed before sleep. However, it doesn't replace crying, and often precedes crying. The *attachment play* creates connection and emotional safety and loosens up feelings that may then often come out through crying and raging.

If your toddler is inviting play before naps or bedtimes, I invite you to follow their lead.

You can also bring in specific forms of *attachment play* to maximise the effects of both connection and release. For example, if they are wanting to play chasing games, you could turn it into a *power-reversal game*, where they chase you and you pretend to be less powerful, and slower and less competent than them. You might keep on pretending to be surprised that they are repeatedly catching you! Or you might play *separation games*, where you offer a kind of peek-a-boo with, *"Where is Hilda? She was here a minute ago!"* And then being surprised when she jumps in front of you!

The more that you can join in wholeheartedly, effusively and lovingly, and the more she laughs (as long as there is no tickling, which can be overstimulating and overwhelming), the more tension she is letting go of through the laughter. This way, she is releasing light fears and other feelings.

It can be common for toddlers to still need to cry before sleep, especially at the end of a busy day, and often that might include the *crying dance* as described above. They need to experience *the balance of attention* between feeling physical and emotional safety in the present, whilst revisiting painful experiences from the past, and expressing the feelings they didn't get to express back then. That often requires us to be what I call an *'emotional shepherd dog'*, staying close with them to communicate to them that they are safe, that we are listening, and that we know that they do have feelings sitting in their bodies to be expressed.

Again, I invite you to closely observe your toddler and follow their lead. They might invite *attachment play* or begin crying during the evening, and it can be easy for us as parents to inadvertently distract them from their play or crying.

If they start initiating play, I invite you to join in. If they start crying in response to something that's happening, I invite you to stay with them and listen to those feelings.

Devon, an Aware Parenting instructor in Australia, shares about how *attachment play* really helped in her sleep journey with her son:

"My kiddo was 14 months when I came to Aware Parenting. I came specifically because I was struggling with his night feeding and frequent waking. The sleep deprivation was tremendous and had accumulated for me to breaking point. Re. breastfeeding, I listened and held the Loving Limit *consistently – it was a challenging couple of nights and I needed a huge amount of support to be able to stay present to him in terms of intellectually understanding the process as well as emotionally debriefing before and after. After that piece he would stir and go straight back to sleep, but the interruption was enough and I would struggle to get back to sleep.*

The key to reducing the 'little wakes' for me was listening during the day and loads and loads of attachment play *before bed. I had a kiddo who loved contingency games, power reversal games, separation games, and body contact games. For an hour before bed (after bath, feed, PJs) we'd play things like him turning on/off the little lamp beside the bed and me pretending to be frightened, or me pretending the book bit me, or me giving him full body massages with silly rhymes and playing peek-a-boo behind pillows or under the blanket). It's worth noting that he and I had very little separation by day – by that I mean an hour or two each week. So even with little disruption and stress, he still needed a lot of undivided attention, play, and listening to feelings right before bed so he could sleep through.*

Loving Limits

Loving Limits, *which are a core practice in Aware Parenting, can become increasingly relevant before sleep for toddlers. We may offer a* **Loving Limit** *if we see that our child has accumulated feelings, and needs our help to let those healing-feelings out.*

A *Loving Limit* is where we say no to the behaviour and yes to the feelings that are causing that behaviour.

For example, they might start hitting us during the *attachment play*, or they might keep bringing us yet another book for us to read to them when they are clearly tired and agitated.

In response to the *hitting*, we might gently hold their hand to prevent them from hitting us, and then let them know, *"I'm not willing for you to hit me, sweetheart, because I'm here to keep everyone safe. And I'm here and I'm listening, and I love you."*[47] Because the behaviour is caused by painful feelings, stopping the behaviour in this loving way is designed to help them express the feelings that were causing the behaviour.

If they keep bringing more and more books, and we see that they are doing that to *distract* themselves from healing-feelings, we might say

---

47 There is no set language for *loving limits* in Aware Parenting. This is just one suggestion. However, it is important to give information about why we are offering the *loving limit*.

something like, *"I'm willing to read you just one more, sweetheart."* And then once we've read that, if they ask for more, we might say something like, *"I'm not willing to read you any more, lovely, because I don't think it's the most helpful thing for you right now. And I'm here and I'm listening."* Again, because the behaviour was trying to suppress feelings, the aim of the *Loving Limit* is to help those feelings be expressed instead.

You'll notice that with both examples of a Loving Limit, we give the toddler information about why we are saying no. This is so that they know that we're not just randomly using power-over them. Giving information is an important part of Aware Parenting.

If we listen when their healing-feelings are naturally bubbling up, this can make the whole process easier. It can be much harder for them to cry with us if we distract them from the emotions so we can get through a bedtime routine, and then try to help them express the feelings later on, when we're all set up and ready.

Crying after a big day, but before being sleepy

Babies and children will often try to express healing-feelings throughout the day and evening, not necessarily just when they are tired. For example, emotions might bubble out after a stimulating day, but before a toddler is tired.

Simone shares her story of how helping her son express his painful feelings after coming home from childcare meant that going to sleep later on was easy, because he'd already released the day's stress. She explains:

"My two-year-old son always has a lot of feelings after a big day at childcare. Before finding Aware Parenting, we would get home and I felt like I was walking on eggshells. I was running around trying to keep him happy as he was always one small thing away from a huge meltdown. He was miserable all afternoon and I had a lot of trouble getting him to sleep at bedtime. Since practicing Aware Parenting, he now comes home and I can tell he has a lot of feelings to express. He often asks to watch TV or pushes me and I put in a Loving Limit: *'I'm not willing for you to push me sweetheart, because I'm here to keep everyone safe. I can see you*

have some big feelings to express, I am here and I'm listening'. After that, he will have a really big release (raging, crying) often for 20-60 minutes.

It's magical, the difference I see in him after this, he is so delightful for the rest of the afternoon: wanting to play, giggle, connect, and it no longer feels like I'm walking on eggshells or trying to keep him happy all afternoon. It's quite the opposite, I'm almost looking for/waiting for an opportunity for him to have a big release so he can get back into balance. After this, he is so easy to get to sleep, no big struggles like before. He just happily goes into bed, lays with me and falls asleep much more willingly and quickly, and sleeps soundly overnight too, without waking. On days he hasn't had a big release, I notice he often wakes overnight too, or earlier in the morning, and is more restless during his sleep. It is so noticeable to see how much his feelings and expressing them in loving arms impacts his sleep."

From a toddler: *Mum, you're taking me to the bedroom and I know that means you want me to nap. I don't know what's going on, but I'm finding it harder and harder to nap. I'm kind of tired, but it's like my body wants to just keep doing things. I move around the room.*

Oh look! Here's Teddy! I really want to play with him. Look at his lovely soft ears.

Oh, and here, over here! These fringes on this cushion look so interesting!

Oh! And what about this! If I bang my drink bottle against the bed, it makes a funny noise.

Oh! And what's this, over here?

You come close to me, and I kind of feel more tired then, but now, here's another thing for me to look at, and I move away from you.

You come close again, and you play this funny game with me, where you pretend you don't see me. I look at you, and you say, "Oh THERE you are!" I look away again, and you say, "OH where is Lee now?" and you pretend to look for me again. I'm here, Mum! "Oh THERE you are!" you say again! I giggle. I stop moving around the room, and I'm here with you. You keep playing the game, and I laugh some more.

I'm not all around the room now, I'm in my body. I can feel inside rather than outside now. We keep laughing together, and then I clamber over you and we play the roly poly game that I like. I feel all close with you, and close with me. Something's happening to my body and I like it. The wind has settled and my sails are calmer. We play the roly poly game some more and we laugh some more. I don't know what's happened, but I do actually feel sleepy now. I climb up on the bed with you and snuggle in. I smile at you, and my eyes close for a little rest. This was nice, Mummy.

CHAPTER SUMMARY

The practice of Aware Parenting changes as babies move through different stages and ages.

From newborn to three months, if you regularly offer your baby an opportunity to express their healing-feelings, they may cry in frequent but short bursts with pauses in between throughout the day. They're likely to have some healing-feelings to express before every sleep. Babies around the world tend to have a peak in crying at around 6-8 weeks.

From three to nine months, babies may need to cry less frequently than they did when they were younger (if they were supported to express their healing-feelings in the first three months) but more intensely and for longer periods each time. It's still typical for babies to need to cry in our loving arms before most naps and sleeps if they are not prevented from doing so.

Depending on the amount of stimulation and stress in the day, and how many feelings have already accumulated, you might find that sometimes they only cry for a few minutes, and at other times (and for some babies in particular), they might have much longer crying sessions, for longer than an hour. There is generally more of a sense of a beginning, middle, and end to a crying session. When they've finished crying in your arms, they might then drift off to sleep, or they might gaze into your eyes.

From about nine months, but depending on when they start crawling, they no longer always need to be held in arms while crying, so our response changes from the crying in arms approach to what I call '*the crying dance*' (not an official Aware Parenting term). Parents often find this phase challenging, particularly in knowing how to honour a toddler's needs for agency and autonomy, alongside support to express their healing-feelings.

In general, as babies move towards the end of their first year, they will tend to need to do less crying to release stress before sleep. Each baby is unique. If there are healing-feelings sitting in their bodies, those are still most likely to bubble up at the end of the day. The later in their life that you started listening to their healing-feelings, the more accumulated feelings they will have to express, and this catching up process can often take some time, i.e. months or even years.

As babies become toddlers, *attachment play* increasingly joins crying as a way to release tension and become relaxed before sleep. It doesn't replace crying, and often precedes crying. The *attachment play* creates connection and emotional safety and loosens up feelings that can often then come out in crying and raging.

Loving Limits can become increasingly relevant before sleep for toddlers. We can offer a *Loving Limit* if we see that our child has accumulated feelings, and needs our help to let those healing-feelings out. A *Loving Limit* is where we say no to the behaviour and yes to the feelings that are causing that behaviour. We might offer a *Loving Limit* if they are in aggression or suppression. I offered some suggestions about the language you might use for *Loving Limits*.

I so deeply trust the unfolding relationship
between you and your baby.

17. Feeding and sleeping

This can be a very contentious topic, so before we start, I am sending you lots of loving compassion, and want to remind you of a few things.

I invite you to listen to yourself and observe your baby and experiment, noticing what the most helpful actions are for both of you. I will also say time and time again, please don't do things just because you read them here. Instead, listen in to yourself, and if something resonates with you, try it out and observe your baby. Are you seeing the same things that I am suggesting that you may see? If not, please go back to the drawing board.

It's very common to feed babies to sleep, and many mothers enjoy breastfeeding to sleep, and likewise, lots of parents like bottle feeding to sleep. As with all of Aware Parenting, I'm *not* telling you that you 'should' do something or that you 'shouldn't' do something. I'm offering you information to see if you resonate, and if you do, I invite you to experiment.

I'm offering the Aware Parenting understanding that babies have an innate relaxation-through-release process to cry with us when they are tired and connected, in order to feel deeply relaxed enough to sleep.

If we feed them at this time, it can have a number of consequences.

Firstly, they will not have the same opportunity to express those feelings, and the pent-up feelings may then mean our baby wakes up more at night.

Secondly, they may start to find it harder and harder to express their feelings to us, even when we do want to listen and are able to, and this may continue into childhood and later years.

Thirdly, they might then find it hard to distinguish between hunger, tiredness, and upset feelings, and may often ask to feed when they are upset or tired rather than hungry.

Self-Compassion Moment

I'm sending you so much love and compassion right now. If you're picking up any sticks, I invite you to put them down. If you're feeling uncomfortable feelings, my heart goes out to you. It's really understandable that you might be experiencing painful feelings and thoughts as you read this. I invite you to reach out for some listening support if you need it.

Eva shares about her experience with breastfeeding and her baby's sleep:

"I clearly remember the day when my daughter was one day old. I felt so incompetent, not knowing how to help her when she started to cry. I called for the nurse and got the following advice. 'If her nappy is dry, she's not hot or cold then it's the breast she wants, just always give her the breast'. And so I did. I thought breastfeeding on demand meant that I must provide a nipple every time my baby was upset.

I also joined a Facebook group which promoted Classical Attachment Parenting, *including co-sleeping, that resonated very much with me, so I took all the rest for granted and to be true. Every day I read posts from other mothers who were crying for help and understanding. They shared that they could not cope with the fatigue and depletion of night-long 'comfort breastfeeding'. I felt more and more anxious as I read the 'sleep expert' comments that they need to keep on going, and that it will pass. I also read other mothers' supporting comments about how okay they were with their five year old tearing the t-shirt off of them every time they wanted 'boobies'. I thought that something was wrong with me, as this totally terrified me.*

My daughter was four months old when her sleep pattern and habits completely changed. I thought it was only related to developmental changes. Now I know that in addition to that, she had so many accumulated feelings of never ever being listened to. I could not put her to sleep just by putting her down in the cot next to me. It was impossible to get her to sleep without being on the breast. She started to wake up more frequently and completely refused to sleep in the cot. We moved to a floor bed when she was five months old, so whenever she woke up during the night I could just 'pop out the boobie' and provide her a 'soothing mechanism' without even opening my eyes. This went on for eight more months. During that time, she continued to wake up at least three to four times every night.

Putting her down to sleep was a minimum of 40-50 minutes that she spent on the breast. I was so fed up. I was extremely tired and over-touched. Moreover I was in physical pain. I continuously had blisters on both of my nipples as she changed her sucking technique. She wasn't even feeding any more, nor sucking properly, but was only snacking on my nipples. I was so desperate that I even tried to substitute my breast with a dummy. She spit it out. I tried rocking her instead of giving her the breast, she just stared at me for hours without falling asleep. I had no more ideas of what to do. She did spit the breast out too, many times. I put it back again and again to her mouth as I'd rather take the pain because I so badly wanted her to go to sleep. I wanted her to have a good sleep, and I also wanted to check out from the day. Just to have a little bit more time for myself.

She was 13 months old when I actively started to listen to The Aware Parenting Podcast. *This inspired me to read* The Aware Baby *and this was my big enlightening moment. OMG she has a massive* control pattern *and probably so much pent-up tension that this is why she needs 50 minutes of snacking to be able to go to sleep. OMG, so my massive night Netflix 'need' to go to sleep is actually a* control pattern *coming from my own childhood. I felt shame and guilt, but also a big determination that I want both of us to have a better connection with going to bed.*

The first night I told her that I understand her upset feelings and that I wasn't going to give her the breast to fall asleep. I told her, 'I'm here, and I'm listening'. She had a big cry. I was having very difficult moments. Lots of judgment came out from my inner voice of 'not being a good and responsive mother'. It was deep for both of us but she eventually cuddled next to me and gently fell asleep. The second night felt a bit lighter, on the third night she did not ask for the breast, nor cried. She hardly cried while asking for the breast after that. Instead, she cried spontaneously when we got to bed.

In the first couple of weeks she still woke up one or two times during the night and she was immediately searching for the breast. In the beginning, I was too tired to change the old habit and it took us again 30-40 minutes to get back to sleep. Sometimes I resisted giving her the human pacifier but she was not able to cry either to go to sleep, so I ended up giving her the breast and taking it away when the pain was so intense that it made me cry. I continued breastfeeding for two more months, as I slowly realised that there wasn't even much milk any more probably for a long while ago. The night waking went down to once a night for a couple of more months.

She is 26 months old now. She hardly wakes up during the night, but if she does, she goes right back to sleep. Since we stopped breastfeeding she developed a couple of other but much milder control patterns *like grabbing my arm or holding my hand as she goes to sleep. With Aware Parenting, I have a much better understanding of what is going on with her. We can easily release the tension with some* attachment play *(e.g. my hand is the 'little hedgehog' wandering all around the bed). We laugh, we connect and when she's ready to release I listen to the feelings as part of our bedtime routine. There is hardly any stress for the both of us around going to bed. Frankly, she runs to her bedroom with a 'let's go to sleeeeep' most nights. We still have a long way to go to catch up with that 13 months (and 37 years in my case) of accumulated feelings. But the healing has started and I experience so much more compassion towards her and myself that I do not even stress about where we are at on this journey."*

Self-Compassion Moment

I'm sending so much love and compassion to you if you've been through experiences like Eva did. However long ago that was, you might need some listening for the feelings you experienced back then. If so, I invite you to reach out for exactly that.

I'd love to share about my past experiences here.

As a teen and young adult, I found it really hard to distinguish between feeling tired and feeling hungry. Whenever I was tired, I wanted to eat.

Once I learnt about Aware Parenting, I realised it was likely that I had learnt this as a baby, from being frequently fed when I was tired and had feelings to express. After some years of inner work, I could then accurately discern the difference between tiredness, hunger, and painful feelings.

Self-Reflection Moment

I wonder if you resonate? Do you find it hard to tell the difference between when you're tired and when you're hungry? Do you often want to eat when you're tired? Do you notice anything similar in other members of your family?

I'd also love to share with you what I've noticed from many mothers whom I've worked with over the years. Listening to healing-feelings (some or all of the time) before sleep, *instead* of feeding to sleep, often brings a number of helpful outcomes.

Mothers often say how much more *connected* they feel with their babies when they're not regularly feeding their baby to sleep. Listening to our baby's deepest and most painful feelings can be incredibly hard to start with. However, the more we listen, and see clearly how much more relaxed and connected they are (alongside doing our own inner work and receiving listening for our feelings), most of us experience more ease in listening, and more closeness.

I've heard many mothers say that they felt close to their babies before Aware Parenting, but after starting to practice it, there came a depth of connection that they hadn't thought possible.

There's a profound intimacy in being with our baby as they show us their deepest feelings, and we really see and hear them.

I can still remember the power and beauty of those experiences with my daughter and son, two decades later.

We might liken this to how we feel in a friendship, where a friend shares painful feelings with us that they might not share with other people, and the deep intimacy it creates. Seeing and hearing another's inner world can be a great honour.

So, let's think some more together about feeding to sleep.

From an Aware Parenting perspective, night feeding is biologically normal during the early months, but offering the breast just to help them fall asleep (even though they are not hungry) is not necessary at any age.

You might recall the early chapters of this book and how we dived in deep to all of this!

> *Self-Compassion Moment*
> I'm sending so much love to you and whatever feelings you feel as you read this. All of your feelings are welcome!

After starting my *Sound Sleep and Secure Attachment with Aware Parenting Course*, Rachel shared with me about the differences she experienced when she swapped from feeding to sleep, to offering connection, play, and listening to feelings before sleep. She said:

"We had a major success last night! My daughter slept from 9pm to 5:15am!! This has never happened. (I did end up nursing her around 5:45 and then she fell into another deep, non-nursing sleep until 8.) Prior to me reading about and starting to implement Aware Parenting, she had only slept five hours at a time once or twice and four hours at a time a handful of times. Most nights, her first wake up would be after two or three hours, and then would be every hour or two for the rest of the night. So, yay! We are making huge progress. I am so happy that I found your course, Marion. It is really changing things for us.

Yesterday, she had a couple of good cries and we really did a lot of play too. In the evening, lots of attachment play. And today, after her good sleep, she was in the best mood pretty much all day. She wasn't clingy at all like she can tend to be, but I still made sure to give her a lot of attention and attachment play. *I have always spent a lot of time with her, but I'm seeing now that the type of focus I give her really matters. When I really focus on her and make the effort to make her laugh as much as I can, she actually goes off and plays by herself!*

And bedtime now is an enjoyable and special time instead of me feeling resentful about how long she takes to nurse to sleep.

You've changed my perspective about bedtime, so instead of thinking that I need to calm her down and getting frustrated that it's not working, I'm following her lead and really loving the bedtime chit chat that's happening. It's so sweet to get this glimpse into what she's thinking about while we're snuggling and giggling in the dark.

One of the best parts is that it takes her less time to fall asleep now than it did with her nursing to sleep every night.

Thank you!! I've only listened to week one of the course so far. Can't wait to hear the rest now. I'm really excited!"

Resentment

If babies are often being fed to sleep, they will be in a kind of light dissociation, which may feel pleasant to them, but because they are not feeling the sensations in their bodies, they will probably not feel deeply connected with us, and we may pick up on that. I've heard so many mothers feeling resentful, even sometimes saying things like, *"It's like I'm a human dummy/pacifier!"* because they are sensing their baby's dissociation, and the urgency to keep dissociating. I've seen this then lead to some mothers giving up breastfeeding because of the resentment and disconnection, alongside the challenges of waking up lots at night to feed their toddlers.

In contrast, I've seen many mothers who practice Aware Parenting continue breastfeeding much longer than they might have otherwise because they're still really enjoying it. This is because their baby is generally present, connected, and relaxed whilst feeding.

Bottle feeding can be experienced in a similar way.

Differentiating between hunger and healing-feelings

Learning to differentiate between when a baby is hungry (a needs-feeling) and when they are trying to express pent-up painful feelings from stressful or traumatic events (healing-feelings) is central to being comfortable to listen to a baby's feelings before sleep or during the night.

In *The Aware Baby*, Aletha Solter describes the main cues to look out for. If you want to dive even deeper into Aware Parenting with a baby, I recommend reading *The Aware Baby* and also my book, *The Emotional Life of Babies*.

Signs that a baby might not be hungry[48]:

- They don't latch on immediately.
- They come on and off frequently.
- They squirm, kick, hit, bite, or grunt loudly while feeding.
- They suck intermittently.
- They fall asleep soon after starting to feed.

Signs that a baby was probably hungry:

- They stay on the breast or bottle.
- They are calm.
- They suck deliberately.
- They feed until they've had enough and then come off, still awake.

I used these principles and practices when my son was a baby. I saw, as he got older, how listening to an even higher proportion of his feelings than we did with my daughter helped him even more to sleep easily and peacefully, be present, make eye contact, cooperate, concentrate for long periods of time, and be gentle with other children and adults, animals, and belongings.

---

48 Some of these can indicate a tongue tie or other issues, so if you are concerned, please reach out to your trusted health professional. There are Aware Parenting instructors who are also lactation consultants.

Candice shares her story of differentiating hunger from healing-feelings, and the effect it had on her baby's sleep. Her story shows clearly that the percentage of healing-feelings we listen to affects our baby's sleep – the higher the percentage, the longer the sleeping intervals. Understanding that our baby could sleep longer if we were to listen to more healing-feelings can bring a sense of power rather than powerlessness, even if we're not able or willing to listen to those feelings at that moment in time:

"I started listening to my second child's tears at five days old. I had already been practising Aware Parenting for 18 months with my first born so I was very comfortable with noticing signs of accumulated feelings. I started to listen to feelings when her sleep became disrupted after only having a feed an hour earlier, or when her suckling became aggravated and off and on. We spent the first six weeks in our home and she was in contact with a body (mostly mine) 97% of the time. She would be in the carrier through the day and she would sleep for 5-6 hours at a time. This was consistent through the night.

I found that I knew to extend the amount of time between her feeding when she began waking at her feeding intervals. During daytime feeds, I began extending feeding intervals by 10 minutes at a time, listening to all the feelings that arose in those 10 minutes. I found that her sleep would return to six hour stretches through the night when I had found the right feeding space. Because we were home all the time I could help her get a lot of her feelings out. When we started going out, people would always comment on how 'chill' she was, as she would just sleep in the carrier, wake to feed and sleep again. I didn't feel sleep deprived in the same way as I did with my first, who woke frequently to feed until I night weaned her at 15 months, despite practising Aware Parenting from three months old (not knowing as much as I did this time).

My now seven month old sleeps for four hour intervals. I am not listening to as many of her feelings as I was in the early days due to going out and socialising, and it shows in her sleep. Especially if we have a couple of busy days. However, it usually only takes two days of devotion to listening in order to get her to sleep for four hour intervals again. The experience with practising crying in loving arms from such an early age has transformed my experience of early motherhood and sleep. And although she doesn't sleep through the night yet (like I was hoping for) I have a very connected, joyful and loving baby because of this."

Like Candice, parents will commonly see clear correlations between the amount of stress/stimulation, the amount of listening to healing-feelings, and the length and quality of sleep. Observing the correlations can give us great clarity and power in knowing what is affecting our baby's sleep and what they need in order to have more restful sleep. In general, the more crying we listen to, and the more intense it is, especially if they complete a crying cycle, the more restfully and for longer periods our baby will sleep.

Self-Reflection Moment

If you're tempted to pick up any sticks at this point, I invite you to put them down. I also invite you to not coerce yourself to do anything in parenting – through 'shoulding' yourself. I encourage you to listen in to yourself. If what you've read does resonate with you, I invite you to drop the guilt stick, if you have not always understood your baby's cues accurately or if you're choosing to feed them when you can see that they're not actually hungry. As always, I invite you to listen in to your 'yeses' and 'noes'. And I also invite you to experiment. You might find that the amazing effects outweigh the challenge of changing core beliefs, doing things differently, and tending to your own feelings.

Some parents may choose to breast or bottle feed before some sleeps, others before all sleeps, and others before no sleeps. Do you feel called to experiment with any of these?

Johanet shares about the difference she experienced when she moved from feeding to sleep to offering a space to listen to healing-feelings before sleep:

"I listened to two of your podcast episodes (I think it was numbers 125 & 126) on baby sleep and it has made such a difference to our 10-month-old girl's sleep. I used to breastfeed her to sleep – or rather, distract her with my boob to sleep – and repeat throughout the night, sometimes up to 10 times (we're co-sleepers). After listening to your stellar wisdom,

her daddy started putting her to sleep – lying next to her, just holding her as she expressed her emotions – and sleeping next to her at night (while I now co-sleep with our five-year-old). Wow, it has made such a huge difference! Thank you sooo much!"

Helping them feel their healing-feelings more freely by changing the timing of when you feed them

It can be harder for babies to express their healing-feelings with us enough to have deeply relaxed sleep if we feed them when they need to cry, or a little while before when they need to cry.

I invite you to clearly observe your baby's hunger cues and always feed them when you think they are hungry, on both sides if breastfeeding and for as long as they want to feed. I invite you to offer your loving presence for your baby to express their healing-feelings when you're clear that they aren't hungry. Feeding can create dissociation, due to the sucking (and in the case of breastfeeding, also the lovely hormones). This mild dissociation may feel pleasant, but it might make it hard for them to reconnect with their feelings again and express them to us until another 30 or 40 minutes passes.

If they have recently fed, the dissociation from the sucking might still be in place, so it might be hard for them to connect with, and express, enough of their healing-feelings so that they can sleep restfully.

You might want to experiment with the timing here. For example, if you want to feed your baby in the evening and then offer to listen to their feelings a while later, holding this spacing in mind can mean that they can then fully feel and express a lovely big chunk of feelings to you and then feel deeply relaxed afterwards.

However, if babies have lots of painful emotions at the surface that they're trying to express, those feelings may still flow out freely, even if we are trying to feed them or have recently fed them.

Spacing between feeds affects night waking

Another important element of the relationship between feeding and sleep is that the length of time between feeds during the day will affect the gap between wake-ups in the night.

You will have seen this in Candice's story, above.

If you're wanting to help your baby sleep longer, you could experiment with this. This would mean observing their hunger cues, offering both breasts at each feeding and letting them feed as long as they want, (or feeding them as much as they want from a bottle). Then, clearly differentiating between hunger or healing-feelings, and then feeding them again when they are hungry, or listening to their healing-feelings if they have healing-feelings to express. This will often increase the gap between feeds in the daytime and thus at nighttime too. Whilst also, of course, always making sure that they are receiving the apt amount of nourishment.

Self-Reflection Moment

Does it resonate with you that babies have a natural inbuilt capacity to heal from stress and trauma through crying in our loving arms when they are tired and all their needs are met? Would you like to experiment with this with your baby? If so, is there a time, such as before a nap or before nighttime sleep, that you're confident that your baby's needs are met, including for nourishment, and that they are comfortable? Would you like to experiment at that point with not doing anything to distract them from their feelings, but simply being still and present with them in your arms or on your lap, and listening lovingly to their feelings?

You might find yourself starting off with doing this just once, and if you see clear evidence that your baby *does* indeed feel more relaxed and more connected as a result, you might want to gradually increase the number of occasions where you listen to their healing-feelings before sleep, and the length of time you listen for.

Taryn shares her story about the huge difference that finding Aware Parenting made to her baby's sleep. Before this, he would only sleep when he had breast in his mouth:

"I'm a Chiropractor. We had our first son at home by ourselves. It was an absolutely incredible birth. Eight hours, straight active labour and my son basically birthed himself. When Arkai came out he let out a massive cry for a good 20 minutes. Everyone was calm for the next 24 hours. After that, the crying began and it didn't stop. He basically cried for the first six months straight. Nothing we did/found helped us and we were going crazy. We thought we needed to stop the crying. He had three very tight oral ties, which we resolved ourselves with Craniosacral and dural tension work and I had extreme oversupply which meant he didn't even need to suck, but after four months the ties had loosened. It was a very traumatic time nevertheless.

By six months, it became apparent that he really was agitated. He never wanted to be put down. He didn't want to be on his back[49], and at this age he began both sitting unassisted and crawling, at the same time. The overwhelming theme of my baby was that he was agitated and wired. He apparently hated being still (we now know that being still would help him feel his feelings) and it was exhausting for us. Not only this, he had developed a control pattern with boobing. He would rarely stay asleep without the boob in his mouth. Exhausting, as you can imagine. We never used dummies.

By nine months he still would wake 6-12 times a night. He never day napped and I thought I was going to lose it. He would stay awake all day, tripping over, crying, etc. I had to put him in the carrier to stop him from hurting himself. He sometimes would sleep in the carrier – mostly not – and if so, not for long.

At 11 months, I finally found Aware Parenting! He's 15 months now. Within the first few months of Aware Parenting, he went to only waking up two times a night! Then he started napping more. Now today, six months into

---

49 From an Aware Parenting perspective, being put on his back was helping him connect with healing-feelings, which were being interpreted as needs-feelings that he didn't want to be on his back.

this journey, he finally let me hold him in loving arms to sleep, for a day nap. Up until this point, he wouldn't let me hold him[50]. He didn't even hug us before we started Aware Parenting! Now he hugs us all the time.

I can't thank you enough Marion! You saved me. You've changed our lives forever. I was so desperate for a loving approach to this. My baby had such a beautiful birth and a completely natural upbringing, and he's so healthy. I just couldn't work out what was bothering him. And now, he's so calm. So different. Again, thank you from the bottom of my heart. But honestly, Aware Parenting changed my life. It's the best thing I've done for myself, my son and my relationship. It's been the hardest yet most rewarding thing I've ever done."

> ### Self-Compassion Moment
> I'm sending love to any feelings you might have after reading Taryn's story. If you've had a similar experience, my heart goes out to you. Even if it was a long time ago, having your feelings heard from those experiences are so important. I invite you to reach out to an empathy buddy or Aware Parenting instructor if you feel called to.

We may see situations like this, where a baby cries a lot even if they experienced a calm birth, no trauma after birth, and are being carried or held most of the time. This often indicates that there was stress in utero. Knowing that babies can heal from this can be really reassuring if we do have a stressful pregnancy.

CHAPTER SUMMARY

It's very common to feed babies to sleep, and many mothers enjoy breastfeeding to sleep, and likewise, lots of parents like bottle feeding to sleep. As with all of Aware Parenting, I'm *not* telling you that you

---

50 From an Aware Parenting perspective, we would see this as the baby feeling and expressing healing-feelings when he was held, which was interpreted as a communication that he didn't want to be held.

'should' do something or that you 'shouldn't' do something. I'm offering you information to see if you resonate, and if you do, I invite you to experiment.

If we regularly feed a baby to go to sleep, it can have a number of consequences. They will not have the same opportunity to express those feelings, and the pent-up feelings may then mean the baby wakes up more at night. They may start to find it harder and harder to express their feelings to us, even when we do want to listen and are able to, and this may continue into childhood and later years. They might then find it hard to distinguish between hunger, tiredness, and upset feelings, and may often ask to feed when they are upset or tired rather than hungry.

Listening to healing-feelings (some or all of the time) before sleep, *instead* of feeding to sleep, often brings a number of helpful outcomes, including that mothers often say how much more *connected* they feel with their babies when they're not regularly feeding their baby to sleep.

From an Aware Parenting perspective, night feeding is biologically normal during the early months, but offering the breast just to help them fall asleep (even though they are not hungry) is not necessary at any age.

The element that can make a huge difference in the feeding and sleeping scenario is learning to differentiate between when a baby is hungry (a needs-feeling) and when they are trying to express pent-up painful feelings from stressful or traumatic events (healing-feelings).

It can harder for babies to express their healing-feelings enough to have deeply relaxed sleep if we feed them when they need to cry, or just before when they need to cry. Another important element of the relationship between feeding and sleep is that the length of time between feeds during the day will affect the gap between wake-ups in the night.

I so acknowledge all that you are doing in taking in this information. I so support you to listen in deeply to yourself and your baby.

18. Naps

Toddlers and naps

Naps can become really challenging with toddlers, and even more so if we have often distracted them from healing-feelings and they have a lot of accumulated emotions.

Ingredients 1 and 3 for restful sleep are particularly relevant here. Toddlers are no longer as tired for naps as they were. Less tiredness can mean it's be harder for their natural stress-release process of crying and laughter to happen. Remember, it's tiredness that makes it easier for babies to feel and release healing-feelings, which is all part of that innate relaxation-through-release response.

I can remember, as if it was yesterday, when I was visiting family back in the UK (from Australia) when my daughter was 18 months old. Up until that time, it hadn't mattered so much about the timing of her naps, but here, when I was stretched and tired myself, and needing a nap myself, it really did. It suddenly became so clear to me that I was finding it so hard to help her have a nap. (If you've read the first part of the book, where I talk about the effect on the social structure of support and whether frequent waking is challenging, you'll see that showing up here!)

I remember the day when I felt so frustrated in response to her not going to sleep, because I was jet-lagged and really needing a nap too. I can clearly picture another day where I fed her in the late afternoon while we were visiting an old friend of mine and she fell asleep, and I knew that would mean a late night for us both. Because I was there without her dad, and was caring for her by myself, all of these experiences became more significant and more stressful for me, because I was needing her to nap and sleep so that I could get my urgent needs for sleep met. It was so clear that the big breastfeeding control pattern I'd given her was making it harder and harder for her to express her feelings with me, and so she was finding it more and more difficult to feel relaxed enough to fall asleep for a daytime nap.

I made the decision then and there that when I had another child, I would make sure I didn't give them a breastfeeding control pattern, so they would easily express their feelings with me, and would therefore sleep easily for naps. And indeed, that's what I did with my son. He and I had a completely different experience, with him continuing to freely cry with me, and having easeful daytime naps, until he no longer needed them – which was around his second birthday.

You might want to follow your toddler's lead with naps and releasing. If they invite play, you might join in with the play. You could always offer a *Loving Limit* if they just keep wanting to play and play and they are clearly tired. If you think that your toddler is distracting themselves from crying, you might say, *"I'm not willing to play any more sweetheart, because I don't think it's the most helpful thing for you, and I'm here and I'm listening."* This might help them express the tears that are sitting below the desire for distraction.

Or, you might find another way to offer a *Loving Limit*. For example, if you are in the bedroom together and they are wanting to play in other rooms in your home, you might close the bedroom door and sit next to it **in the room with them**. If they indicate that they want to leave the room, you could offer the *Loving Limit* and listen to their feelings: *"I see that you want to play in the other room, sweetie, and I'm not willing to do that now, because I don't think that's the most helpful thing for you. I'm here with you and I'm listening."* This may also help them feel and express the feelings sitting in their body so they can feel relaxed enough to nap.

AnnMarie did my sleep course many years ago, and shared her aha moment about naps:

"In order to really listen our child, we need to really listen to ourselves. Wow, wow, wow! What a gift this reminder is dear Marion!!! Thank you for this beautiful course. I think my biggest success has been by honing and deepening my understanding of the concepts of release, relaxation, and connection. I would get so frustrated and at times angry with myself and my daughter trying to 'get' her to nap. I thought that she was just 'refusing' to nap. As a new mom, I just didn't understand her needs. As I

started taking Marion's courses, I understood that the releases, whether they were through crying or through wanting to play, were essential to my daughter's relaxation...which as I embraced her wanting to play on my lap and laugh a little in my arms, helped to get more connected... which helped us BOTH relax...which then led to her sleepiness for a nap! It is like MAGIC!"

Giving up the day nap

This can be such a tricky time for parents, and if you're in that stage now, I'm sending you so much love. Again, I invite you to trust your child and observe them. Remember the experimental process! You might find that on the days where they don't nap, your child gets much more tired in the evening. You may then cooperate with their natural relaxation-through-release process, and listen to the tears and tantrums that flow out more easily as a result of them being more tired.

Their increased tiredness will mean that it's easier for them to access accumulated feelings and thus to have a bigger and more intense cry in the evening. You'll then probably find that they have a more restful and longer sleep. They might also nap more easily the next day.

On the other hand, they may be so sleepy on days that they don't nap that they fall asleep in the late afternoon or early evening without crying.

This might happen while sitting in a high chair, coming home in the car, or breastfeeding – as happened for me with my daughter, as I shared above. They might then awaken later, still needing to cry, but the late nap may offset their usual bedtime by several hours.

To prevent this from happening during the transition period, some parents find it helpful to avoid doing certain things in the late afternoon, including car rides, other movement activities, and breastfeeding, because they might lull their child to sleep temporarily, and suppress the crying.

Ashlee shares about the experience she had with her son and his nap with Aware Parenting:

"We are living and travelling in our caravan with our son Miller who has recently turned two. We had been to the boat harbour that morning to see some dolphins and then to the maritime museum to tour a navy boat. We had an amazing morning with a very excited but centred child and had some lunch back at the van. In the afternoon, we decided to take some washing to the laundromat and wash our dog. Miller was getting tired after a big day. He was having some days where he would have a lunch time nap and others where he missed his nap. We assumed today was a day he would miss his nap too. However, on the way home he fell asleep. I sat in the car for half an hour with him and answered a call from my mum which woke him up. He was visibly upset. I took him into the van to his dad while I got a few things out the car and his crying escalated.

From there Miller released feelings for an hour. He had a huge cry which involved tears, yelling, and flailing his body. He hurt his foot in the process and wanted an ice pack so I got him one. He was then crying and upset over the ice pack. Everything was wrong with the ice pack but if I moved it away he wanted it. It wasn't about the ice pack! It was about releasing the emotions and energy from his body. At times, he was trying to hit, pinch, and bite us. We put Loving Limits *in place to keep everyone safe and to help him release the tension and frustration.*

Towards the end of the hour, he began to return to calmness again. After some cuddles, he put the ice pack on his foot and looked up with a precious smile and said, 'I feel better, Mummy.' We cuddled on the bed with Daddy and it turned into a game where he would freeze our faces with the ice pack and give us kisses over our face to melt us. We had a happy and calm little man for the remainder of the day, and he slept through that night – which he doesn't normally do. The following day he was so calm and happy. We know we are doing what's helpful for our son, listening to his emotions when they arise, no matter how big or small."

From a child: *Daddy, this giving up naps thing is so hard, isn't it? I just can't go to sleep any more after lunch like I used to. I try to squeeze up all my tiredness but it just doesn't work. And then my body goes kind of* *wild later on. I feel tired, I feel wild, I feel so much. I don't know what to do with myself. Everything my brother does bugs me. I want to lash out. I start running towards him, ready to bash him. But Dad, what's this? You get in between us and you stop me from hitting him. Aarrrrgggh.... But I WANT to hit him Dad! And now I want to hit you. But you stop me, and suddenly, all these strange feelings in me go through a funnel towards you.*

RAAARRRRRGGGGHHHH. It's all coming out. I am the loudest biggest fiercest lion and my loudest ever roar is coming out towards you. You hold my hand, stopping me from hitting you, and it all comes out. I roar and rage and rage and roar, and it's like all the jumbles of the day are coming out of me. I keep going and going, until there's none left. When I stop and open my eyes, I'm still in your arms, but I'm all soft. I smile at you, and you smile back. A bit later, we eat dinner together. It's yummy, but I'm so tired. Can I go to bed now, Daddy?

CHAPTER SUMMARY

Naps can become really challenging with toddlers, especially if they have a lot of accumulated emotions. That's because they are no longer as tired for naps as they were. This is relevant to both ingredients 1 and 3 for restful sleep. You might find *attachment play* and/or *Loving Limits* helpful to bring the needed laughter or tears.

If they are giving up their day nap, their increased tiredness in the evening will mean that it's easier for them to access accumulated feelings and to have a bigger and more intense cry in the evening. You'll probably find that after a big loud release, they then have a more restful and longer sleep. They might also nap more easily the next day.

They may be so sleepy on days that they don't nap that they fall asleep in the late afternoon or early evening without crying, and then awaken later, still needing to cry, but the late nap can make their usual bedtime much later. To prevent this from happening during the transition period, some parents find it helpful to avoid doing certain things in the late afternoon, including car rides, other movement activities, and breastfeeding, because they might lull their child to sleep temporarily, and suppress the crying.

I'm so willing for you to experience even more ease with naps and the process of giving up the naps.

19. Your own inner work

Doing our own inner work as a parent is vital if we are to practice Aware Parenting.

In relation to sleep, there are three key ways that our inner work makes a big difference.

The *first* is related to our baby or toddler's experience of safety and closeness.

Because they need closeness to feel safe and thus relaxed enough to fall asleep, how we feel in our body when we offer that closeness will affect the level of safety they experience.

If we are agitated, stressed, scared, or dissociated, and we are holding them or lying next to them, our emotional state will affect the extent to which their body experiences that they are safe to go to sleep.

If we are scared or stressed, it's likely that they will intrinsically pick up on the possibility that there is something in the environment that is a threat. This will mean it's harder for them to feel relaxed enough to fall asleep.

The *second* is related to their experience of the *balance of attention*, which is also about how safe they feel in the present moment.

They need to know that they are safe in the present in order to revisit experiences from the past, so they can feel and express those feelings when they are tired.

If we are stressed, overwhelmed, agitated, angry, or dissociated, they are likely to sense that there isn't the safety in the present moment to revisit those past experiences and to express those feelings through crying and raging.

If so, they are more likely to move into dissociation, which will affect the quality and quantity of their sleep.

> ### Self-Compassion Moment
> *My heart goes out to you however you feel when you read this. I invite you to refrain from judging yourself when you reflect on being in these states. In the DDC, it's common for most of us as parents to feel stressed, overwhelmed, and all kinds of other uncomfortable feelings. This is an invitation for more self-compassion rather than judgment.*

In addition, we don't need to feel completely calm and 100% present in order for our baby or toddler to know that they are safe in the present moment, and free to feel and express painful feelings that bubble up to be released when they are tired.

However, valuing our own needs and being willing to have them met will mean we are more likely to be present, because we won't have as many needs-feelings bubbling up, and will be less likely to need to dissociate.

In addition, regularly feeling and expressing our own painful feelings to an empathic listener leads to us having less of them bubbling away at the surface, especially when we are tired, and less of a likelihood that we need to dissociate. This will mean that our baby or toddler will probably be more willing to express their healing-feelings to us when they are tired.

The *third* is that it is a natural part of the process that when we listen to our baby, child, or teen's feelings, or join in with their play, our own feelings from the past will bubble up to be heard, often from when we were the age that they are now. These feelings can include sadness or grief, frustration or outrage, confusion or overwhelm, fear or terror.

Having those feelings lovingly heard can bring about profound healing and transformation for us. However, if they are too much for us to be with, and we don't receive the support from someone who is able to be lovingly present with those feelings, two things might happen. We might either avoid offering a listening space for our child's feelings, or offer it, but not really be willing for them to express those feelings, because we are not able to be with the emotions that bubble up in us as a result.

If Aware Parenting resonates with you, one of the first things I recommend is finding a supportive listener with whom you regularly connect, taking turns to share, with the listener offering their loving and empathic presence. Once you find one, and are used to sharing together, I recommend gradually finding a few more.

We are meant to have the support of a whole community. Having several empathy buddies is a small drop in the ocean compared to what we would have if we lived in a healthy and supportive culture.

Having the support of a counsellor or psychotherapist can also help, especially if they're familiar with Aware Parenting, and particularly if the feelings that are coming up in you are really big, or if you feel terror or dread.

Another way to support your inner work is to connect with an Aware Parenting instructor, who can also help you with the practical application of Aware Parenting for restful sleep, and with your own feelings and needs.

If you're familiar with inner work and comfortable with listening to your own feelings, reflecting on your own experiences with sleep and feelings can be helpful too, such as with elements of *The Marion Method* including the *Inner Loving Presences*, the *Inner Loving Presence Process*, and *The Willingness Work*.

Self-Reflection Moment

If you'd like to, and you feel the emotional safety and resources to do so, I'm going to invite you to reflect on your past experiences. If you have an empathy buddy or are working with an Aware Parenting instructor, you might want to share your responses with them.

- Do you know anything about your time in utero, your birth, and your early days as a newborn? If so, which of those might have been stressful or traumatic for you?
- Do you know where you slept as a baby and toddler?
- Do you know any details about how much you slept?
- Are there any family stories about your sleep as a baby or toddler?
- Did you have a dummy, soft toy, blanket, or other item to help you sleep?
- How has your sleep been as an adult?
- Have there been times as an adult that you've found it hard to go to sleep or woken up in the night and not been able to get back to sleep? How did you respond? What was going on for you at that time?
- Do you see any links or themes between your sleep as a baby and toddler and what you are experiencing now as an adult?
- What is your first impulse when your baby shows signs of tiredness?
- Are you seeing that in a different light now, having read what you've read?
- How do you feel, reading what you've read so far?
- What resonates with you?
- Is there anything you're unsure about or need more information about?
- What do you sense your next steps are?

Lia (who is now an Aware Parenting instructor) shared about the inner work she was called to do after she first started listening to her baby son's healing-feelings. She wrote this right at the beginning.

"I believe that children are born knowing intuitively what they need to heal. I strive to parent in a way that respects that. Today is a momentous occasion. Ori slept through the night last night! It's been a little over one week where we've been implementing Aware Parenting's 'crying in arms' approach (where a child is lovingly held and listened to while they cry

after all immediate needs have been met). I have not been feeding Ori to sleep. We are a co-sleeping family, and while I am a huge fan of co-sleeping, it doesn't mean that you are immune to frequent night wakings, so we have been struggling with that just the same!

I had never seen Ori sleeping so relaxed. The cactus arms are usually a good sign! [Note from Marion: Lia shared a picture of her son with his arms above his head, something I see often with babies and children sleeping in warm environments with Aware Parenting]. Since we've started listening to feelings, Ori's been crying much more during the day. Like having a proper cry once or twice a day before his naps and always with either Joris or myself holding him. He sleeps so well after and is so relaxed. Quite a few times, the crying has been quite intense, with a lot of squirming and squiggling and back arching and his cries are LOUD. Especially when I'm holding him and it's right in my ear.

There was clearly a backlog of emotions, and he did have traumatic birth experience, which I think a lot of the feelings were about. The process isn't easy for me. I am so tempted to shush and sing and bounce him to stop the crying. However, it has gotten easier, now that I see how relaxed he is after the cries. It's revolutionary! Crying in arms also made so much sense to me because many times clients will cry during a kinesiology session (and I have cried during many of my own), which I think can be a beautiful part of the healing process. I listen without trying to fix, bounce, shush them or offer them food – so why do we treat children differently? Well, hearing babies cry can trigger a lot. It's not easy, because of culture and conditioning. The first time I let him cry freely while holding him (knowing he wasn't hungry, sick or needed a diaper change), I was sweating profusely and had to blast the air conditioning. It definitely triggered a survival response in me. I felt adrenaline course through my veins. Panicked, doubtful thoughts raced through my head, "Maybe he has an ear infection. Maybe this is crazy. Maybe something is really wrong." I've had a night the past week where the crying lasted more than an hour and I felt my anxiety increase. I had a good cry myself the next day to Joris, a bit of a release myself. I realised then it really wasn't about Ori, but about re-parenting myself and reaching another level of truly being comfortable with emotions.

Since then it's gotten a lot easier. I'm able to hold space for Ori and breathe and really feel into my heart space, like I do for clients in my kinesiology practice.

We live with my parents and it's been very hard for them to understand, although they do try. I'm realising that it can be so challenging when we are conditioned to see feelings as something very wrong, and culturally we learn that we are not acceptable when we feel or express our feelings. It's a work in progress for me to understand for myself, and when I'm frustrated in relating to others, too. Why do we spend so much energy trying to stop the crying? Why is it seen as so wrong? It was, and continues to be, a paradigm shift for me. When we understand the reasons why babies cry – that in addition to communicating needs, they also cry to express feelings and to release stress and tension – it makes beautiful sense. And encourages us to support this amazing wisdom of our bodies.

I saw something very beautiful on Marion's website: "I am here with you. I am listening. I love you exactly as you are." I remember these words as Ori is crying. I whisper them to him. They became my mantra.

And the peaceful sleep we are both enjoying aside, the crying has made us closer. Ori's sharing and me listening is an intimacy that I never would've imagined. I want him to always feel that he will always be loved exactly as he is, and that it is always safe for him to come to me with those big feelings. He is so much more relaxed and sleeps so deeply.

It's night and day compared to all the months prior where he's had a restless sleep, woke easily (floorboards creaking were our nemesis) and frequent wakings. The difference is remarkable.

We've gotten rid of our white noise machine, which I know people love but personally I couldn't stand it. It felt like sleeping in an airplane!

I am grateful to have such a healthy, beautiful and funny snuggle muffin."

Self-Compassion Moment
I wonder how you feel, after reading Lia's story of starting to practice Aware Parenting. I'm sending loving compassion to whatever you're feeling.

To your inner baby:

I'm sending love to all of your feelings.

I'm sending love to you and however you felt before you went to sleep.

I'm sorry that you grew up in a culture where your painful feelings were not welcomed.

I welcome your feelings at your own pace and timing.

I love you, however you feel.

I will always stay with you when you are crying.

I will never leave you alone when you're upset.

I will stay close with you when you're falling asleep.

I trust your own timing with sleep.

I'm here and I'm listening.

I love you exactly as you are.

CHAPTER SUMMARY

Doing our own inner work as a parent is vital if we're practicing Aware Parenting. I recommend regularly receiving loving support for your feelings.

I also invited you to reflect on your own experiences with sleep and feelings.

I so support you to be deeply compassionate with yourself and all of your feelings.

20. The process of helping your baby feel relaxed enough to sleep

Whether your baby is a newborn, or a two-year-old, I'm here to support you as you start, or continue, your Aware Parenting sleep journey.

First of all, I'd love to offer you some general suggestions. They are simply starting points. As you develop your own Aware Parenting sleep practice, you'll discover what is most supportive for you and your family.

You might think that there are a lot of elements here, but as you practice, I imagine you will find that those that you find helpful become second nature to you.

Then I'd love to offer responses to common sleep issues and what you can do.

1. Thinking: hold the theory clearly in your mind

The three things needed for sound sleep:

- to feel tired (sleepy);
- to feel connected (*closeness creating a sense of safety*); and
- to feel relaxed (*by releasing any healing-feelings present*).

The two reasons for crying:

- for communication; and
- for healing.

The two types of feelings:

- needs-feelings; and
- healing-feelings.

The two ways babies heal from stress and trauma:

- crying with our loving support while they make vigorous movements; and

- *attachment play* (less common for young babies).

2. Feeling: have your own feelings heard

Having an empathy buddy listen to the feelings that show up for you when you think about:

- listening to your not-yet-crawling baby cry in your arms when all their needs are met;

- finding the *balance of attention* so your mobile baby can cry with your loving support while you do the *crying dance*;

- joining in with *attachment play* with your toddler; or

- offering a *Loving Limit* if your toddler is asking for lots of things before bed, and then listening to their healing-feelings.

Or, you might need to share about other stresses in your life, and painful feelings from non-parenting related things. If you're feeling overwhelmed, frustrated, or numb, letting out some of those feelings will be really helpful for both you and your baby.

When you don't have any extra time, that might be as quick as leaving a quick voice note in a voice-messaging app. Even leaving a minute or a few minutes of messages, knowing that you are going to be lovingly heard, can make a huge difference to how we feel and how much emotional energy we have to support our baby in the going to sleep process. If you have a partner, sharing with them that you're going to help your little one feel relaxed enough to sleep and connecting in with a hug or some warm support can also bring more energy and emotional spaciousness. Perhaps the two of you might do this together as a team?

The more your feelings have been felt and expressed, the easier it will be for your baby to feel relaxed when they are sleepy, both through the physical communication of safety they receive from your body, and because they will feel freer to have a cry with you if they need to.

3. Presence: connecting in with yourself and helping yourself become present

To help our baby feel connected with us and with their healing-feelings, we need to be relatively present and connected to ourselves and our own body.

Presence is the antidote to dissociation.

I know how hard that can be in a busy day, *and* I invite you to find small things you can do to help yourself with this. It might be dancing around the kitchen for a song or two, doing some yoga with your baby, or simply connecting in with your breathing and noticing your sensations whilst you're cooking dinner. This can make a huge difference.

Finding ways to stay connected with, and respond to, your sensations and needs throughout the day can really help.

For example, that might be having a big bottle of water close by so you can drink whenever you're thirsty, and going to the toilet as soon as you notice the need to go, even if that means carrying your breastfeeding baby with you. Sinking in to the sofa when you're sitting down and holding your baby, and being willing to relax in to that support, can make a huge difference.

The more connected you are with your body and your needs, the more your baby will feel your presence.

One of my mentees shared with me that after focussing on nourishing her needs for a week, her baby, who had been sucking his thumb for a few weeks, and crying with his dad but not her, started freely crying in her arms again.

You might want to listen to a short *Inner Loving Mother* meditation, if you're familiar with *The Marion Method* work.[51]

---

51 See Resources for more information on the *The Marion Method*.

Jacqui sent me a message about how focusing on her own presence was the missing piece for her with Aware Parenting and sleep:

"Marion! I've reached out so many times about my now 14 month old's sleep – I've met with Nic (Wilson, an Aware Parenting instructor and Marion Method Mentor in Australia) and devoured this latest sleep series you've done on the podcast. I felt like I was missing something while listening to my son's feelings as it just didn't seem to be helping and Nic reminded me to be totally present and honestly this was the last thing that needed to click for me! Now he's sleeping at least an hour for each nap – none of them needing me to feed him – he cries in my arms for 10 mins or more and then I put him down and he does these beautiful long naps and longer stretches at night. I'm so, so, so thankful for all your resources and Aware Parenting. I told my friend about our success and she tried supporting her daughter to sleep through listening lovingly and willingly and she was blown away at how well it worked for them both."

4. Preparation: preparing yourself physically and emotionally

This might mean going to the toilet, having a snack and a drink, and setting up the environment if you know that you're going to offer your little one your presence to express their healing-feelings. For example, if you have a pre-crawling baby and you're going to be listening to their feelings in your arms, this could be creating a really comfortable place for you to sit, with your back supported and pillows around you, or a stool for your feet so they can lie along your legs on their back with their head at your knees, so you can look at each other.

If you have a toddler and you're going to be doing *attachment play* and playing with *the crying dance*, that might be setting up lots of pillows on the floor so you can both be comfortable.

As you continue practicing Aware Parenting, over time you'll find what really supports you and your baby the most. That is likely to morph as they get older.

5. Tired: watching for tiredness signs

You know that they are tired when you can see tiredness signs. You might have already done things you wanted to do before their nap or nighttime sleep, such as feeding/food, nappy change/offering potty, changing their clothes, etc.

It can be hard for many babies to express their healing-feelings soon after being fed. You'll probably find that your baby will be able to more easily feel and express their feelings if you feed them a while before you sense they will be getting sleepy (so that they have moved through any dissociation created by the sucking and they are back to being present with their sensations and emotions again).

If you haven't done the things you wanted to do before helping them sleep, like changing their clothes, you might find that they want to cry whilst you do those things.

I invite you to not distract them or try to rush them through those things, but to be present with them and with their healing-feelings *while* doing those things. For example, if you're in the bath with them and they start crying and they're not hungry, you could hold them and listen to their feelings. You might even trust that the things you are doing are reminding them of past experiences and helping them connect with feelings from then so they can release them.

6. Connected: offer them closeness and connection

Remember that the more connected and present you are with yourself, the more they will feel deeply connected when you're with them.

You might want to focus on closeness and connection during the time before sleep. For example, if it's the evening and you're cooking dinner, could you have your baby safely on your back in a carrier, or lying or sitting somewhere safe and close so that you can see each other and you can talk to them as you're cooking? Once they're older, could you have your toddler in a learning tower or safely standing on a stool at a kitchen counter next to you, helping to make dinner?

Offering cuddles and warm touch whenever you can will provide a sense of connection. Slowing yourself down – whenever you notice that you're rushing or in your mind and not present – can make a big difference for you both.

After a bath or shower, would you like to snuggle up with them in a towel? I invite you to connect in with your love for them. Perhaps you'd like to look in their eyes and really see them. I invite you to hold them, have them on your lap, or lie down next to them before sleep.

7. Supporting them to feel relaxed

Notice where you might be inadvertently distracting them from their innate relaxation-through-release processes

Your baby might be trying to cry and you might be changing positions, singing songs, shushing, bouncing, jigging, rocking, or feeding, trying to avoid their tears. Your toddler might be inviting play and you might be trying to 'calm them down'. They might be agitatedly asking for a million things and you just keep on giving them all the things, thinking that they are expressing unmet needs, when they're actually trying to distract themselves from expressing the very healing-feelings that will lead to deep relaxation.

Instead of distracting them, follow their lead

If you are holding your baby in your arms or on your lap and they start low-grade crying, I invite you to simply be still and present with them. You might say things like, *"I'm here with you, and I'm listening. I love you"* Offer them eye contact, remind yourself that they are safe and all their needs are met, and keep listening.

If your baby or toddler is inviting play, I invite you to join in with them effusively. For extra effectiveness, add *attachment play*, such as peek-a-boo games or power-reversal games, e.g. where they are the more powerful one and they push you over and you pretend to fall over and be mock-surprised. If they are laughing (as long as there's no tickling), keep going. This is because the laughter is releasing feelings and tension from their bodies and will help them feel more relaxed and more able to sleep.

If your toddler is starting to pinch, bite, or hit, I recommend offering them a *Loving Limit*. This is where you do the minimum possible to stop the behaviour e.g. holding their hand that is about to hit, and saying something like, *"I'm not willing for you to hit me, sweetheart, because I'm here to keep everyone safe, and I'm right here and I'm listening,"* and then listening to the healing-feelings. Or, you might respond to these behaviours with *attachment play*, such as power-reversal games.

If your toddler is asking for one thing after the next and still isn't happy, or is trying to distract themselves by doing lots of things, or wants you to read them lots of books, or to keep on playing for hours, you can offer a *Loving Limit*, this time with the empathy first: *"I'm not willing to read you another story, sweetheart, because I don't think it's the most helpful thing for you, and I'm right here and listening,"* and then listen to the feelings.

Keep following their lead

If your baby is still crying with you and you're confident that all their needs are met, keep listening to their feelings.

It's normal for babies to need to cry for big long spells, to move their arms and legs vigorously, and even to sweat. Their crying might become very loud and intense. This is normal and natural too. All these are ways their body knows how to release stress and tension. They might kick with their legs, and the crying will probably intensify if you offer contact with your hands and their feet, so they can push against you. They might arch their back.

I invite you to trust that their body knows what to do, and to remember that your role is to support that innate wisdom.

If they start to nod off in your arms, and you think they might have more healing-feelings to express, you might want to change their position and say something like, *"I'm still here, and I'm listening, if you have more to tell me."*

This is a bit like squeezing out the emotional toothpaste – helping them to finish expressing a whole chunk of feelings and completing the whole crying cycle. This is most likely to result in deep relaxation and restful sleep.

If at any time you feel concerned that they might have an unmet need, you could offer them whatever you think they might be needing, e.g. feeding. They will let you know whether that was a need or not if you observe them closely.

To make that observation: if when you take that action, such as feed them, they are clearly calm and relaxed, present and able to make relaxed eye contact, it's likely it was a need. But if they appear tense, agitated, and avoid eye contact, it's likely that they did need to cry to express healing-feelings, and you've now distracted them from those feelings.

Your toddler's play might turn into crying. Simply be there with them, offering your loving presence, and a loving phrase such as, *"I'm here with you. I'm listening. I love you."*

Your toddler might keep on trying to hit or bite. I invite you to keep offering the *Loving Limit; "I'm not willing for you to hit me, sweetheart, because I'm here to keep everyone safe, and I'm right here and I'm listening,"* and keep listening to their feelings. Do what you need to do to keep them and yourself safe, e.g. putting pillows in between you. Again, I recommend aiming for the emotional toothpaste tube squeeze. Stay close, offer your loving presence, and listen to as many healing-feelings as you can.

The longer and more intense the laughing and crying, the more stress and tension they are releasing from their body and the more relaxed they will feel afterwards, which is likely to influence their sleep more, especially if you listen all the way through to completion.

Notice whether they're becoming more relaxed and present

If you're holding your baby crying in your arms, you might notice that their muscles are becoming more relaxed and they melt into your body more. If your mobile baby is moving around on the bed or floor with you, you may feel them melting in to you more. If your toddler is laughing or crying with you, you might notice them becoming more cuddly, loving and present. They might complete the whole crying cycle and then gaze into your eyes.

This will give you information and reassurance that what you are doing is supporting their natural release and relaxation response and is helpful for them.

If they complete a whole crying cycle without you stopping the crying before they've finished, you are likely to see the most difference in their levels of relaxation and quality of sleep.

8. Keep connected: stay close with them as they fall asleep

If your baby is in your arms, or you're lying down next to your toddler, you might want to wait for about 10-15 minutes after they've fallen asleep before placing them down or leaving (or you might want to stay there, if you want to rest, or sleep, or enjoy the cuddle!). You might want to connect in with your own breath, your own presence, and your love for them as you do that.

You might also listen in to your own feelings, and give yourself empathy for how you're feeling now, and how the process was for you.

9. If they wake up soon after

If they wake up soon after falling asleep, it tells you they probably had more feelings to express.

If it's a daytime nap and you can tell that they're still tired, or it's during the evening or night, and they obviously need more sleep, you might want to stay close without moving them much, hold them if they're not yet crawling, and offer more loving listening. You might find they return to crying again, as if the sleep was a quick rest before they expressed the next chunk of feelings so they could complete the crying cycle. Knowing this can make a huge difference, meaning you're way less likely to feel frustrated if they have just woken up soon after.

It is also likely to mean that you might feel called to focus more on helping them complete a whole crying cycle before they go to sleep the next time, knowing that they are then less likely to wake up after a short time.

10. Your feelings

If painful feelings came up for you during the process, perhaps you'd like to talk to your partner if you have one, message/phone/video call your empathy buddy, message the Aware Parenting instructor you're working with, or do some journalling. The more you get to feel, express, and have your feelings that show up at these times regularly heard, the more you will be able to keep listening to your baby's healing-crying and offer them your presence and *attachment play* on an ongoing basis.

11. Observation

I invite you to notice any differences between how they were *before* listening to their feelings, and how they are *afterwards*.

Increased relaxation can be seen in the following ways:

During sleep:

- Relaxed muscles
- Melting into your body (different from clinging or dissociating)
- Not moving around much (but also not needing to always be in one particular position)

- Relaxed and open hands

When awake:

- More eye contact
- More smiling
- Face more open and luminous
- Concentrating for longer periods
- More happy vocalisations
- Less screeching and whining
- Less agitation
- More affectionate and loving

The more of a difference you see, the more it will give you reassurance that what you are doing is helping them feel more relaxed and sleep more peacefully. This is likely to help you be more willing to keep practicing Aware Parenting, and to feel calmer yourself while you're listening to healing-feelings.

CHAPTER SUMMARY

To support your baby to sleep, you can focus on thinking (holding the theory clearly in your mind), feeling (having your feelings heard), presence (connecting in with yourself), preparing yourself physically and emotionally, watching for tired signs, offering closeness and connection, and supporting them to feel relaxed through listening lovingly to their crying.

You are likely to see the most difference in the quality of their sleep if you are able to listen right to the end of the crying cycle.

I'm so willing for you to understand exactly what is going on and precisely what your baby most needs.

21. Specific suggestions for particular situations

If you are feeling unsure

It's so understandable that you feel unsure when you first start listening to healing-feelings when your baby is tired. I really recommend having the support of an Aware Parenting instructor if you want more support.

Going at your own pace – and only doing what feels right to you – is so important.

Rebecca shares how she gradually built up the amount of time she listened to crying in arms, and how she felt comfortable to listen to more as she saw the clear effects on sleep:

"I wasn't practising Aware Parenting until our daughter was eight months old. We were doing 'Classical Attachment Parenting', but without knowing about the power of releasing big feelings. At that time, I was really exhausted, because for a few months, she had been waking 5-10 times per night. I then bought The Aware Baby, *where I read about crying in loving arms. My biggest trauma from my own childhood was being left alone to cry, so it was hard for me to be with her when she cried. I had done everything to make her stop crying. I had thought that only then were all her needs met.*

Still, Aware Parenting resonated with me. The first day I was able to hold four minutes of crying before I was too afraid that I might cause harm and offered the breast, the next day, eight minutes, the third day, 30 minutes, and from then on up to an hour. Very often I read bits from The Aware Baby *during the crying to reassure myself that what I was doing was healing for her. And although I did only a little amount of letting her express her feelings, after about three days she didn't wake 5-10 times, but only one or two times per night, which left me with an open mouth (don't know how you say it in English: I couldn't believe what was happening). I was sooo happy that she could get more sleep that was more restorative and that also we didn't start the new day like zombies."*

You are finding it hard to differentiate between hunger and tiredness and healing-feelings

This is so common! I want to remind you of a few things that might help you have more clarity.

As babies' stomachs get bigger, they can have longer spacings between feeds, as long as you are giving them a full feed by offering both breasts and supporting them to feed as long as they want.

If the intervals between feedings don't increase over time, especially during the early months, it's possible (and likely) that you're feeding them when they have healing-feelings to express.

You might want to observe them clearly, and if they regularly come on and off the breast, suck only intermittently, or fall asleep almost straight away, it's likely that you're feeding them when they're not hungry.

Your baby already has a breastfeeding *control pattern* and is used to breastfeeding to sleep

You might find it helpful to remember that they learnt to suppress their feelings from you (without picking up any guilt sticks, and having compassion for yourself) and so, if you choose to breastfeed them to sleep less often, or not feed them to sleep at all, you are actually helping them reconnect with their innate relaxation-through-release response.

You might want to let them know that you aren't going to feed them to sleep, and instead, you are going to listen to their feelings. Babies understand so much, and communicating to them what we are going to do can help them know more about their world.

You might also experiment with moving the timing of feedings so that you're sure that they're not hungry. They will probably have a backlog of feelings so there might be quite a lot of crying at first, depending on how old they are, and how much stress and trauma they've experienced.

Your baby has a dummy to go to sleep

I invite you to tune in to what you really want to do and are willing to do.

So much of Aware Parenting is freeing ourselves from the effects of our conditioning, so we can see the needs of our baby (and ourselves) more clearly. Doing things because we want to and because this resonates with us as being most helpful, rather than doing it because we think we should or we've been told it's the way to do things, are very different experiences. If you'd like to move ahead with Aware Parenting, one option is to hold your (pre-crawling) baby when they're tired, not giving them the dummy, and listening to their crying instead.

Depending on how long they've had the dummy and how many healing-feelings it's been suppressing, you might still want to give it to them after you've listened to some of their feelings before sleep.

On the other hand, offering a dummy could lead them to think that you don't want them to cry, so you might choose to stop offering it altogether. Most babies adapt quickly to this change and make use of the opportunity to release accumulated feelings at bedtime.

Your baby might be teething

Many parents are told that if their baby is crying, it must always be because they are physically uncomfortable. Teething is often one of the common perceptions of the cause of crying.

From an Aware Parenting perspective, most babies will feel mildly uncomfortable when they are teething.

We might see common signs such as a red cheek, drooling, more clinging, and more wakefulness at night. It is likely that a baby might have some healing-feelings to express from the mild discomfort, overwhelm, and confusion (because they don't understand what is going on from them).

However, it is rare that the teething would be painful enough to cause long and large bouts of crying.

As always with Aware Parenting, we invite parents to do what they can to support their baby to feel more comfortable, such as offering a chewing ring and supporting ease from the discomfort in ways that fit with their values.

However, I've found that in general, babies who are brought up with Aware Parenting and who have a relatively large percentage of their feelings heard don't seem to need to do a lot of healing-crying when they are teething.

Of course, there might be some babies with specific teething issues where this may be different.

The beauty of regularly listening to crying in arms also means that we can clearly tell the difference between healing-feelings and a pain cry (which is often higher pitched), so we will be able to tell when a baby is actually in physical pain.

It seems likely that for babies with lots of accumulated feelings, teething might help them access and express other healing-feelings that have been sitting in their bodies.

For some babies, they might not be teething at all, but simply healing-crying, which, is not being understood and is being interpreted as physical pain.

As with all of Aware Parenting, I invite you to deeply listen in to your own intuition and observe your baby if you think teething is causing crying. Then you can get clarity about what they really need.

Your baby sucks their thumb whenever they are tired, and falls asleep sucking their thumb

You may wonder about the difference between thumb-sucking and dummies.

It's important for us to remember that thumb-sucking is something babies choose to do with their own body when they don't feel the emotional safety to cry. In contrast, a dummy is something that we put in a baby's mouth to stop them from crying.

The first is their choice, the second is ours.

It's can be hard to help a baby who sucks their thumb when they are tired to express their healing-feelings instead.

First, I recommend focusing on meeting your needs and having your feelings heard more, because one of the reasons babies may suck their thumb is due to us not being as present as they need to express their feelings to us. Alternatively, thumb-sucking can often begin when babies are placed in a cot for a nap or in the evening while they are still awake. You might also observe whether you are inadvertently distracting them from their feelings at other times. Changing those practices can help babies be more willing to express their healing-feelings when they're tired.

Attachment play *can be helpful to loosen up the feelings underneath thumb-sucking.*

For example, you might pretend to suck your thumb, make loud noises, and pretend to be surprised each time you pop it out of your mouth. You could pretend to suck their thumb, and generally be playful in relation to their thumb-sucking. If they take their thumb out of their mouth and start crying, you might experiment with gently holding their hand in your hand and offering them empathy. If they desperately want to put their thumb back in their mouth, I recommend letting go of their thumb, because they're telling you that there isn't the *balance of attention* and they don't feel the emotional safety to cry. In which case, I invite you to keep working with your own feelings and presence, as well as with *attachment play.*

You're listening to healing-feelings before sleep but your baby is still agitated and waking up a lot

There could be at least three things going on here.

1. Percentage of feelings

What I've discovered in my own journey as a parent and Aware Parenting instructor is that the majority of us will *vastly underestimate* how many healing-feelings that babies have.

Although you are listening to healing-feelings, it's possible that your baby has plenty more to express, and this is affecting how relaxed they feel.

Very commonly, and particularly as first-time, first-generation parents practicing Aware Parenting, we will listen to a certain amount of a baby's healing-feelings and think we are listening to a much higher percentage than we actually are.

This was the case with my daughter. I thought I was listening to nearly 100%, but as she became a toddler and I understood Aware Parenting more, I realised that the figure was probably closer to 50%.

Sleep is one of the most sensitive barometers to accumulated feelings. Even if you're listening to 50% of their painful feelings, that other 50% will still be sitting in their bodies, affecting how relaxed they feel at night.

However, we don't need to listen to 100% of a baby's healing-feelings for them to be able to sleep restfully. In fact, I don't think that anyone, as a first-generation parent practicing Aware Parenting in the *Disconnected Domination Culture*, will be able to listen to 100% of a baby's feelings.

However, the higher the percentage we are able to listen to, the more relaxed they will feel at night.

You might be listening to 50% of their healing-feelings, but there is still 50% of the stress and tension sitting in their body. Increasing the amount of listening we do, often by also increasing the amount of emotional support we receive, can help them feel more relaxed at night. Making sure they complete a whole crying cycle can make a huge difference too.

2. Spacing of feedings

Another influence on the amount of night wakings is the gap between feeds during the day.

If your baby is older than three months, and you are giving them small and frequent feeds, that pattern is likely to be similar at night. You might like to experiment with feeding fully from both breasts (or bottle feeding similarly) for as long as your baby wants and observing your baby's hunger cues. This is likely to lead to longer intervals between feeding during the day. This can support your baby to also be able to sleep at least that long at night (and often for a couple of hours longer), as long as they don't have a lot of accumulated feelings.

3. A need for closeness

When babies are at the age of peak separation anxiety (between eight and 15 months), they sometimes have a greater need for skin-to-skin contact at night.

If they are sleeping separately from their parents, this need for physical connection could cause night awakenings. Even a co-sleeper next to the parents' bed might not be close enough.

Also, if the parents have new stress or trauma in their lives, the baby's attachment needs and night wakings can increase, even when the parents support bedtime crying. (Remember their need for safety to be able to sleep.)

Your baby is waking up more and more as the night goes on

This is very common and generally means that a baby has accumulated feelings that are sitting at the surface and making it hard for them to feel relaxed. Their wise body is communicating that there are some healing-feelings that really need to be expressed.

Listening to more and bigger healing-feelings before sleep, with them competing a whole crying cycle can often change this.

Your baby wakes up in the night but seems happy and won't go back to sleep

If this happens, it's likely that healing-feelings have woken them up but they're not yet experiencing the *balance of attention* to feel and express those feelings. You could experiment with sitting up in bed, bending your knees and holding them with their back along your legs and their head at your knees. (See the diagram at the end of the book.) That way you can offer eye contact and closeness and you might find that they are more easily able to connect with any feelings that might have woken them up. If the night waking happens frequently, then focusing on listening to more feelings before sleep (as well as before and after naps) is likely to help.

However, in some cases, a baby might be waking up because of a need for more connection, especially if they aren't getting much during the day, or are separated from their parent/s during the day.

You're listening to feelings but your baby wakes up soon after you place them down somewhere

This can often mean that they didn't get to express a whole chunk of healing-feelings and complete the crying cycle.

This can happen when you think they have finished crying when they haven't yet, or when you stop the crying by feeding them when they're not hungry, or use other distractions. If this is the case, you could make sure that when they are starting to drift off after crying with you, you change position, and offer your loving presence, and a loving phrase such as, *"I'm still here and I'm listening, if you have more feelings to tell me."* Rather like the previously mentioned emotional toothpaste tube, you are supporting your baby to express their healing-feelings until they feel a sense of completion, so that they can feel deeply relaxed.

It's this finishing the crying cycle that often makes a big difference to the quality and quantity of sleep. We can liken it to sharing a painful story with a friend, but not getting to finish the end of it, falling asleep, and then waking up, wanting to tell them everything.

You're wondering whether to listen to healing-feelings during the night

This is such a personal decision, and depends on how it would be for you to listen to crying during the night. Some parents decide to do this as well as supporting healing-crying in the evening, while others just focus on the daytimes and evenings.

Sometimes, it appears that a child really does need to express the feelings in the middle of the night, or at a specific time during the night, particularly if those are emotions from a particular point of time during their birth.

Amanda shares her family's story, which did include listening to healing-feelings during the night:

Around the time of my child's second birthday, I realised I was overwhelmed by exhaustion. Throughout my daughter's first year of life, she slept in two-to-three-hour intervals, which dwindled to just one hour as she grew older. Numerous nighttime breastfeeding sessions and the evening ritual of bouncing her to sleep were physically and emotionally draining me. I had been practicing Classical Attachment Parenting *from the time of my daughter's birth, and in my mind, that meant always 'soothing' her when she cried. I found myself increasingly overwhelmed and in search of support.*

I came across Marion's work and discovered Aware Parenting. It was an instant connection for me, and I felt such joy in learning all about Aware Parenting. My husband and I agreed we would unite and create a safe and supported space to hold our daughter's feelings before bed and at night and lovingly tend to the breastfeeding control patterns. *We also started exploring* attachment play *during the awake hours. The first week, my daughter cried and raged for hours in the night. We held her, listened to her, and gave her love and empathy. Finally, when she fell asleep, she slept so deeply that she woke up rested and relaxed. Aware Parenting taught me the profound value of deep listening, the importance of holding space for children's emotions, and my willingness to do so! I also learned that my own feelings need to be listened to so that I can sleep well, and I have since made that a priority in my life.*

I went on to joyfully breastfeed (in the daytime) for another two and a half years and had a graceful weaning when we both felt ready. My daughter is a peaceful sleeper and my whole family continues to thrive as an Aware Parenting family."

If you're confident that they're not hungry or uncomfortable in other ways, and you are willing to listen in the middle of the night, you might simply offer your loving presence and listen to their feelings.

You want to co-sleep with your baby and young child

With Aware Parenting, there are so many different ways that everyone can get their needs met. I've heard of so many different combinations of bed-sharing from parents. I invite you to experiment until you find what's a fit for you.

When my son was born, he and I co-slept with his sister and their dad. We had moved a single bed from another room and had it next to our queen-sized bed, so it became a massive bed. Because we'd listened to a lot of our daughter's feelings, she didn't stir in the night when our son woke up. I focussed on listening to our son's feelings during the daytime – I was aiming to listen to as close to 100% as I could, because I wanted him to freely express his feelings to me, after giving my daughter a big control pattern *as a baby which made it hard for her to express her feelings to me. Listening to this large percentage of his feelings meant that he rarely needed to cry during the night and he generally slept in a very relaxed and restful way. I loved that we could all be close together overnight. Like the children's nursery rhyme, "There were four in the bed...", one by one, they left the bed that I'm sitting on right now as I write these words! First, their dad left, when we separated. Then my daughter left for her own bed, and then my son left for his. I absolutely loved co-sleeping. I still had the massive bed all for myself (plus a few dogs!) for quite a few years, until we moved the single bed to my son's room when he moved into the granny flat in the garden when he was nearly 18.*

Candice shares about her experience with co-sleeping:

"I have a seven-month-old and a two-year-and-three-month old. I found that because of listening to feelings from five days old with my seven month old, she needs much less contact with my body than the 27 month old needed at the same age[52]. I find it so gorgeous to have that closeness with both of them through the night. And I find it restores my love for them both if we have had any tricky times through the day. My 27-month-old actually sleeps better off my body now that they're both in the bed. Although there definitely were some big feelings for both of us in the adjustment to sharing my time between two. I missed and still miss her as much as she misses me. I think it would have brought on even bigger feelings for us both if we had more separation while sleeping."

Sara shared her story with closeness and sleep for multiple siblings. I love her story because I think it invites each family to take their own path, and to support each child with their preferences and timing in relation to moving into their own bed:

"Over the years, we've had countless different sleeping arrangements. Each baby and toddler has needed/preferred different things, so we've just catered to that in the moment. My first slept independently by choice before his sister was born. My second asked for a bed in her big brother's room before my third was born. My third was sleeping in my bed until my fourth was born, he stayed with me until bub was about four months old and then he asked to sleep with his dad (who slept in a bed in another room).

---

52 This can be because being in a particular position can be a *control pattern.*

My fourth had her own bed next to mine before my fifth was born and she stayed there until bub was about 12 months old, then she asked to share with her big sister. That didn't last long though and now hubby has a queen bed that he shares with Miss 3 and Mr 6 is in his own bed in their room. Miss 8 and Mr 10 have their own rooms and beds, but Miss 8 will still often hop in with her dad. Mr 21mths and I bed-share. We joke that our house is musical beds, and it really is, sleeping arrangements change sometimes monthly. As the kids grow and their needs change, we've always just done whatever works. I've never changed anything in preparation for a new baby because it's hard to know what will work until you're living it. When I've had a toddler and a newbie in bed, I sleep in between baby and toddler or in the 'c curl' position so the toddler can't accidentally hurt the newbie. They just kind of don't wake each other. It is so hard when your toddler chooses to sleep elsewhere, I've definitely cried every time. I'm a 'cross bridges when you get to them' kind of Mum and it's worked well for us."

You're practicing Elimination Communication/nappy free/natural infant hygiene

If you're practicing Elimination Communication, you might notice that there is an extra reason why a baby might wake at night: to eliminate (wee or poo).

I practiced EC from when my daughter was eight months old and with my son from when he was a newborn. When my son woke to wee, I offered him his little potty, he would wee in it, and he would go back to sleep again if he was feeling relaxed. If he had healing-feelings to express, he wouldn't go back to sleep again until he had expressed those feelings through crying with me.

With my daughter, I wasn't really clear about differentiating out all the different needs and responding in an attuned way to whichever of these it was until she was about ten months old. However, with my son, I would always aim to respond to what he actually needed. If he needed to eliminate only, I would offer him the potty. If he woke up at night, I would generally offer him the potty first, then see if he had any feelings to express (by whether he was ready to return to sleep straight away). When he was hungry, I would feed him.

You like routine

Whilst observing your baby's cues, you can still bring rhythm and routine into your lives. You might start to see a pattern to their sleeping and can subtly adjust it so that it fits with your family life. Over the years, I've seen parents who love routine practice Aware Parenting, and parents who love none, and everywhere in between.

We can each tailor our Aware Parenting practice to our own unique family situation.

CHAPTER SUMMARY

This chapter offered suggestions for a number of specific scenarios, all of which invited you to listen in to your own feelings and intuition. I invited you to learn new information while being compassionate with yourself for not knowing the information previously, experiment with the new ideas, observe your unique baby, and listen in to your own experiences, making changes where you think they are necessary. The focus throughout was on connection with your baby, and compassion for yourself.

I offered the following phrases:

- *Please observe your baby and what they are communicating to you, and trust yourself and your observations.*
- *It's so important to go at your own pace and only do what feels right to you.*
- *I invite you to tune in to what you really want to do and are willing to do.*

- *This is such a personal decision, and depends on how it would be for you.*
- *With Aware Parenting, there are so many ways for everyone to get their needs met. I invite you to experiment until you find what's a fit for you.*
- *We can each tailor our Aware Parenting practice to our own unique family situation.*

Your baby is unique, and so are you.
I so celebrate you, honouring both of your
uniquenesses in your sleep journey.

22. Common sleep questions and answers for parents of babies (ages 0–2)

In this next section, I answer questions from parents about sleep. Please hold in mind that to deeply understand what is going on in any specific family, I would ask parents to fill in a pre-consultation questionnaire. This provides more details about the baby's behaviour and past stress and trauma history, as well as about the parents' understanding of Aware Parenting and what they've done so far.

You might want to only read the questions that are similar to yours. However, I do also invite you to read all the questions and answers at some point in time, even if they don't seem relevant to you, because they will probably help you understand sleep from an Aware Parenting perspective even more than you do now.

Because I don't have that detailed information about your family, my answers are generalisations. It's important that if you want more information about your own family situation, you mull over the responses, see if they resonate with you, experiment, and come to your own conclusions based on what you observe.

I also encourage you to consider working one-to-one with an Aware Parenting instructor for tailored support and advice.

The questions and answers are in categories: going to sleep; waking up; theory questions; and our own feelings, and within that, they are in chronological order, starting with newborns through to two-year-olds.

Going To Sleep

Bouncing cradle for next baby?

Q ~ Would you advise against using a sling cradle at any given point? (It bounces up and down). We used it for a bit for our daughter and now have a new baby on the way. But now that I'm familiar with Aware Parenting, I wonder if it's a bad idea? That it quickly becomes a *control pattern* and that baby needs movement during sleep? Is that right or not?

A ~ Hi lovely, yes, bouncing cradles and hammocks can help babies bypass their feelings to go to sleep, and if they are used a lot, can lead to movement *control patterns*, where babies need movement during sleep but also when they have feelings during the day. This can lead to toddlers who move around a lot when they are upset. If you want to hold your baby, listen to her feelings, and *then* put her in the sling cradle once she is asleep, it would be much less likely to become a *control pattern*.

How to support my four-week-old without breastfeeding to sleep?

Q ~ My baby is four weeks old and I'm breastfeeding all the time and haven't started listening to any healing-feelings before sleep. I breastfed my first child to sleep. I don't know how to get a baby to go to sleep without breastfeeding. Shall I sing to her and rock her instead?

A ~ I hear that you've only experienced breastfeeding to sleep, and I think you might feel amazed to witness the process of crying in arms before sleep. When your baby is tired, you could hold her and offer her your loving presence, without feeding, rocking, jiggling, or bouncing her. Simply be as present as you can in your own body and with her. It's likely that she will cry to release some healing-feelings and then fall asleep when she has expressed a chunk of them. I'm sending you lots of love in your experimenting process. I invite you to go at your own pace, listening to her feelings when you are confident that all her needs are met.

Six-week-old falling asleep in a baby carrier

Q ~ I have a six-week-old daughter and have just found out about Aware Parenting. I'm wondering about baby carriers. Is it okay for my baby to fall asleep in it or will it create a *control pattern* for movement?

A ~ I love that you've found out about Aware Parenting! As a form of attachment-style parenting, Aware Parenting recommends as much closeness as you can offer your baby, and a baby carrier is a beautiful way to meet that need as well as your own needs for more ease in also doing other things. You ask if it is okay for your baby to fall asleep in it, and I want to remind you that this is about understanding what is happening in each situation and then making your own decisions based on that information. You will probably find that if she *sometimes* falls asleep in the carrier, it won't create a *control pattern* for movement, if she is still getting to express her healing-feelings regularly, including before sleep. However, if she *often* falls asleep in it without crying to express healing-feelings, then it is likely that movement could become a *control pattern* and it will become harder for her to express her healing-feelings to you.

If you don't want that to happen, one option could be when you see that she's getting tired, to stop moving and sit down, offer her your loving presence, and ask her if she has any feelings to express to you. This might also be an opportunity for you to have some rest! You might loosen the carrier if she seems to need that to experience the *balance of attention* to express those emotions. Once she's let out the feelings fully and falls asleep, you might choose to then tighten the carrier up again and continue with your day. That way, she still has lots of closeness, you have ease and rest, and she can express her healing-feelings to you and have restful sleep.

Feeling frustrated and resentful when six-week-old cries before sleep

Q ~ My six-week-old keeps having big cries before her naps and sleep and I am often feeling frustrated and resentful. What can I do?

A ~ I'm sending you so much love and compassion. I really hear how frustrated and resentful you often feel when she is crying before sleep. The very first thing I would recommend is to have your frustration and resentment heard by a loving listener, such as another parent also practicing Aware Parenting, or an Aware Parenting instructor. Having our own feelings heard is essential if we are listening to our baby's feelings, and makes a huge difference to how we feel. It's normal and natural for our own feelings to bubble up when our baby cries in our arms, especially if we're also tired (which is also when we're less able to suppress our feelings). These can be feelings from our unmet needs, such as for support or sleep or community, and they can also be unexpressed healing-feelings from our own infancy or childhood.

Alternatively, the frustration and resentment may be coming from what you're telling yourself about the crying. It would be understandable if you were telling yourself things about her big cries, such as, *"Why is she crying so much? Why does she have all these feelings?"* If you are judging yourself or your parenting, that will also lead to painful feelings. I wonder if any of these resonate with you? You might feel very differently if you choose to remember that this is her innate wisdom in operation, and she is expressing her most heartfelt feelings to you, because she feels safe with you. Remembering too, that listening to her feelings in this way will help her heal from stress and trauma, will help your bond with her be strong, and will help her sleep more restfully. I wonder how you feel when you read this? I'm so willing for your experience to shift in beautiful ways.

Am I distracting my six-week-old by changing her position?

Q ~ If my baby (six weeks old), is crying and I change the position that I am holding him and he stops, would that be considered a needs-feeling rather than a healing-feeling since he was probably just uncomfortable? Often I will feel like he has some feelings to express and then hold him requesting some eye contact and he will stop crying and engage in deep connected eye contact – making me feel like it must be connection he is needing rather than a need for emotional release? I'd love clarity on this.

A ~ I love your question. This is a practice that requires us to keep observing to understand these nuances. I invite you to experiment and observe him. Unless a baby has had a traumatic birth and has a lot of big healing-feelings to express, it can often be quite easy to distract them from their feelings by changing position. If you were already holding him and being present and still with him and he was crying, he would already be experiencing connection with you. However, the deep connected eye contact sounds as if he is really present with you at those times. You might find that talking with him and letting him know that you are there and are listening if he has any feelings to share with you might support the *balance of attention* if he does have healing-feelings to express at that time. Ultimately, only you will be able to tell through your observation and experimentation whether him stopping crying is because his needs are met, or because he's completed expressing that chunk of feelings, or he's dissociating. I'm so willing for you to enjoy the experiment!

Sleep deprivation from three-month-old making it difficult to listen to toddler's feelings before sleep

Q ~ I'm feeling so sleep deprived with my three-month-old baby waking every hour that I just don't have it in me to listen to my toddler's feelings before sleep.

A ~ Oh sweetheart, my heart goes out to you. I imagine you are absolutely exhausted. In addition, caring for a baby and toddler is such a lot, particularly without a village of support. We really aren't meant to parent in nuclear families. I want to remind you of that. First of all, I would recommend doing whatever you can to receive more emotional and physical support. You having your needs met and your feelings heard more will increase your emotional capacity to listen to your baby's feelings. If you are then listening to more of your baby's healing-feelings, they will be able to sleep for longer, which will help you be more likely to have more capacity to listen to your toddler. You might even find that you can listen to both of their feelings at the same time. If you have a partner, or a friend or relative who is open to Aware Parenting, could they help with any of the listening to healing-feelings? I'm so willing for you to receive more support with this! So much love to you.

Four-month-old is crying a lot before sleep

Q ~ We have a four-month-old who cries a lot, particularly before he goes to sleep. We have just started Aware Parenting a couple of weeks ago. We hold him in our arms and listen to him cry. Before naps, he usually cries for 15-30 minutes before each sleep. In the evening it takes a lot longer. We usually give him a dummy after an hour of crying because we want him to get more sleep and we find listening to the feelings really hard. We sometimes worry that he is not getting enough sleep because of the amount of time he is crying.

We also know we should only let him cry in our arms if all his needs are met. Is sleep a need that has to be met before allowing him to cry in our arms? Would you recommend us taking him to bed earlier, before he shows any sleep signals, to make sure he gets sufficient sleep throughout the day?

We have not seen any significant decrease in the amount spent crying since starting this method. Is this normal?

Can we expect his crying to decrease after a while or is it possible that he will always need to cry this much?

A couple of months ago he was restless and he kept himself awake with his arms. We decided to swaddle him before he goes to bed, and that is what we still do now. What is your view on swaddling? Can restricting movement of his arms give him stress or will it only be comforting?

We only use the dummy in the evening to help him go to sleep. We worry that he might not get enough sleep otherwise, and that we ourselves will not be able to endure his crying for weeks or months. Any thoughts on using a dummy this way, allowing him to cry for an hour in our arms but then also helping him fall asleep?

A ~ I'm sending you both so much love and compassion, reading about the questions you have. Aware Parenting is so different to other paradigms and there is so much to learn, isn't there? I'm so glad that you're diving in deep to ask questions. I imagine that you might have two needs here: one, for information (which I trust will get met here). Second, I imagine that you both have feelings bubbling up here, and I would see that as a vitally important need to attend to. Do you feel able to set up times where you take turns in sharing your feelings with each other?

I wonder if you find it helpful to know that before sleep is one of the most common times for babies to express feelings – this is part of their natural relaxation-through-release process, so that tension is released from their bodies and they can sleep more peacefully.

Your son is doing the most natural and healthy thing to be doing before sleep! He is deeply connected with his innate wisdom.

It is also really normal for the 'cry before evening sleep' to be the biggest one, for several reasons – they are often more tired, so they can more easily express more and bigger feelings, they've had a whole day of experiences to heal from, and they are preparing for a longer stretch of sleep.

I hear that you're worried that your baby won't get enough sleep if you don't give him a dummy. The more stress and tension he releases, the more relaxed he will be, and the more sleep he is likely to get. Once you experiment more, you will probably discover that actually, the more healing-crying he does with you, the more restfully he will sleep and the longer he will be able to sleep.

The dummy will actually prevent him from sleeping as restfully and restoratively as he can.

I hear that you're also giving him the dummy because of how you're feeling when he's crying. The most important thing is being compassionate with yourselves for how much you are able to listen to, and having your own feelings heard so that you are able to listen to as much of your baby's feelings as you can. I have a few other options to offer before you do give him a dummy – I wonder if any of them resonate? Could you take turns listening to his feelings, with the other parent going to another room whilst that happens? How about you and your partner expressing your feelings to each other so that you feel more comfortable with your baby's feelings? You might even find that the more you get to express your feelings with another adult and the more you see a difference in your son's sleep and other behaviours, that you will feel relaxed during his crying in arms and may even come to enjoy it. Alternatively, how about putting on some headphones so that you can be with him and his feelings but are less stressed yourself? Or can you think of anything else that will support you to be able to listen to his feelings and not give him a dummy?

With Aware Parenting, we're aiming to communicate to our baby that we welcome their healing-feelings. The more we distract them from their feelings, including with a dummy, the more they are likely to receive the message that we don't want to hear their feelings, and the harder it will become for them to express their emotions to us, including when they are tired.

I also hear that you haven't seen a decrease in the amount of time spent crying and you wonder whether this is normal, and whether it will decrease after a while. In response to this, it is very normal and natural for all babies to cry every day for many months, if not longer, and that there is often the most crying in the early months (with a peak at about 6-8 weeks) – when babies are expressing feelings related to being in the womb, being born and any birth trauma, and the overwhelm of being out in the world compared to how it was for them in the womb.

Each baby differs in how much they need to cry, depending on how much stress they experience, particularly during and immediately after birth, and how sensitive they are. I wonder if you remember all the times where you distracted him from his healing-feelings before you knew about Aware Parenting, and whether you can imagine that now he is catching up on expressing those feelings. Most of us are not able to listen to 100% of a baby's healing-feelings, and the percentage we are able to listen to also makes a difference in terms of how much they cry each day.

However, it's important that you are seeing tangible differences in him since you've been listening to his healing-feelings. For example, does he seem more relaxed in his body? Does he make more relaxed eye contact in the day? Does he seem happier in general?

And, yes, over time, if we are listening to a high percentage of feelings, their need to cry lessens after the first several months, as they've expressed feelings related to their birth and in utero, and are less likely to feel overwhelmed. However, they will still need to cry regularly, especially if they've experienced more stress, such as going out and being in a busy place.

You ask whether sleep is a need that has to be met before crying in arms. In Aware Parenting, it's the other way around.

We can trust babies know how to sleep, and that they need to *feel tired, connected, and relaxed to sleep* – and crying in arms is their innate process to help them feel deeply relaxed, which is why they cry before sleep. We can deeply trust them. Your son is so innately wise and is doing exactly what his body knows how to do. His crying before sleep helps him feel deeply relaxed so he can sleep restoratively.

From an Aware Parenting perspective, we would *not* recommend swaddling at this age, because it can lead to powerlessness and then dissociation. In addition, at this age, vigorous arm movements are often part of the stress-release process, specifically releasing the frustration that babies experience while trying to reach and grab objects (related to their hand-eye coordination). I wonder if these answers bring you clarity?

Four-month-old crying before sleep

Q ~ Us again! We have been letting our four-month-old son cry in our arms before every sleep for over a month now. We have not seen much improvement in the amount of time spent crying or sleeping. He still cries for 15-30 minutes before each sleep during the day and 45-90 minutes in the evening. I think he cries because of a trauma or tensions that could not be released before, I don't think it is only the stress of the day itself that makes him cry this much and this heavily. Do you know a way to know the reason behind his crying?

While I hold on to the intrinsic value of letting our son cry to release tension, my wife is more worried about the amount of sleep that he gets and the fact that he cannot sleep when he signals to us that he is tired.

She now suggests we lay him in his bed and sit beside him, holding his hand and talking to him. She hopes that this way, he will be able to get to sleep faster and we can avoid the standard delay we now have between him being tired and actually sleeping. What do you think of this method, where we stay by his side as he cries very heavily in his bed? Thank you very much!

A ~ Hello again! I'm glad to hear how you are all getting on. It is common and natural for every baby to cry this kind of amount every day for many months. I wonder if that's helpful for you to know? As for not seeing a difference in his sleep, are you seeing any difference in his levels of relaxation, his muscle tension, his eye contact, how much he smiles, how much he melts into your hugs?

If you don't see any difference at all in any of these things compared to before you started practicing Aware Parenting, I would suggest getting some support from an Aware Parenting instructor. If you don't see any difference after implementing this approach for at least a month, I would recommend that you also take a look at the amount of current daily stress in your baby's life.

If you are concerned that crying in arms might not be helping him, another option is to stop listening to his healing-feelings for a period of time – such as 24 hours – and to see if you then see a difference in him compared to now – when you are listening to those feelings – in terms of his agitation, sleep, tension and eye contact.

The wonderful thing about Aware Parenting is that we can experiment and observe our babies, and they will show us what is helpful and what isn't.

As for knowing a reason behind his crying, it's normal for all babies to have a lot of healing-feelings, from their time in utero, their birth, and daily overstimulation. Some parents can ascertain the cause by giving attention to their own thoughts and feelings. If we notice ourselves thinking about the birth whilst they are crying, it's possible that the crying might be related to their birth. Another way is to observe them –

for example, back arching whilst crying is often a way that babies heal from birth experiences. By revisiting what they experienced (this time whilst crying in our loving arms) they can heal from those experiences. The more stress or trauma babies experience, the more feelings they will have to express to us.

As for your wife's concern that your son cannot sleep when he signals to you that he's tired, I would see what's happening very differently – **that he is completely connected with his natural and innate healing process.** Babies need three things to sleep – *to feel tired, connected, and relaxed.* Most young babies will have healing-feelings to express through crying in arms before *every* sleep. This isn't something wrong – this is their natural release-and-relaxation-process in operation. Your baby is showing you what he needs when he's tired to become more relaxed, and you are giving him that.

Rather than seeing this as a delay to speed up so he can go to sleep faster, I see this as an essential part of him doing what he naturally knows how to do so he can feel more relaxed to sleep. His body is so wise.

As for lying down next to him and holding his hand, I would recommend as much closeness with him as you can have whilst he is crying. If he can cry freely and loudly whilst in your loving arms, that is helping him feel relaxed. You can trust him. I wonder if this helps with clarity and reassurance for you and your wife? I'm sending you all lots of love.

Four-month-old still crying in arms before sleep

Q ~ I started to listen to my baby's feelings when he was six weeks old. I spent hours and hours with him in my arms, him crying and sleeping. All these hours spent like this were fine with me. I was confident it was the right thing. I never suspected illness or anything like that. He was seen by a paediatrician recently and he is doing great. Now, the thing is, he still cries a lot! I know there is not a linear way to healing but I start to lose confidence I think. He can never go to sleep during the day without crying. Recently he started to cry in the mornings as well. Up to a month ago or so he was sleeping more in the mornings and the crying of the day would start in the afternoon. I just need to know it won't be forever. When he is happy, he is very playful and alert, a joy to be around. I want more of that! We did have a traumatic birth, unfortunately. Even though I was happy and positive we experienced 60 hours of labour, an epidural, slipped ventouse, and forceps. Should I be concerned? Am I right to trust him completely and to listen to him as often as it feels like he needs it? Will it truly get easier someday soon?

A ~ Oh sweetheart, I'm sending you so much love. You have been listening to so many healing-feelings. I really hear that you are wondering if you should be concerned and for how long this will go on for. I imagine it was reassuring to hear from the paediatrician that he is well.

Your son is likely to have a lot of painful feelings to express from his birth and listening to all those feelings will be helping him heal. However, because of the ventouse and forceps, you might also look into some physical therapy of some kind to see if his neck or skull are feeling uncomfortable in any way.

I invite you to trust yourself – and to follow your instinct if you think there is anything else to check out physically, e.g. with your diet if you are breastfeeding. However, it is normal and natural for babies to have a *lot* of feelings to express, especially if they experienced a traumatic birth. These early months are also high in overwhelm and overstimulation for babies.

In addition, the fact that he is just crying before he goes to sleep, which is a baby's innate wisdom to release tension so they can sleep more restfully, suggests to me that his crying is absolutely healing-crying.

It really will get less, sweetheart. Are you getting any support? Do you have an empathy buddy to share your feelings and concerns with? You are doing so much – and receiving physical and emotional support ourselves is so essential. The information that jumps out at me the most is how happy, playful, joyful, and alert he is. To me, that clearly suggests that all his needs are being met and the amount of listening to his healing-feelings you are doing is really beneficial to him. Does that resonate with you?

Four-and-a-half-month-old's 'sleep regression'

Q ~ I have a four-and-a-half-month-old and we started crying in arms a few weeks ago. We have been struggling with the four-month 'sleep regression' and waking multiple times overnight. My little one will constantly try to suck on his hands, and grab my hands and clothing to suck on whilst crying in arms. We do sometimes feed to sleep and when I pop him down, he will wake and cue that he is still hungry. I am torn with the feeling of not responding to this need; however, I know he isn't hungry. I do reassure him when this happens and try to sit with him through this, however sometimes the worry of not responding to him if he is hungry turns into me offering him a feed again and we repeat the cycle. I love the ideas of Aware Parenting and this approach makes the most sense to me out of anything I have come across.

A ~ Hello lovely! From an Aware Parenting perspective, what other paradigms call 'sleep regression', we see as generally an accumulation of feelings that wake babies up to be expressed. Your baby sucking on his hands and your hands and clothing matches that interpretation and indicates that he might be trying to suppress his emotions at these times. This can happen if we have inadvertently stopped our baby from expressing their healing-feelings, often because we thought they were indicating unmet needs.

If you feed your baby from both breasts for as long as he wants and he falls asleep, and then you pop him down and he wakes up and signals he wants more feeding, it is likely that he is not hungry and that feeding has become a **control pattern.**

Does that resonate with you? If we feed babies when they have healing-feelings to express, they learn to interpret those feelings as hunger, and then to signal to feed when they feel those same feelings, which can appear to mean that they are hungry. And as you say, you are clear and confident that he isn't hungry. You can really trust yourself, sweetheart.

I hear that you're worried that he might be hungry even after you've fed him, and so you feed him again. You will be able to tell whether he is hungry by how he feeds. If he is agitated, comes on and off the breast, sucks intermittently or disinterestedly, or falls asleep soon after starting to feed, that would confirm your sense that he isn't hungry after all.

I wonder if it resonates with you that by breastfeeding him when he had feelings to express, he is now interpreting those sensations of feelings to indicate hunger, and so is asking to be fed. I wonder if that will help you have more confidence in your knowing that he isn't hungry? Are you willing to trust your sense that he isn't hungry, and to simply hold him in your loving arms and listen to his feelings instead? Then, you can later observe him. When you listen to more healing-feelings, you will probably find that he wakes up less often. You might also find that he does less to try to suppress his feelings when he's crying in your arms. This will give you reassurance that you are reading his cues accurately.

Presence with my five-month-old and his crying

Q ~ I notice that when I'm present, it helps my son relax more into sleep when I hold him. But sometimes I'm really present and that seems to help him cry more. What's going on here?

A ~ I so honour all the presence that you're offering your son. When you are present and he relaxes into sleep when you hold him, that tells you that you were meeting his needs for closeness and physical and emotional safety, and he didn't have many healing-feelings to express, so he went to sleep. However, at five months old, most babies will have healing-feelings to express to us when they are tired. Your beautiful presence helps him feel physically and emotionally safe with you so he can express his healing-feelings and afterwards feel deeply relaxed. You might find it helpful to think about times you are with a friend who is deeply present when you have painful feelings to express, and their presence helps you feel and express those feelings even more. Does this resonate with you, lovely?

Unsure about five-month-old's tiredness cues

Q ~ Before coming across Aware Parenting, I read that you can tell a baby is tired when you can't settle their cries with a feed, and if they're fussing, sweating and arching their back. Now I'm confused. What does Aware Parenting say about these things? Do you think they are tiredness cues?

A ~ Hello lovely! From an Aware Parenting perspective, we would see all of these as signs that a baby is trying to release stress and trauma from their body through crying in arms. Babies might be tired when they're crying, but that's because the tiredness is helping them release stress through crying with us, rather than because the tiredness is painful in itself.

If we feed them and they are still crying, it's likely that they were not hungry in the first place, and they were trying to cry to heal. If they're arching their back while crying, that's often a sign that they are revisiting, and healing from, their birth experience. If they are sweating, that is often a part of the natural release process, as they release stress and tension from the fight or flight response.

There may be times where there are other reasons for these behaviours, but they are often signals that a baby is doing exactly what is most helpful for them – to release stress from their bodies so they can sleep more restfully. I wonder if that resonates with you?

Is patting my six-month-old a *control pattern*?

Q ~ I often listen to my six-month-old baby's feelings before sleep. However, sometimes he doesn't seem to need to cry and he just wants to play unless I can calm him. I gently tap him on the back or bum, like a heartbeat rhythm and sometimes a gentle shooshing sound. He falls asleep quickly. Are these tappings and shooshing going to create a *control pattern*? I'm doing it to calm him rather than stop emotions. In other words, is it creating a *control pattern* if you're just trying to get them to sleep when they don't need to release feelings as opposed to doing it to keep them quiet? Is the assumption with Aware Parenting that if they're not falling asleep when tired and seemingly happy/relaxed that they must need to cry? That techniques such as patting, sshhh sounds, etc. don't contribute to that relaxation process but they're just a *control pattern*?

A ~ I so celebrate all the feelings that you're listening to! And yes, from an Aware Parenting perspective, if a baby of six months is clearly tired, and we're holding them, and they're not falling asleep by us simply holding them in our arms, it generally means that they have some unexpressed feelings that are preventing them from feeling relaxed enough to fall asleep. If we regularly do anything to bypass those feelings, such as tapping or shooshing, it could become a *control pattern.* Does that bring the clarity you're looking for?

Six-month-old sucks her thumb before sleep and won't cry with me

Q ~ My daughter sucks her thumb whenever she's tired, and won't cry with me. What can I do?

A ~ I'm sending you so much love, sweetheart. Thumb-sucking is a symptom. So, I have three initial suggestions for you to explore: how you feel when you imagine listening to her feelings; whether your own feelings are being listened to; and whether you are unwittingly distracting her from her feelings at other times, e.g. through feeding her when she isn't hungry. Often these explorations can support us to help our baby to be freer to express their healing-feelings to us. As for responding to her in the moment, I invite you to bring your loving warmth to melt her freeze, so it can turn into tears if necessary. You might want to bring presence to your own body first, and to offer her gentle present touch, perhaps to her hand or her arm. You might then want to follow that up with *attachment play*, perhaps putting your own thumb in your mouth and pulling it out and making a 'pop' sound along with a joyful face. Or perhaps you may pretend to try to suck her thumb. In the play, you might find that she smiles and takes her thumb out of her mouth. That tells you she's already feeling more of the warmth and the connection.

Once she has taken her thumb out (we do not recommend taking a baby's thumb out of their mouth), you might play with a gentle and nuanced *Loving Limit,* by putting your thumb in the centre of her palm. When I have played with this, I've imagined a loving connection from my heart, through my arm and my hand, through to the baby's hand, to her heart.

I would focus on really feeling that connection rather than on 'getting her' to cry, or stopping her from sucking her thumb.

If she then starts to cry, you can trust that she is feeling that warm connection and the *balance of attention* to feel and express her feelings. However, if she is trying to get her thumb back in her mouth, I would suggest taking your thumb out of her hand, because she is communicating that she isn't feeling the *balance of attention* yet. If you still have the willingness to do more *attachment play*, I would then go back to that. Even if she doesn't take her thumb out of her mouth, the warm presence and play will be making a difference to her.

Seven-month-old sucks thumb with mum but cries with dad before sleep

Q ~ We have a seven-month-old who has very different experiences falling asleep with me vs. my husband. We hold him and allow him to cry/ express his feelings, giving eye contact, physical touch, and reassuring words without rocking or shushing. With me, he will sometimes cry for maybe a minute or two, but will typically suck his thumb immediately, remaining calm and and falling asleep within 10 mins or less. At bedtime with my husband, my son loses it completely, he doesn't suck on his thumb but will cry intensely for 20+ minutes, flailing and pushing away from my husband with his feet. When he does finally sleep after crying intensely with my husband, it does not seem like the beautiful relaxed state described after a release. He is hiccoughing. He does all the same things I do, but I think my son is crying out for me (I'm the primary care giver), and when I have gone into the room in the past, the moment he is in my arms, he sucks on his thumb and falls asleep almost immediately (without rocking/shushing/etc.).

A ~ I so honour all that you and your husband are doing in listening to your son's feelings. What the three of you are experiencing is a dynamic I have seen thousands of times over the last two decades – I wonder if you find it helpful to know that? I would love to respond with my thoughts and I would also love to preface it with a couple of things – 1. the most important place to access your information about what to do next is to listen to yourselves and observe your son; 2. I would recommend a consultation with an Aware Parenting instructor to dive deeper into this. You ask why he is not crying much with you. It is very common for babies to find it harder to cry with their mothers, particularly if we are breastfeeding, because we will generally veer on the side of thinking that our baby is hungry when they have healing-feelings to express (of course we want to make sure that they aren't hungry). That suppression of emotions through breastfeeding often means it then becomes harder for them to cry with us, especially if we are holding them in a similar way to how we hold them when feeding them to suppress their feelings. But it's not just about breastfeeding. If we are with them more than their dad (or other parent) and are inadvertently distracting them from their feelings in other ways too, they will come to find it harder to cry with us. One thing you could do if this is the case, is to focus more on differentiating between hunger and a need to express feelings.

Another option could be connecting in with whether you really are willing to listen to big cries? Do your own feelings show up? Are there fears or concerns there for you? This is why having our own empathy buddy is so important. The more we feel truly comfortable with our baby's feelings and the more willing we are to listen, the more likely they are to be free to express their feelings with us. Does any of this resonate? I love how clearly you are observing his behaviour, and yes, him sucking his thumb is a *control pattern*, which is an invitation to experiment with these suggestions.

As for the second part of your question, I think it is so important for you and your husband to get to express your feelings and share with each other about how you feel. If you then are willing to experiment, you might want to try out different things. What happens if you hold your baby and he sucks his thumb? How does he sleep that night? How much eye contact does he make the next day? How is he when he wakes up? How relaxed are his muscles? Then you could experiment with your husband holding him and you sitting right next to them, perhaps touching your son's hand, to give you reassurance that he is feeling your loving presence *and* the support to express his feelings. What happens after that in terms of all of those observations?

We can only really get reassurance from observing a difference. If you clearly see that he is more relaxed in his body, makes more eye contact, sleeps more peacefully, and concentrates for longer after crying with his dad, that might give you reassurance that the crying with his dad is healing. Then you will feel more comfortable to clearly tell him that daddy is going to listen to his feelings, knowing that that is the most helpful thing for him.

What I have found in working with parents over the years is that when they have that reassurance, this becomes such a wonderful way for everyone gets their needs met. The baby gets to express their feelings, feel more relaxed in their body, *and* to be securely attached with their dad, knowing that their dad welcomes all their feelings. The dad receives the confidence that he makes a huge difference and gets to bond deeply with his baby. The mum gets to have time just with herself for her needs to be met or to be present with an older child.

By the way, it's common for babies to hiccough or have some sighs after crying in arms has finished. It's all part of the completion of the healing process. The important thing is to notice how he is after that. That's generally when the deep relaxation comes.

Seven-month-old has no routine

Q ~ We have no routine and never have. We feel like there's so much conflicting input out there – feed-play-sleep, feed to sleep, listen to feelings, listen to feelings only for baby to fall asleep then wake, cry, sleep and repeat! I know that while we're trying our best with our daughter's needs my husband and I are not meeting our own needs at all, it seems impossible when the only decent daytime naps are when she's asleep on me after a feed. How do others approach some sort of routine? I guess I've been aiming to just follow our daughter's lead, but I know it just isn't working.

A ~ I'm sending you so much love and I'm hearing how hard things are. And there is so much conflicting advice out there, isn't there? My first suggestion is to connect in with yourself to see what approach resonates with you the most. If it's Aware Parenting, I would recommend not reading about other approaches while you are experimenting with it, so that you can fully practice it and can clearly observe the effects.

Next, I would recommend receiving some listening from a loving listener, such as an Aware Parenting instructor. It's so vital to have our feelings heard if we are listening to our baby's feelings, and when things are really hard, that's even more important for us. Once you're feeling a bit more emotionally clear and spacious in yourself, I would invite you to listen to as much crying as you can before your baby goes to sleep. Most babies will have healing-feelings to express to us before each sleep. The higher the percentage of feelings you listen to, and the more fully and intensely your baby expresses her healing-feelings, especially if she completes the crying cycle, the more she will feel deeply relaxed and the more she will be able to sleep even when she's not on you. If the longer daytime naps are only on you after a feed it suggests that she may have some more feelings to catch up on so she can feel more deeply relaxed. Listening to more, and supporting her to complete a cycle will mean she will be more likely to be able to stay asleep without being on you.

Do you feel able to listen to her healing-feelings before sleep and then to see how that affects how relaxed she is when she's sleeping? The more relaxed a baby is, the more we can support them to find a rhythm that also works for us too. Does this help? So much love to you.

Breastfeeding babies to sleep

Q ~ What are your thoughts on breastfeeding babies to sleep?

A ~ Hello lovely! It's such a common thing to do, isn't it? From an Aware Parenting perspective, babies have an inbuilt relaxation-through-release response, which is to cry in loving arms when they feel tired and connected; that way they release tension from their body, heal from stress and trauma and naturally feel more deeply relaxed. If we feed a baby to sleep, we are not making the most of that natural process.

This can have a number of effects if we do it frequently:

- they might have more and more accumulated feelings, leading to more restless sleep and more waking up as well as other effects during the daytime;

- they might find it harder to express their painful feelings to us;
- they might not know the difference between hunger, upset feelings, and tiredness; and
- they might not get to heal from stressful and traumatic experiences.

I support every parent to do what most resonates with them – and if Aware Parenting resonates with you, you might like to experiment with the differences between breastfeeding your baby to sleep and listening to their healing-feelings before sleep, and what you notice in their sleep and other behaviour as a result. Through your own experimenting, you can then make a decision based on what meets your baby's needs and your needs the most. How do you feel and what do you think when you read this?

How to help a baby relax if he never expresses feelings through crying?

Q ~ How do you help a baby to relax if he never releases any feelings through crying? We're trying through *attachment play* and lots of connection time, but he never let his feelings come out and we're exhausted. He's waking up more than eight times during the night.

A ~ Oh sweetheart, I hear how exhausted you're feeling, and I'm sending you lots of love. I'm also really celebrating all the *attachment play* and connection you are offering. If your baby isn't expressing any feelings, I invite you to observe whether there are times when you're inadvertently suppressing his feelings. For example, perhaps you are feeding him when he's trying to express his feelings, or jiggling, or bouncing him, or distracting in other ways. It's so easy for us to do these things without even noticing, since they may have been things that were done to us, or actions we've seen done to babies so many times. Have you tried holding him in your arms when he's tired and telling him that you're there and listening? Ideally, doing this at least half an hour *after* feeding him will help him be more able to connect with his feelings, while giving you confidence that he's not hungry. Does any of this resonate?

If you're already doing all of these things, the next invitation is to see if you and your partner have some of your own big feelings bubbling at the surface. When we are suppressing *our* feelings, our babies will feel that and will often wait until we have done our own inner work. Having our own feelings heard by a loving listener can make a powerful difference, helping us be more present, which supports our baby to be comfortable to express their healing-feelings to us. If things still don't shift, I recommend having some 1:1 support from an Aware Parenting instructor. Big love to you all in this process.

Seven-month-old arches her body backwards when crying in arms

Q ~ I've recently started doing Aware Parenting with my baby. I used to always feed her to sleep, and now I've started to listen to her healing-feelings before sleep. I tried the position that you have in the back of *The Emotional Life of Babies* [note from Marion: it's also at the back of this book] but unfortunately she pushes off me with her feet quite hard and throws her body back in an arch off my knees, so I stopped doing it. However, I'm holding her in the cradle hold and she always thinks I'm going to feed her to sleep like I used to and that doesn't seem fair. I don't know what to do. Any suggestions?

A ~ I so celebrate your willingness to listen to your daughter's healing-feelings before sleep. I wonder if you find it helpful to know that her pushing off you with her feet while she's crying, and arching her body back, is all part of the physical process of healing through crying? It might be that she's revisiting her birth experience (since back arching often is) and healing from that. The pushing with her feet is part of her feeling a sense of power, which is part of the moving out of the fight or flight response. Even if it isn't her revisiting her birth, the physical action of her legs and arms is part of the release process. I wonder if you could put a pillow on your lap, and have a pillow behind your back, and return to the position I suggested, so you are supported while you support her when she's pushing and arching, so that she is safe? If this resonates with you, I invite you to experiment with it and notice afterwards whether she feels more relaxed when she's had a full body release like that. This process is always about experimenting to find what works most effectively for you and your baby. If that doesn't work, I invite you to experiment with other positions.

Is my nine-month-old too young for *Loving Limits* before a nap?

Q ~ I've been getting to know Aware Parenting for a little while. We've had some really traumatic events; her birth was traumatic and I'm a newly single mum. However, I am really committed to trying to listen to as many feelings as possible. My mum bought us a gentle sleep consultant (definitely not cry it out) as I have always struggled with her sleeping, particularly naps. But none of it sat right, as I still really want to co-sleep and I haven't done any of it but I feel like I wasted her money. My mum is staying with us lots at the minute to help me so she is seeing me constantly struggling and doesn't understand why I won't follow their advice. I am moving away from feeding to sleep and listening to lots of feelings at night and she is sleeping better in the night. But in the day, no matter how long she's been up when I take her into bed, she is just happy and crawling around. How do you set a *Loving Limit* with a baby? She obviously can't understand me saying it's time for bed now darling, even if I've drawn the curtains, I play 'asleep', etc. She would be happy just crawling around on the bed for the rest of the day. I don't want to stop her as I know her moving around could be letting out the feelings. But it would go on forever! I've been in there for over two and a half hours before, it's not until I rock her or feed her that she will go to sleep. Help!

A ~ I'm sending you so much love, hearing about the traumatic birth and the separation. What a huge amount you have been through. My heart goes out to you. I wonder if you have some empathy buddies for support with your own feelings, sweetheart? I so hear how tricky it is with your Mum and following the gentle sleep consultant's advice. As for the naps, if your daughter is clearly tired, and is clearly avoiding expressing feelings, you could offer the *Loving Limit* by gently preventing her from crawling around everywhere, if the crawling is clearly her distracting herself from her feelings. The moving around is very unlikely to be a way she's letting out feelings. I invite you to experiment with crawling beside her, and preventing her from distracting herself. You will probably find that helps her connect with her feelings.

How do I listen to feelings of nine-month-old twins before sleep?

Q ~ We have nine-month-old twins. How do I listen to their feelings before bed? One starts crying and then the other one starts too.

A ~ I'm sending you so much love. Being with the healing-feelings of one baby is a lot, and with twins, even more! The wonderful thing is, that we can really trust our babies. If one of the twins starts crying, and you are there and present with them both, and the other one starts too, you can trust that they are both feeling the *balance of attention* to express their healing-feelings to you. It's important that they can be close with you, for example, perhaps you're sitting on the floor on a soft carpet or rug, and they can crawl to you for closeness, and you can support both of them in whatever way is possible. That might be one arm around each of them, or one on your lap and the other cuddling up next to you. You can offer them your loving words, such as, *"I'm here with you both. I'm listening. I love you."* If they seem to have feelings in relation to sharing you, such as both wanting to be on your lap, you could offer them empathy, *"You both want to be on my lap. I so understand. I'm here and listening. I'm here with you both."* You said "we", so I imagine there are two parents. Whenever you can, having 1:1 time with each baby expressing their healing-feelings to one parent can be deeply healing too! You can deeply trust your babies and yourself!

Is it best to decouple feeding from naps and bedtime for 11-month-old?

Q ~ Is it best to completely decouple the feed from naps and bedtime? For example, feed straight after breakfast/lunch/dinner instead? I've definitely noticed that sometimes it seems like my baby is going to have an emotional release cry, then I feed her (as she normally feeds at that point and I think she'd be hungry otherwise, or at least upset as she's used to that connection/comfort) and then afterwards she's too tense to nap but the crying doesn't come.

A ~ As you've observed, breastfeeding is wonderful, *and* it also creates dissociation, because of the sucking and the hormones in the milk, so it may be much harder for her to access her feelings for some while after feeding. So if you're wanting to support her to feel and express her healing-feelings instead, not feeding her close to when she's tired will help her be more able to stay connected to those feelings so she can express them to you. This might mean lots of clear observation so you are really confident that you're differentiating between when she's hungry and when she has painful feelings to tell you. Love to you both!

Breastfeeding, crying, and sleeping (12-month-old)

Q ~ I have been nursing my 12-month-old daughter to sleep since birth during the day and at night, and holding space for her crying only when she initiates it herself. Diving deep into Aware Parenting and I've gotten to know that nursing to sleep is a *control pattern*, so I am trying to figure out how to keep breastfeeding her and also help her to sleep without my breast, for her naps and at night.

A ~ I so honour your willingness to both listen to your daughter's healing-feelings and also continue your beautiful breastfeeding relationship. I wonder if you find it helpful to know that there is no one way to do this. There are many different options, and I invite you to listen in to which way resonates with you and to experiment with it. One way you could go about it is to observe her, and to notice when you are really clear that she is asking for the breast to suppress feelings, and to start listening to her feelings at those times, when you are really clear that she isn't hungry. If you want to gradually stop feeding her to sleep, you could choose times where you have plenty of emotional spaciousness in yourself to listen to her feelings, and let her know that you aren't going to feed her to sleep and that you are there to listen instead. She will probably have quite a few accumulated feelings, so it might take some while for her to catch up with those. To start with, you might find that her feelings are closer to the surface in the evening before sleep, and after she wakes up from a nap.

Parents often find that the breastfeeding relationship becomes even closer and even more wonderful once more crying is listened to. They often feel less resentful and continue breastfeeding for longer because there is so much presence and connection during the feeds.

Crying before sleep once baby can crawl

Q ~ What happens when you go from crying in arms to a baby who can crawl? What does the situation look like? Do you lie next to baby or do you sit up next to baby? And what if the baby crawls away, do you lift the baby back to his place in the bed?

A ~ Things really change in terms of crying in arms before sleep once a baby can crawl, don't they? Each family will find their way with it. I talk about the shift to what I call *'the crying dance'* (which isn't an official Aware Parenting term). I see this as a bit like a partner dance, like the Tango, where we are following our baby's lead, staying connected, and seeing how close we need to be in order for them to still feel the physical and emotional safety to cry with us.

If they crawl away and are still crying, we can still stay present and listening, trusting that they know the exact distance that is healing, and will come closer if they need to. If they crawl away, and stop crying, I suggest following beside them, talking with them, and staying close so that they can stay connected with their feelings. If they try to leave the room, I would close the door and sit with them in the bedroom or wherever you are, offering a *Loving Limit – "I'm not willing for you to leave the room, sweetheart, because I don't think it's the most helpful thing for you, and I'm here and listening."* In other words, we're sensitively finding ways to ensure that the baby feels connected to us and to their healing-feelings. I wonder if this resonates with you?

12-month-old has always gone to sleep in the pram or car

Q ~ I've pretty much always helped my son go to sleep in either the pram or the car. Now that I know about Aware Parenting, I know that it's a *control pattern* and that I'm distracting him from his feelings through movement. How do I help him go to sleep without these?

A ~ Oh, I love that you understand this, and so support you in these next steps you're making. Instead of putting him in the pram or in the car, I would invite you to simply hold him or lie next to him when he's tired. You might first chat and perhaps do some *attachment play*. Then you might find that he moves into crying and raging with you. I invite you to see it all as an experiment, and to follow his lead wherever possible. For example, he might get really playful, and you might play peek-a-boo type games with him. I trust that you will find a new way together, based on his own innate relaxation response.

13-month-old pulling my hair whilst breastfeeding to sleep

Q ~ My 13-month-old likes to pull my hair and rub it between her fingers while breastfeeding to sleep. I can't stand it, I'm aware it's likely a *control pattern*, and I just continue to redirect her hand and ask her to please not pull my hair. Does this sound reasonable?

A ~ Hello lovely, oh I really hear that you really can't stand it and that you're aware that it's likely to be a *control pattern*. If you're not enjoying it, and you're clear that she has healing-feelings at that time that she's trying to express, then it's clearly not meeting either of your needs. I wonder if you would like to feed her at a different time, perhaps a bit earlier, and then listen to the painful feelings that her pulling your hair and rubbing it between her fingers is trying to suppress. That way you could both get your needs met. You can prevent something that you can't stand, and she can express the feelings that are bubbling up when she's tired. Does this resonate for you? I'm so willing for you to both get your needs met.

14-month-old refusing to go to sleep in his cot

Q ~ For the past week, my 14-month-old boy has been refusing to sleep in his cot. Previously we had no issues, but now he will start screaming when put in his cot, even if he's already asleep. We have spent a lot of time listening to him, explaining that we're still around, etc. I've also tried lying on the floor next to his cot, with my hand on him to let him know I'm still there with him, but he's just inconsolable. There have been a few nights where it has taken two to three hours to get him to sleep and it's really wearing us all down. Any advice would be much appreciated, thank you.

A ~ Hello lovely, I'm sending you so much love. There could be a few different things possibly going on here: closeness, agency, and accumulated feelings. I wonder if you'd like to play around with them to discover which one it is.

Closeness: It's normal for babies and toddlers to want closeness when they're going to sleep. I wonder if you might put a mattress on the floor where you could both lie down together next to each other and see what happens then. Or would you like to do this in your own bed?

Agency: Similarly, his need for agency might be coming in here – it's natural for toddlers to want to be able to do things, and to feel frustrated or powerless in response to being restricted in a cot where they can't get out. The mattress or bed experiment could also help you see whether that is happening for him.

Accumulated feelings: The third possible factor is accumulated feelings. The fact that you say he's inconsolable suggests that he's expressing some big feelings from the past, using his natural healing and relaxation process. I wonder if that resonates with you? If so, you could simply be right there with him, again, on the mattress or bed or whatever other way you experiment with for closeness, listening to his painful feelings, and supporting him with this healing process that he's going through. In doing this, it will also help him sleep more restfully. I'm so willing for you to get clear about what is going on for him.

Can I co-sleep with a baby and a 14-month-old?

Q ~ I'm expecting another baby in a few months but still co-sleeping with my first baby who is 14 months old. We have been night weaning for a few weeks now. I'm not really sure how I can manage two babies in one bed. I would like to begin to transition my son into his own bed now but when I think about putting my son in his own room I'm bombarded with overwhelming thoughts and feelings like, "He will feel alone and abandoned and unloved." I read the saying, 'If it doesn't feel right then it might not be right,' but I'm sort of wondering what other option I have now with a second baby coming so soon.

A ~ Hello lovely, I so hear that you don't know how you will manage with them both in one bed, and that you think your toddler will feel alone and unloved if you put him in his own bed in his own room. I love how you are listening to what doesn't feel right for you and him. I wonder if you would like to make your bed into a really big bed. Depending on the size of your room, that could mean putting a single bed next to the big bed you already have to make a giant bed. Having two mattresses next to each other on the floor is another choice that many families love. I think you will find that your toddler being able to feel your closeness at night will help him in this huge transition he's about to go through. In addition, the more of his healing-feelings you can listen to before the baby is born, the more deeply he will sleep and the less likely he'll be woken up by the baby. I wonder if any of this resonates with you? I'm so willing for you to find a way that's a fit for everyone in your family.

15-month-old distracts himself from feelings before bed

Q ~ I try and let my 15-month-old have a cry with me whenever he needs it which is generally at bedtime. I get him ready in his pyjamas and sleeping bag (he sleeps in our bed), nurse, then we have a bit of a play on the bed and I usually let him know that we are now getting ready for bed. At that stage he is so tired that he barely can keep his eyes open. And when I take him in my arms he will start crying (great, I want him to), but he keeps finding ways (pointing at things) to distract himself from crying. Then I let him go and he babbles and plays for a little longer and I try again. Then the whole thing kind of repeats itself until I eventually reach my limit where I just don't have the capacity to listen anymore and I offer him to nurse again which obviously calms him and after that he is fine and lays with me and maybe takes 15-20 minutes to fall asleep. Any suggestions on how I can handle this situation differently?

A ~ Hello lovely! I so honour all that you're doing with your son before bed, and yes, I have a suggestion – I wonder if it will resonate for you? Perhaps you might find it helpful to remember about *Loving Limits*? When he's distracting himself, you could offer one of these – for example, *"I see that you want me to look at that, and I'm not willing to do that right now, because I don't think that's the most helpful thing for you, and I'm here and I'm listening."* It's our role to help our lovelies stay connected with their feelings, and it's so normal that we get frustrated if they keep distracting themselves from their feelings and we don't offer a *Loving Limit*. I wonder if you'd like to play with this to see if it helps him express his feelings more easily, and if you also observe how that affects his sleep and other behaviour? You might also find that feeding him a bit earlier on will mean that his healing-feelings are more accessible and he can cry more freely with you.

18-month-old fights sleep

Q ~ Our son has had a really great start, we had a home birth and breastfed and co slept until a couple of months ago. Since that time, he has had lots of feelings at bedtime. We slowly transitioned him in with his brother to help with connection but he often stays awake for an hour after his brother. He fights sleep and throws himself around. We try to settle, rock, and hold him. Eventually he falls asleep but we find it very frustrating. We do lots of play and connection but I feel like we are missing something as he is very unsettled and often wakes in the middle of the night also.

A ~ Oh I so hear how frustrated you have felt and I'm sending lots of compassion to you. I wonder if it resonates with you that the settling and rocking is likely to be suppressing his feelings that are trying to come up before sleep, and that rather than him fighting sleep, it might be that you are (in the most loving of ways) fighting his natural relaxation process. I so trust your sense that you're missing something and I wonder if it's the crying and tears? I wonder if, after the play, you might find that naturally the feelings start to bubble up for him, and perhaps get located on a pretext for a cry. Children are so wise, and will often find a situation to hang their feelings on, so they can let them out. Aware Parenting can

377

invite you to be an emotional detective, looking for times where your son is inviting *attachment play*, or trying to cry to release stress. Our role is to watch for those invitations and support them in that. Does this resonate with you, lovely?

18-month-old awake until midnight

Q ~ I'm wondering what is the Aware Parenting perspective is on sleep regression? For the past two weeks my 18-month-old won't go to bed until around 11pm/midnight. He won't nap until 3-4pm most days. Some people have suggested trying to cut the nap out so that he goes to sleep earlier in the night, but it is very difficult to keep him awake and he just becomes overtired and doesn't go to bed early anyway. I want to trust him that he knows his own body but my own needs for sleep are not being met. I read online that sleep regressions are common at 18 months, but I can't recall reading anything in Aletha Solter's book so far, so I was curious what the Aware Parenting perspective is on them. I'm also unsure if this stage will pass on its own or if I should be intervening somehow?

A ~ Hi lovely, oh I so hear that your own needs for sleep aren't being met. My heart goes out to you. And I love your question! In Aware Parenting we don't have the term 'sleep regression' – instead, we see that when a baby or toddler is taking longer to go to sleep, it can often be a sign of accumulated feelings. Additionally, we don't have the term 'overtired'. Instead, when children start getting antsy and crying when they are tired, an Aware Parenting approach would be to move in close and support the expression of those healing-feelings. Then, there is the timing of his nap. Is he showing signs of tiredness earlier than 3pm? Have you tried moving in with closeness and seeing if he has feelings to express? If he doesn't have a nap, I wonder if you see invitations for crying in the evening when he gets tired, such as he isn't happy with anything you offer, or he starts to cry over small things? If he's really tired, because he's missed having a nap, he's likely to be able to access his healing-feelings more easily and have a bigger and more intense cry, which will then help him feel more relaxed and sleep more restfully. Watching out for ways you might be inadvertently distracting him from his feelings could be another way in. The more relaxed he feels, the more likely this sleep pattern will shift.

18-month-old, new sibling, and co-sleeping

Q ~ I'm about to give birth in a few months and I have an 18-month-old. They will be so close in age. How can I co-sleep with both children? How can I create a better sleep arrangement with two kids under two? My son is having difficulty sleeping with his dad, as I have co-slept with my son since birth. I just can't see them both sleeping in the same bed in the beginning together, I know I won't be able to support each of them at the same time.

A ~ There are so many ways to go about this, so I invite you to explore what you would really love to do. I have seen every single option in families. One beautiful way can be to have two beds or two mattresses together, so there is lots of room for everyone. You might have another room with another bed set up, so you and your partner can play around with the different arrangements as time goes on. The most important thing to remember is to listen in to yourself and do what really resonates with you, rather than doing what other people tell you to do, or what you might have internalised about what you 'should' do. There are so many ways for you to all get your needs met and I'm so willing for you to find one that you really love. One of the factors that will make the biggest difference is your son expressing the highest percentage of feelings you can possibly support him with before the baby is born. The more that happens, the more relaxed he will be in his body, the more restfully he will sleep, and the less he will be woken by his new sibling. Big love to you all.

22-month-old distracting herself from feelings before sleep

Q ~ My daughter takes a long time falling asleep, usually 1-2 hours both day and night. When she is tired, I usually follow her lead and play a little (wild and silly), sing a little and then I set a *Loving Limit* and say that it's over now, and if she needs it I listen to her. She rarely gets angry or upset, she just finds something else to entertain herself with. Like she keeps wanting to talk about things, wants a toy, the duvet on and off and that's how it goes in circles, even though I try not to agree with it and I hope for a big cry – which rarely really comes. She gets frustrated and finally sleeps. But it doesn't seem right the way she falls asleep. And when she finally does sleep, she sleeps restlessly by moving around a lot in bed in her sleep and she often wakes up and cries after one hour's sleep. She is really unhappy and with a frustrated cry – and she wakes up easily from the slightest sounds too. Do you have any suggestions on how I can help her? Should I set a *Loving Limit* sooner? Should I decide that then we take the duvet away as she constantly takes it off and on so she might be able to cry over that?

A ~ Hello lovely, oh I so deeply acknowledge all that you are doing and how long it's taking. I celebrate that you can clearly see all the ways that she still has accumulated feelings – the restless sleep, the waking up crying or waking up from the slightest sounds.

And yes, I would trust your sense here – it's our role to help our child feel connected with their feelings, so if they're doing a lot to try to distract themselves, we can help them in this situation by offering *Loving Limits*. If you are clear that this is accumulated feelings and not needs, and then when she asks for another toy, you could offer a *Loving Limit: "I hear that you want a toy, sweetheart, and I'm not willing for you to have that right now because I don't think that's the most helpful thing for you, and I'm here and I'm listening."* Or when she wants to keep moving the duvet, to find a way to gently offer a *Loving Limit* there. The aim is for her to find what I call an emotional coat hanger[53] to hang her feelings on, so she can express them and then feel relaxed enough to sleep. She needs your help with this. I wouldn't take the duvet away. With the *Loving Limit*, we're aiming to stay really close to the true situation that they are presenting. I so trust that you experimenting with *Loving Limits* will bring about a beautiful shift with sleep.

P.S. It took me years of practicing to really embody Loving Limits. It's really common for that to be the case for us, because of growing up in the *DDC*.

---

53 This isn't an official Aware Parenting term, but it's a way I describe when a child finds a pretext to let out healing-feelings.

Helping nearly two-year-old feel comfortable with dad putting him to bed

Q ~ How can I help my (almost) two-year-old to become comfortable with having dad put him to bed? It's been me doing it for two years – my partner is starting to try and chip in more, but my son struggles to let him do it if I'm around. Even with connection and play before bed he still only wants me. Is there anything to help this if we haven't had time to build connection before bed (on those days that are – finish work, pick up from daycare, race home, dinner, bath, and bed)?

A ~ Hi lovely, I so acknowledge what a huge thing it is that you have been supporting your son to sleep for nearly two years. I wonder if you feel called to offer your son a *Loving Limit: "I hear that you want me to put you to bed tonight, sweetheart, and Daddy is going to put you to bed tonight because I am going to xyz"*, and then listen to his healing-feelings. Or his dad could do something similar: *"I so hear that you want Mummy to put you to bed, sweetheart, but I'm putting you to bed tonight because Mummy is going to do xyz, and I'm here and I'm listening"* – and then listen to his feelings. If you can see this as a helpful opportunity for your son to express healing-feelings he's been holding in, and if you observe he's actually more relaxed and happy after expressing emotions like this, it's likely to give you reassurance that this is helpful and not harmful to him. So much love to you all.

Waking up

Is my six-week-old waking because he needs closeness, or because he has healing-feelings to express?

Q ~ I realise that in *Classical Attachment Parenting* the ideal is to 'contact nap' with your children. I have a four-and-a-half-year-old, a two-year-old and a six-week-old. I usually have the baby in a carrier but sometimes my back hurts and I try and put him down to sleep (in our queen bed that we sleep in together overnight). Sometimes he is happy enough to sleep in there for an hour or so but often the moment he realises I'm not there next to him he will cry and then stop as soon as I picked him up or lay next to him. Is this just normal baby behaviour (need-feeling to not be alone/for physical presence) or could this 'restlessness' be considered a symptom of unexpressed healing-feelings?

A ~ I'm sending love to you and your back and I so support you in finding ways that are a fit for both you and your baby. I so deeply acknowledge you and all that you are doing, not only caring for your baby, but your other two children too. In case you find it helpful to know, we don't use the term 'contact nap', in Aware Parenting. It's possible that your baby is waking because he is needing the closeness with you, but it's more likely that he didn't get to complete expressing his healing-feelings before sleep and that his sleep is more superficial as a result. I invite you to experiment with listening to as many of his feelings as you can before each nap and sleep, and to support him to complete the whole crying cycle. Then observe whether, after 10-15 minutes of him going to sleep, you can then place him down and he stays asleep. I'm here with you, cheering you on!

Four-month-old has 'sleep regression'

Q ~ Our baby is currently going through a four-month 'sleep regression' and we have found it really hard. He used to sleep through the night and wake up happy. Before bed we would offer a lot of connection and he would generally fall asleep in our arms and sleep through. In the past few days he has been waking around 1am and then waking every hour after that until morning. When we tell this to people and look for support, we are being shamed for the fact that we aren't sleep training and are being told that he should no longer be contact napping and should know how to self-settle. My baby co-sleeps with me and having him close just feels right. Each time he wakes, I give him a cuddle and he fairly quickly goes back to sleep, but staying asleep is the problem. Is there anything different I should be doing or will he get past this sleep regression on his own if we just keep giving him all of our love, support, and closeness?

A ~ I'm sending you lots of love, hearing how hard you're finding this, not only with his waking, but also in your experience of being shamed for not sleep training. I want to let you know that I so celebrate all that you are doing with co-sleeping and how much that you are deeply listening in to what resonates for you. I also acknowledge all the connection you've been offering him before sleep. I wonder if you find it helpful to know that 'sleep training', 'contact napping', 'self-settling', and 'sleep regression' are all terms that aren't included in Aware Parenting. In Aware Parenting perspective, there are three things that babies need for sound sleep: to feel tired, to feel connected, and to feel relaxed. If a baby is tired and connected – as your baby is – but is not relaxed, and keeps waking up, it's generally because they have unexpressed accumulated feelings.

By four months, if we didn't know about Aware Parenting, the feelings a baby has from being in the world have often accumulated to a point where those feelings are waking them up more and more often. This is because they are trying to release those feelings so that they can feel more relaxed.

From an Aware Parenting perspective, listening to a baby's healing-feelings before sleep supports them in being able to stay asleep for as long as they need, or until they are actually hungry. I wonder if any of this resonates for you? If it does, you might experiment with changing what you do to help him to go to sleep. If you're rocking or feeding him to sleep, it's likely that those actions are distracting him from the healing-feelings that are waking him up later on. The more of those emotions he expresses before going to sleep, the less likely he will need to keep waking to try to express them then. You really can co-sleep and breastfeed and have restful sleep!

Six-month-old waking up crying

Q ~ I have recently come across Aware Parenting and I love it! Our six-month-old was waking every two hours to feed, was quite easily settled and went back to sleep. Now, we have no issues with getting him to sleep at the beginning of the night, however, it's the wakings that we struggle with, he has only slept for longer than a three-hour stretch a few times. He has recently been waking in quite a tizz, heavy crying and agitated body and then harder to get back to sleep. The nights are very long at the moment. How can I support him to have longer stretches of sleep?

A ~ Hello lovely! In general, when a baby's stomach gets bigger, he can take more milk at each feed and go longer in between each feed and sleep for longer. If we don't realise this and keep feeding them at approximately the same intervals, we might then be interpreting their healing-feelings as needs-feelings and feeding them when they have healing-feelings to express. Then their unexpressed feelings start accumulating and accumulating. This is very common, and is why babies can start taking longer to get to sleep and become more restless in their sleep. This could be what is happening when your baby is waking up crying. It sounds as if he is waking to express some healing-feelings to you. Does that resonate? You might want to observe him even more closely during the daytime to discern whether you are feeding him when he isn't hungry but has healing-feelings to express. Also, holding him in your arms and listening to his feelings before he goes to sleep is likely to mean that he catches up on expressing them then, and so will be less likely to be woken up by feelings that are bubbling up to be expressed later on. I wonder if this resonates with you?

Seven-month-old wakes up after crying in arms

Q ~ I'm interested to learn more about managing crying in arms, co-sleeping, and naps. My baby always falls asleep on me after crying in arms and I end up either transferring him to a sling to carry him on me or waiting for him to wake up. In the evening he sleeps earlier than I do so I usually have him on me until I go to bed. I would like to have some time in the evening or during his naps when he sleeps separately but he has never done this and I'm not sure how to do it. Perhaps just putting him down next to me when he is deeply asleep? I worry that this will cut his sleep short and he will wake after one cycle. I don't want to leave him in a separate room.

A ~ Hi lovely! I hear that you're worried that if you put him down next to you when he is deeply asleep that this will cut his sleep short and he will wake up. If you have listened to as much crying as he needs to do, then waited for a while until he's moved into deeper sleep, and then place him down next to you, you're likely to find that he stays asleep for as long as he needs to sleep. If he wakes more quickly, it's likely because he has more feelings to tell you, in which case you could listen to more if you're willing, and in future, to make sure you support him to complete the whole crying process before falling asleep. Does this resonate with you?

Eight-month-old is waking early

Q ~ Currently I bed share if my eight-month-old wakes after her second feed or if her second feed is in the early morning (4 am onwards) as she seems to need more closeness. However this probably isn't sustainable for us as a family in the long term.

A ~ Hello lovely, I'm hearing that this isn't sustainable for you as a family and I'm sending you lots of love. Is it the waking up, the feedings, or the bed sharing part that isn't sustainable for you as a family? If it's the bed sharing part, I wonder if you've thought of playing around with the bed set up for your family? Sometimes there can be surprising ways for babies to get their needs met for closeness. It's very normal for a baby of that age to need closeness in the daytime and at night. As a form of attachment-style parenting, Aware Parenting advocates meeting a baby's attachment needs while also doing what you can to meet your own needs. Does that resonate for you?

If it's the waking up twice at night that isn't sustainable, you might want to explore what's going on for her that she's waking up twice at night.

Listening to more of her healing-feelings in the evening and before she goes to sleep is likely to mean that she can sleep for longer during the night. In addition, is the closeness meeting her needs for connection, or is she clinging on in a way that suggests she's dissociating from her feelings through those actions? If the latter, it might be that she's dissociating from her feelings in the daytime or evening, which is why she's doing it again in the night. I imagine there are a few things to discern here. I'm so willing for you to get really clear about what's going on so you can all get your needs met for sleep and closeness as a family. I recommend a consultation with an Aware Parenting instructor if you're not finding clarity.

Do I need to listen to feelings at night (10-month-old)?

Q ~ My baby is 10 months old and had a traumatic birth, with separation and medical intervention. I began listening to healing-feelings three months ago, starting with five minutes and gradually building up the listening time. I am slowly but surely seeing the improvement in reduced wakes at night. Will the more feelings that are listened to in the day/before bed continue to reduce the wakes at night or is more night listening required?

A ~ I'm sending so much love to you and your baby, hearing about the traumatic birth you both experienced. And I so celebrate you gradually being able to listen to more feelings. And yes, in general, the higher the percentage of healing-feelings that you listen to during the day, and particularly before sleep, the more and more relaxed your baby will feel in the night, thus they will wake up less and less. However, some babies do seem to need to cry in arms at night to heal a particular part of their birth experience, e.g. if something significant happened at 2am, they may always wake up then to heal from the experience through crying in arms. However, many babies *do not* need to specifically heal from birthing experiences at nighttime and will gradually catch up on expressing accumulated feelings by crying in arms before sleep. I invite you to keep experimenting and observing, to see which is the case with your baby.

'Self-settling'

Q ~ How can I help my baby learn to 'self-settle' when she bed-shares part of the night?

A ~ In Aware Parenting, we see what is called 'self-settling' in other paradigms as teaching babies to dissociate from feelings. Rather than doing this, I would suggest offering your baby closeness when she wakes up, and an opportunity to express her feelings then. Or you might want to focus on listening to more feelings during the day, particularly before naps and sleep, which will help her be less likely to wake up when bed-sharing. Does this resonate with you?

'Resettling' my six-month-old

Q ~ I'd love to know how to tackle a resettle, day and night. Once they have a release and then fall asleep, if they wake up after one sleep cycle crying, do we just hold them until/hoping they would fall back asleep? I usually would feed my baby back to sleep or give the dummy and rock her back to sleep. But then I struggle with short daytime naps.

A ~ Hello lovely, if your baby often wakes up after one sleep cycle, it might be that she isn't getting to express a whole chunk of healing-feelings and to complete a crying cycle before going to sleep, particularly if you are feeding her or giving her a dummy to go to sleep. Have you played with inviting more healing-feelings when your baby is moving towards sleep, by changing position, lovingly looking in her eyes, and saying something like, *"I'm still here and listening, sweetheart. Do you have any more feelings to tell me?"* And yes, instead of feeding, giving her a dummy, or rocking her if she still wakes up, you could simply hold your baby in your loving arms, being present with her, and see if she has more healing-feelings to express to you. If you're wanting longer daytime naps, maximising listening to healing-feelings before her nap will often be most likely to help.

Do I need to turn the light on at night when listening to my seven-month-old baby's feelings?

Q ~ Often I feed my son back to sleep, but sometimes, when it's clear that he has got some emotions that are waking him up, I lie next to him and hold his hand while he cries. I don't know whether that is enough emotional support for him. Do I need to sit up and turn the light on?

A ~ I'm sending you so much love. Listening to crying in the middle of the night can be so hard, especially if we're feeling really tired. Your question is related to the *balance of attention*. Your baby needs to know that he is physically and emotionally safe in order for the crying to be healing. As long as he's got lots of physical connection with you, I imagine he is feeling that. However, I find that many parents like to have a very low light, so that their baby can see their eyes if they need to. A red light that is blue-light-free can be helpful here. That way he can see you if he needs to, but it's less likely to wake you both up, and there's no need to sit up in order for him to feel connected with you. I wonder if that's a fit for you?

Is feeding to sleep/night feeding my eight-month-old biologically normal?

Q ~ My friends tell me that that feeding to sleep and night feeding are biologically normal and that I shouldn't stop that for my eight-month-old son. How would Aware Parenting address this?

A ~ These are common perceptions, aren't they? There are two separate issues here: feeding to sleep and night feeding. I invite you to listen in to each of these for yourself and to what resonates for you. Does it resonate with you that it's biologically normal for babies to be fed to sleep? Or does it resonate with you that babies need to feel tired, connected, and relaxed to go to sleep, and that crying in arms is the innate biological process they have to release stress and trauma from their bodies before sleep? If it's the latter, would you like to experiment with this? For example, you could feed your baby for naps and before sleep for a period of time, such as over a 24 or 48 hour period, and observe him. Then you could aim to listen to his healing-feelings before sleep for the same length of time. Then you could notice the differences in those two different situations, especially in terms of his eye contact, muscle tension, and sleep.

Then I would ask you the same question, in terms of what resonates with you, in relation to night waking. The wonderful thing about this one is that we don't need to do anything differently at night. For example, if listening to healing-feelings resonates, you might experiment with practicing that before sleep and then observe to see whether your baby starts sleeping for longer stretches at night. If he does, that would give you the evidence that he doesn't have a biological need to wake up at night to feed then. Through deeply listening to yourself, experimenting, and observing your baby, you will discover your own answer.

From an Aware Parenting perspective, breastfeeding a baby to sleep when they are not hungry is not necessary for them at any age.

Nine-month-old always teething

Q ~ My nine-month-old seems to be always teething, that's why she doesn't sleep much and keeps waking up. What's the Aware Parenting take here?

A ~ I'm sending so much love to you and your daughter, hearing that you're not getting much restful sleep. From an Aware Parenting perspective, teething can affect sleep. The mild discomfort of teething can mean they don't sleep as restfully as usual. However, sometimes, wakefulness diagnosed as being caused by teething might not be fully accurate. If a baby seems to be consistently wakeful at night, without showing those typical signs of teething during the day, it may be that they have accumulated painful pent-up feelings that are waking them up lots, rather than uncomfortable gums. In addition, when babies are teething, they will commonly experience painful feelings too – such as confusion, overwhelm, and powerlessness. So it's also normal that they will need to do more crying in arms to release those feelings. If they're not doing that, or not enough of that, they will also be even more wakeful.

As for whether to listen to healing-feelings while the teething is happening, this is really a personal choice.

With Aware Parenting, we first do what we can to reduce discomfort as much as possible. That might include giving a baby cold or hard things to chew on to bring relief. However, we can also trust babies and their innate body wisdom. If after doing what we can to reduce or eliminate physical discomfort, they choose to cry in our loving arms when all their needs are met, we can then listen to the healing-feelings. This may well help them move through the teething more easily, with fewer accumulated feelings. Have you ever stubbed your toe when you had lots of feelings bubbling, and had a big rage or cry, and then felt much calmer and more comfortable afterwards? Sometimes, when babies do crying in arms while teething, it can actually help the teething be easier.

In general, I've found that the higher the percentage of healing-feelings a baby gets to express, the less challenging teething is for them.

Shall I wake up my 10-month-old?

Q ~ They say, "Never wake a sleeping baby". So I didn't – until sleeping became a problem. I became desperate and took some sleep training advice (didn't know about Aware Parenting yet) about waking your baby around the same time every morning and waking him up if his naps take longer than one hour. I really would like to know the Aware Parenting approach on this. Do I wake my baby at the same time every morning or do I let him sleep until he wakes up by himself?

A ~ Hello lovely, Aware Parenting is all about deep trust in babies, and recognising that babies know exactly what they need. From an Aware Parenting perspective, we wouldn't recommend waking up a baby if they are sleeping. We really can trust babies! However, if there is an important reason, such as your baby is having a late nap in the afternoon and that means he will go to be really late and you won't get much sleep that night, then I would invite you to wake him up so you can get the sleep you need. Aware Parenting is about both parents and babies getting their needs met. I'm so willing for you to both get your needs met.

10-month-old waking three times a night and I want to reduce it

Q ~ My 10-month-old is waking three times a night and I know she's not hungry every time. I always used to feed her to sleep, but as I've got more confident with Aware Parenting, I stopped doing that about a month ago. Before that, she was waking up about seven times, so I am so pleased with how things are going. What shall I do next? I think she is probably only hungry once during the night now. I'd like to drop the feeds to twice at night, and then to once.

A ~ I so celebrate all that you've done already as you've got more confident with Aware Parenting. There is no set way of doing this next step, and lots of choices. Which way resonates with you? You might want to focus on increasing the amount of healing-feelings you listen to during the day, especially before her nap and before sleep in the evening. The more painful emotions she expresses, the less feelings will be there to bubble up at night. And/or you might want to listen to some feelings during the night. That will depend on when you're most confident that she's not hungry and when you have most willingness to listen to her crying. For some parents, that might be the first wake up, especially if she wakes fairly soon after going to bed and you know she's not hungry. Other parents find it easier to listen once their baby starts waking up more and more frequently, because they can be sure that it isn't hunger, because the gap is much shorter than the hunger spacing they are confident about. Over time, you night want to stretch out the time gap of when you're willing to feed her. I wonder which of these most call you right now? I'm so willing for it to all go smoothly and easily for you.

No crying with 12-month-old when on holiday

Q ~ We are away and we are staying in a hotel room with people on all sides. I haven't allowed any cries before bed or in the middle of the night and I feel overwhelmed and exhausted. I feel like we've taken ten steps back and our nights have gone back to how they used to be before not feeding to sleep, waking 5/6/7 times and being on the boob for a long, long, long time. I'm feeling so resentful and frustrated when he wakes in the night, and am starting to resent breastfeeding. I am in a vicious cycle!

A ~ Oh sweetheart, I'm sending you so much love and compassion. I so hear that you are overwhelmed and more exhausted than ever. My first suggestion would be to reach out for some emotional support, so you can share your resentment and frustration. I'd also love to offer compassion to you in the situation of being away. I think it's so natural to feel uncomfortable to listen to feelings in this situation and my heart goes out to you. I wonder if you are hiring a car whilst you are away? I used to find that when on trips away, driving somewhere private and listening to my children's healing-feelings in the car was really helpful when staying with people. Is something like that possible for you? I also hear the frustration and resentment and am so willing for things to shift for you soon, either finding somewhere where you can listen to your baby's feelings, or once you get home again, listening to his feelings more again. Big hugs!

13-month-old using my body as a dummy

Q ~ At the moment our biggest challenge is sleep. We co-sleep and my 13-month-old son has never really slept more than 2-4 hours in a row without waking up and wanting boob. I also feel he uses my body as a bit of a dummy, often from about 2-4am he just wants to suckle to keep himself asleep. It also doesn't feel like he drops into a deep sleep as every time I try to get out of bed to leave him asleep it's not long before he wakes up. Up until now I've been okay to go along with it and prioritise his sleep and need for connection, however it's starting to take a toll. It's quite exhausting and can lead to frustration. It impacts my relationship with my partner and impacts time to myself. I feel I need to start making some proactive steps to assist his sleep. Any advice would be appreciated.

A ~ I'm sending so much love to the exhaustion and frustration that you're feeling. And I so honour all that you've done to prioritise his sleep and connection. Listening to his healing-feelings will also help him feel connected and will help him sleep more relaxedly and more restoratively. I wonder if you find it helpful to remember, when you're feeling frustrated, that you supported him to feed when he had healing-feelings, and you also have the power to support him to express those feelings through crying instead. If that resonates, I wonder if you are willing to listen to him crying with you before sleep rather than feeding him to sleep? If you feel the energy and willingness to do so, you might also want to listen to his feelings in the night when you're clear that he isn't hungry. The more relaxed he feels, the more he will be able to sleep, which means you will all get your needs met more. He wants to sleep restfully as much as you want him to. So much love to you.

16-month-old waking three to four times a night

Q ~ Our 16-month-old is still waking 3-4 times a night and requiring our assistance to fall back to sleep. Is this normal? Is it normal that he has NEVER slept through either? I mean not even close (from newborn - 12 months he woke almost every 1-2 hours) it's soooo so hard not to get angry at this point, I'm so tired.

A ~ I'm sending you so much love. I really hear how tired you are. And I so hear how hard it is for you to not feel angry, after all that you have been through. My heart goes out to you. I wonder if you find it helpful to know that your son doesn't want to be waking up this much either, and that he wants to sleep peacefully as much as you want him to. If he was waking every one to two hours, it sounds like he had quite a lot of unexpressed feelings bubbling up and waking him up. (Either that, or perhaps he was feeding at similar gaps in the daytime.) Did he have a stressful birth or time in utero? Did you know about Aware Parenting back then? When did you start listening to his healing-feelings? The more unexpressed healing-feelings a baby has, the more those feelings will wake them up at night, to be released through crying.

Rather than seeing something as normal or not normal, I love to discover what is going on for each individual baby or child. Does it resonate with you that he is waking up because of unexpressed and pent-up feelings? If so, I would recommend fully encouraging and supporting him to release through both *attachment play* and supported crying before sleep. You might also want to look at what assistance you are giving him to fall back to sleep. Are you giving him the opportunity to cry with you at those times? The more he gets to express pent-up feelings in the evening and before sleep, the less likely it is that those feelings will wake him up at night. And if he is still waking up at night, you might listen to his crying then.

If the night waking continues even after you are listening to his feelings before sleep, you might want to gradually increase the gap between the beginning of one feed and the beginning of the next during the night. In her article[54], *"The Crying-in-arms Approach for Helping Babies Sleep Through the Night,"* Aletha Solter recommends an approach of offering increasing intervals over three weeks. Please note this is only for older babies of at least six months old. She recommends three-hour intervals for the first week, four-hour intervals the second week, and five-hour intervals in the third week. If the baby wakes up before this amount of time, you can be lovingly present with her and listen to any crying she needs to do with you. Aletha Solter says,

"Most babies begin to sleep through the night before the five-hour interval is reached. However, I don't recommend total night weaning because some babies may still need one night feeding past the age of six months. Please note that this approach is only for babies who are co-sleeping. If your baby sleeps alone in a separate room, the reason for night waking may simply be a need for closeness."

19-month-old wakes up every hour from 3am onwards

Q ~ For context, I have a 19-month-old son and we've been practicing Aware Parenting for five months and listen for his feelings daily. Before Aware Parenting he would be up every 45 minutes and now he wakes up 3-4 times a night (so much better now). I started night weaning him a month ago, hoping he would start sleeping through the night, but he still wakes up every hour usually from 3am onwards. So now he sleeps well until the early morning and then keeps waking up until he fully gets up at 6.30am. I've been trying to listen for feelings during those hours but he doesn't go there and just wakes up fully. So now I 'give in' and just give

---

54 You can find this on The Aware Parenting Institute website, www.awareparenting.com

the boob cause I'm afraid he will get up and not fall back asleep. Would you have any awareness on how to support him so he could sleep longer stretches in the early morning?

A ~ I so celebrate all the listening to your son's feelings you've been doing for the past five months. I love hearing that he's feeling so much more relaxed in his body now and how that's helping him sleep much longer. As for how to support him so he can sleep longer stretches, I would suggest aiming to listen to more feelings during the day, and particularly before he goes to sleep at night. The more he gets to release through laughter and play, and crying and raging before bed, when his body will be naturally trying to do that, the less he will need to wake up at night to try to express the feelings then. Does that resonate?

How can I prepare my 19-month-old for one night away from me?

Q ~ I'm going for a retreat at the end of the year for one night and it is the first time I've been apart from my son at nighttime. Normally we co-sleep and I'm still breastfeeding him 2-3 times a night. He will stay home with my partner who is very hands on and has no problem putting him to sleep. But I do worry about how he will go when he wakes up and I won't be around. My plan is to keep my son informed about it (I like to talk to him when he is asleep so it all sinks in to the unconscious as well), and to keep talking about it with my *Listening Partner* and friends so I won't have any big feelings around it when the time comes. I'd love to hear ideas on how to support him and minimise any stress. Maybe some *attachment play* games about separation? Thank you!

A ~ I'm sending love to you and to the worry you're feeling about being away from him for that night. I love your idea of separation games. I wonder if you might also want to do two things:

1. Focus on listening to more healing-feelings before sleep, so that he is waking up less at night by the time you do go away;

2. Experiment with him sleeping for parts of the night just with your partner, so your son can be releasing feelings with him whilst you're

still in the house and he can be without you at night for shorter periods. That way, I imagine he can also catch up on some of the crying that isn't coming out at the moment. I imagine that might be the *balance of attention* he needs to be able to express the feelings that are waking him up. That way, you can also work slowly towards being way the whole night and gauge how he is with it all. I imagine this might be a beautiful opportunity for him to express some big feelings with your partner, especially if breastfeeding is a bit of a *control pattern*. I wonder if either of those resonate with you? I'm so willing for it all to go really well for you all!

19-month-old co-sleeping daughter wakes up the minute I do

Q ~ My daughter is 19 months old and sleeps pretty well during the night but will wake up the minute I do. I don't make any noise or movement. She isn't ready to wake up as some mornings it's 5am and she's only had 9 hours sleep and she usually has 10-11 hours. She does have her own big bed but I haven't moved her in there yet. Could transitioning on her own bed allow her to sleep better without my disturbing her?

A ~ Hello lovely, I'd love to offer two thoughts. One, is that it is normal for toddlers to be attuned to our presence. Their attachment needs are still so strong at this age and they still need so much closeness. So waking up when we get up and they don't have that closeness any more can still happen because of that. Their accumulated feelings can also have an effect here, especially if breastfeeding has been a *control pattern*. If this has been the case, then being in particular positions in relation to us can then be a *control pattern*, meaning that when we move away, the feelings that have been suppressed bubble up. Or her waking could be a combination of these two causes. You might find that listening to more feelings before bed helps with the second part of this – you could experiment to see if it does. The more crying and raging she does with you, the less likely it is that she will wake up because of the second reason. Does any of this resonate with you? I wouldn't recommend moving her to her own bed when she's either needing closeness or more emotional releases. There are many other ways for you to both get your needs met, and I am so willing for that for both of you.

Stopping feeding 19-month-old to sleep

Q ~ I am sensing that now is the right time to stop feeding my 19-month-old to sleep. He is starting to show signs of not needing my breast anymore. Up until now he has been on my breast until almost asleep and then I place him in his bed and stay with him until he is asleep. Last night after feeding him and him appearing to be almost asleep I lay him down in his bed and he got straight up and reached over wanting to be cuddled. I cuddled him for a short while and put him back in his bed. Again he sat up and reached out. This time I said, *"It's sleep time now and I'm here with you."* He started getting upset and eventually started crying. I kept repeating, *"It's sleep time now, I'm here, I'm listening and I love you,"* while leaning over and cuddling him. About 20 minutes later he was quite distressed so I picked him up and held him and he fell asleep in my arms then he went down in his bed. Today for his nap I didn't offer my breast but held him and he fell asleep in my arms before laying him down in his bed. I am not sure if I'm doing this correctly? Last night was the first time I really listened to crying while using Aware Parenting language. Was not picking him up but assuring him I was with him, the right thing to do? Whenever I pick him up, he stops crying straight away, so am I not meant to pick him up and hold him? I'm confused what crying in arms is if that is the case.

A ~ Hi lovely, it's such a big and new practice, isn't it? I so acknowledge all that you're doing. First of all, I'd love to respond to your question about picking him up. If we have often breastfed our babies when they had feelings to express, it can get harder for them to express their feelings when they are in our arms, being a similar position to where we have suppressed their feelings. Does that resonate with you? In addition, the term 'crying in arms' refers to non-mobile babies. Once they can crawl to us, they don't necessarily need to be in our arms for crying to be healing. Having closeness and our loving presence is often enough for toddlers to feel safe enough to heal through crying with us. However, they *do* need to be able to choose to be close with us if they want to while they're crying. Since he's in a bed and not a cot, it sounds like he can make that choice. But as always, I invite you to check in with yourself. When you were leaning over and cuddling him, did you feel a sense of connection between you? If you have generally fed him to sleep, he has some accumulated feelings to express which are probably what you were seeing when he was crying with you. Again, I invite you to listen in to yourself and to him. Did you see a difference in his sleep that night after crying with you, and did you see any difference in his behaviour the next day? The more we see differences, the more reassurance we receive. Love to you both.

20-month-old waking up 10 times a night

Q ~ My 20-month-old baby has never slept through the night, he wakes up 10 times during the night, yet he would sleep by himself more than two hours during the day. Am I wrong if I wake him up after a maximum 2.5-hour nap?! Otherwise he will sleep even worse during the night or wake up super early in the mornings. What do you suggest I do?

A ~ Hello, lovely! I'm sending you lots of love, imagining you waking up 10 times during the night with him. What are you doing with him before sleep? When toddlers are waking up that much at night, it's often because of accumulated feelings. Does he get to have crying sessions with you before bed? If not, my suggestion would be to look for ways you might be inadvertently distracting him from his feelings and thus his natural relaxation-through-release response before bed. Does this resonate with you? As for waking him from his nap, if that is helping him have more sleep and that is helpful to you, I so support you in doing what you need to do. Your needs are so important.

Theory Questions

How do we help them feel calm?

Q ~ I'm confused about do we need to help them regulate, e.g. with breathing interventions, or just let them go until they're finished and eventually they naturally learn to regulate?

A ~ Hi lovely, I'm sending love to the confusion. I want to let you know that in Aware Parenting, we don't use the term 'emotional regulation', because in some other paradigms, it is sometimes used to mean what we regard as dissociation or suppression. With Aware Parenting, we trust that their bodies are innately wise, and when they get to fully express their feelings all the way to the end, they will be really deeply relaxed. I've seen it thousands of times and it's a level of relaxation we're not used to seeing in this culture. So we don't need to teach them to become calm, instead we are invited to learn how to support them use their innate wisdom to become completely relaxed. Does this resonate with you and bring clarity? Much love.

How do babies who are left alone sleep well and long?

Q ~ What is the explanation that children who are not raised based on Aware Parenting sleep well and long? I have seen it many times. In my work in daycare (with one to three-year-old children) where the children are put to sleep for the first time in the institution in the pram and cry hysterically (I will never let that happen again!) one to three times – and from then on, always seem to be able to fall asleep easily and sleep for two to four hours. And among friends where the children get pacifiers, are rocked in prams, etc. (all the known *control patterns* you can give children) and who sleep between two to five hours during day naps! And the whole night like seven hours at four months old! What a luxury! And some sleep in their own beds too. But how can that be from an Aware Parenting perspective? And why are my children still waking up at night when I am listening to their feelings?

A ~ Hello lovely, I so hear that you have been thinking about this, and I have a few answers.

1. People often confuse relaxation with dissociation. This is why people often think that a baby or child who has stopped crying when they are jiggled or rocked or given a dummy is now actually feeling relaxed, when from an Aware Parenting perspective, they are not relaxed but are in a mild form of dissociation. With the children at your daycare, it is likely that they are dissociating rather than feeling relaxed.

2. Paradoxically, sleep itself can also be a form of dissociation. Perhaps you've noticed yourself feeling sleepy when offering a

child *attachment play*. This is because big feelings are coming up, and sleep is a way to dissociate from them. For some babies and children, this can be the case, and might also be what you're seeing.

3. Some children who use *control patterns* that aren't related to a parent's body will actually wake up still, but they will not cry or call out and instead will dissociate again by repeating the *control pattern*.

4. As for your children not sleeping that long: I so celebrate all the listening to feelings you are doing. I find it helpful to remember that because all of this is so new for most of us, we will only be able to listen to a percentage of our child's feelings, and whatever percentage we are *not* listening to, they are holding in their bodies, and this affects how relaxed they are, which also affects their sleep. However, because they have closeness and because you do listen to their feelings, if they wake up at night, they do not do what you are talking about with other babies and children who simply stay quiet and go back to their *control patterns*. Instead, your children let you know that they have unmet needs or healing-feelings. Also, their *control patterns* are more likely to be related to our bodies, such as breastfeeding, which means they will let us know they have awoken, which a baby or child who doesn't get closeness at night and who has a *control pattern* not related to our bodies is less likely to do. How do you feel when you read this? Does it bring clarity? Big love.

Our own feelings

Feelings towards own mother

Q ~ I'm struggling with feelings about and towards my own mum. The more I listen to my boy cry and rage, the more memories I have of feeling so alone with my emotions as a child and having no one to listen to me. I was always labelled a bad sleeper as a child and teenager, and still struggle with insomnia but I now really remember just not wanting to go to sleep because I felt so alone. My mum often talks of how I was a terrible sleeper as a baby and how I exhausted her, and I can't help but feel angry when she says this now.

A ~ Hello lovely, I'm sending so much love to all the feelings you are feeling now, including the anger you feel when you hear your mother say how you exhausted her. My heart goes out to little you, who felt so alone with your emotions and didn't have anyone to listen to her. I wonder if you find it helpful to know that it's really normal and natural for us to have big feelings show up from our own infancy and childhood when we practice Aware Parenting? In fact,having these feelings heard is a core part of practicing Aware Parenting. That's why I highly recommend at least one empathy buddy, and/or working with an Aware Parenting instructor. As we listen to our child's feelings, we can also get to express the feelings we felt as babies and children. Lots of love to you and all of your feelings. I'm so willing for you to have them heard in beautiful ways.

> ### Self-Reflection Moment
> What are you thinking, and how are you feeling, after reading these? Did you have any aha moments? Did any feelings bubble up for you? I want to remind you how big this process is, getting free from our conditioning in relation to sleep. It's so normal for this to be a big process for us!

SECTION 2 SUMMARY

How are you feeling after reading this whole section?

This was a big section, and I imagine that if this information is new for you, that you might want to return to it several times, and that each time you do, new things will jump out at you or make sense, or fall into place.

Please remember that this is a huge step to take and is literally undoing generations of conditioning. Please be gentle with yourself and remember both to put down any harsh sticks and get plenty of emotional support and listening for your feelings. This really is a vital part of practicing Aware Parenting!

I'm here with you as you continue to take in this information.

PART 3

Children (2–12 years) and sleep

23. The three ingredients for restful sleep and what you can do to help your child sleep restfully

Please note that in the other sections of the book, the word 'children' is used to refer to babies, children, and teens, but in this section, I use the word 'children' to refer to the age group of 2 - 12 years.

Our responses to our child will obviously change as they make that journey from two to 12!

Here again are the three ingredients for restful sleep:

i.   to feel tired (sleepy);

ii. to feel connected (*closeness creating a sense of safety*); and

iii. to feel relaxed (*by releasing any healing-feelings present*).

i. To feel tired (sleepy)

Common signs of tiredness in children include:

• yawning

• losing interest in activities

• difficulty concentrating

• losing coordination

• lying down

What this means in practical terms

Observation

Once we observe that our child is sleepy, we can then move to the next two ingredients, i.e. offer them connection if they still need it while going to sleep, and follow their cues when we see opportunities for them to release tension through laughter, crying, or talking.

As a form of attachment-style parenting, the aim in Aware Parenting is to support independence at each child's own unique pace and timing, by sensitively responding to their burgeoning confidence and competence.

If we generally respond aptly to their sleepiness cues when they are younger, we can trust that they will listen to their own sensations of tiredness as a result. Through observing them, we'll see when they know how to take responsibility for going to bed themselves when they are tired.

If we often distracted them from their healing-feelings when they were tired as babies or younger children, it's possible that they also learnt to dissociate from their sensations and feelings of tiredness.

If that's the case, we can focus on supporting them to fully reconnect with the sensations of sleepiness in their bodies. There are many ways we can do that.

We might help them understand the difference between sensations of hunger and sensations of tiredness. This can be through conversations together, sharing about how we experience sleepiness, and how they might notice it in themselves. We might play games which help them listen to the sensations of tiredness in their bodies. We may even explain about how we responded to them when they were younger and talk about the possible results of that, without judging ourselves when we tell them the story.

> ### Self-Compassion Moment
>
> *I invite you to drop any self-judgment or guilt sticks here, and to be compassionate with yourself. This is particularly vital if we do share this kind of information about our past responses with our child. If we are judging ourselves and feeling guilty, they are less likely to be free to express the feelings they feel when they hear the information about how we responded to them in the past. Whereas, if we've felt and expressed any sadness to a loving listener before we share this information with our child, we are likely to offer them an open space to freely tell us how they feel.*

This philosophy continues throughout their childhood and into adulthood. If we're willing to hear their feelings in relation to what we did or didn't do to them in the past, without judging ourselves or becoming defensive, they will be free to heal from any hurts or ruptures. This is a profound gift of healing that we give them. Many children and adults are not able to have healing experiences with their parents because the parents judge themselves and aren't able to hear their child's experience without feeling guilty or becoming defensive.

ii. To feel connected (*closeness creating a sense of safety*)

In the *DDC*, we are taught that children 'shouldn't' need closeness, but as you'll remember from the early chapters about our hunter-gatherer ancestors, it is absolutely normal for children to need to be close at bedtime in order to feel safe.

Closeness supports children to feel safe to fall asleep without dissociating. Our emotional state will also affect how safe they feel when we are close with them.

> I'm not going to suggest any particular age that a child can go to sleep without closeness (and without dissociating), because each child is unique in their timing of when they feel safe enough to do so.

This invites us to observe each individual child and recognise their own pace and timing of when they no longer need us to be with them when they are falling asleep (once they feel safe when alone).

> ### Self-Compassion Moment
> *If you left your child to sleep alone before they were ready, or if that happened to you as a child, and you're feeling painful feelings, I'm sending you so much love. I invite you to reach out to your empathy buddy or other loving listener, to share your emotions and have them lovingly heard.*

Highly Sensitive Children[55] often need closeness while going to sleep and through the night for a lot longer than other children (and are generally ready for sleepovers at a later age too). This is because of their nuanced sensitivity to stimulation. They are picking up more information and so are likely to experience not feeling safe at night until later than other children. From an evolutionary perspective, we can imagine that they were of great service to the community, being able to pick up on possible danger before anyone else.

Children who have experienced a lot of change or trauma may need closeness while going to sleep for more years too, because they are still learning that they are safe now. Other factors related to closeness and safety can affect this timing. For example, the distance of their bedroom from the living areas and other bedroom/s and whether it is on the same level (if you live in a home with more than one storey), and whether they are sharing a bedroom with a sibling or grandparent, or a dog or cat.

Over time, children become increasingly independent at their own timing and pace, and they will naturally get to a point of not needing to be close to us to feel safe and be able to fall asleep without dissociating and sleep restfully.

However, the need for closeness generally reduces gradually. On some evenings, they might want to go to sleep alone in their own room, whereas at other times they might prefer us to be in their room as they fall asleep, and on yet other nights, they might want to go to sleep in our bed with us.

---

55 This term and concept is from the work of Elaine Aron.

The more connected with them we are, and the more we trust their unique pace and timing, the more we will be able to sensitively support them with this process.

A child who is newly able to go to sleep without us physically touching them might still want to know that we are in the next room, or close by. It's likely to be a long while before they would feel safe enough to be comfortable and relaxed to fall asleep if there were no-one at home with them.

You might find it helpful to see this whole process as a gradual movement towards independence – and the embodiment of them knowing that they are strong and safe.

Once they no longer need closeness with us to go to sleep without dissociating (i.e. unless *control patterns* are clearly getting in the way of them listening to their tiredness cues), Aware Parenting invites us to trust their timing of when they want to go to sleep.

In her book *Attachment Play*, Aletha Solter explains that children can learn to take responsibility for when to go to bed sometime between six and twelve years of age (page 111).

What this means in practical terms

Opportunities for connection

Cuddling, massages, and holding a child's hand can all meet needs for closeness, and each child will have different ways that they prefer to feel connected. *Attachment play* can also really contribute to a deep sense of embodied connection and safety, particularly types of play which include lots of body contact, such as rough and tumble games.

Even once a child is able to go to sleep without closeness, filling up their cup with connecting with us during the day, and particularly in the evenings, can help them feel an ongoing sense of connection – and thus safety in their bodies – to fall asleep without our physical presence.

Joss, a Level 2 Aware Parenting instructor in Australia, shares about her journey with her children's sleep:

"I always knew that I wanted to co-sleep with my children and we slept together from the night my first child was born. It made so much sense to me from an evolutionary perspective that closeness and connection whilst falling asleep and during the night would support my children's needs best. I realised that as a child I longed for that myself and found it really healing for us to be together. It is so natural for children to want a loving caregiver to be with them whilst sleeping and at particularly stressful times, it was so clear to me that having me close supported much deeper relaxation, emotional safety, and attachment.

We had lots of different arrangements in the first few years of having two children. I slept in between both of my children right from the night my second was born. In that way, I found it easiest to respond to both in the night, to ensure their needs for close connection were met and to be available to feed when required without getting up. At times, my partner would sleep with us, and at times he would sleep in another room, sometimes with my older child if he was disturbed by the baby crying. But I would initially listen to her feelings in the day and at bedtime and feed when she woke during the night to minimise disruption for everyone else. I really loved co-sleeping (and really missed it when they chose to move into their own rooms).

We co-slept for many years and they chose for themselves when they wanted to be in their own room. This really met their needs for choice and agency and, even then, there were times when they were sick or had big feelings and wanted to sleep with me again for a night or two. I know it added an extra layer of deep connection and trust between us for them to know I was always available for closeness and support in this way."

Self-Compassion Moment

I'm sending love to you however you feel when you read this. If you feel sad when you reflect on choices that you made in the past, I invite you to share those feelings with your empathy buddy. I'm here to remind you that whatever happened in the past, it is possible to repair ruptures and foster more profound and deep connection with our children. It's also never too late to help them feel a deep sense of support, connection, and safety in their bodies, thus affecting their ability to sleep restfully and peacefully.

iii. iii. To feel relaxed (*by releasing any healing-feelings present*)

Tantrums and crying with our loving support continue to be two of the key processes to bring about deep relaxation and restful sleep, especially in early childhood. However, play and laughter also become much more common ways to support relaxation as toddlers become young children. I'll share more about *attachment play* in the next chapter. As they move into later childhood, children increasingly release their painful feelings through talking about their experiences.

However, it's still natural that an older child will sometimes need to cry or rage with us before they go to sleep.

Talking never fully replaces the powerful healing and relaxation processes of laughter and crying.

Please note: Young children can sometimes feel scared and resist sleep because they fear that they won't wake up again, especially if they have heard expressions like 'putting a dog to sleep' and 'putting a child to sleep'. In that case, the child would need accurate information to feel safe. You might also choose to change your language so that they clearly understand the difference.

If a child is sucking their thumb or a dummy, or always wants food or drink when they are tired, or always snuggles in under the crook of our arm in a particular position, or rubs the skin on our hand while going to sleep, these are signs that these have become *control patterns* for them. Those behaviours may be helping the child temporarily bypass feelings that are bubbling up when they're tired. If they go to sleep that way, it's likely that those feelings will bubble up again later, causing agitation, wriggling, restlessness, or night waking.

What if an older child no longer needs closeness with us to go to sleep, but often uses a *control pattern* to suppress their healing-feelings, such as reading or screens? Here, we are invited to support them to reconnect with their body and feelings so they can feel more connected and relaxed and can also respond aptly to their sensations of tiredness.

Holding a long-term context that our intention is for our child to become a teen and then an adult who is deeply connected with, and responsive to, their own sensations of tiredness, and their needs for connection and safety, and who is willing to express their feelings through talking, crying, or laughing – can be really helpful.

Remembering this can support us to refrain from trying to force or coerce them to go to sleep when *we* want them to.

What this means in practical terms

Following your child's lead, whether it's with play and laughter, crying and raging, or talking about their day

We can *trust* that our child knows what they need to feel relaxed, even if they learnt to override it when they were younger. The innate wisdom is always still there, even if it's become a bit hidden.

If they start getting playful before bed, we can join in with them, using *attachment play* principles to maximise the power of their play and laughter. As they get older, they might simply use humour, and likewise, we might respond in humorous ways.

If they start crying over something small, we can trust that this is a *'broken cookie moment'*[56] and listen to the big feelings that the small thing is giving them a pretext to feel and express.

If they are asking for lots of different things and none of them is actually meeting their needs, it's likely that they need us to offer them a *Loving Limit*, e.g. *"I really hear how much you want to wear the blue pyjamas, but they're in the washing machine, sweetie. I'm not willing to take them out, because they're all wet. And I'm here and I'm listening."*

Or perhaps they're doing everything they can to distract themselves from their feelings. In which case, we can be that *emotional shepherd dog*, staying close, offering connection and *Loving Limits*, *"I'm not willing for you to go back to the playroom now sweetheart, because I don't think that's the most helpful thing for you, and I'm right here and I'm listening,"* and listen to the crying or raging that will probably follow.

Or maybe they're asking you to read them another ten books, and you see that's a distraction too, because they are so tired, so again you can offer a *Loving Limit*: *"I really hear that you want me to read you another book, darling, and I'm not willing to read any more, because I don't think it's the most helpful thing for you right now. And I'm here and I'm listening."*

As they get older, they might have *control patterns* which don't require us, such as eating or using screens, and we might respond with *attachment play*. However, if our child is trying to dissociate through food or screens, we have a slightly different approach concerning *Loving Limits* compared to with most other *control patterns*.

Why we don't recommend *Loving Limits* with food

In Aware Parenting, we don't generally recommend using *Loving Limits* with food, except in particular situations, including breastfeeding

---

56 When a child's feelings have accumulated, they try to release them through small pretexts. The term 'broken cookie' comes from one such example: when there is only one cookie left in the jar, and it is broken, and the child starts crying about the broken cookie.

(because it's the mother's body), or if the child has issues with weight or illness. This is because our aim is to help children be deeply connected with their innate body wisdom in relation to food.[57] In addition, they might experience a *Loving Limit* with food as arbitrary and authoritarian. However, this can be challenging if our child has already learnt to suppress their healing-feelings with food before sleep. We will often need a lot of listening to our own painful feelings if we see our child regularly wanting to eat to suppress feelings when they're tired.

However, not offering *Loving Limits* with food doesn't mean not doing anything when we observe them using food to dissociate from their feelings. They still need our support.

There are lots of things we can do to help children with food *control patterns*, including:

- Moving close with connection and warmth;
- Offering *attachment play*[58], e.g. giving them a non-food item and pretending to insist that it is food, when it's actually a hat, or a sock;
- Giving information;
- Role modelling the relationship with food we want them to have;
- Inviting them to listen in to their sensations and what their body is communicating;
- Inviting a pause, e.g. that they hold the food or cutlery in their hand and tune in to how they are feeling;
- Helping them release their painful emotions in other ways and at other times;
- Using *Loving Limits* in response to other *control patterns* that they have.

---

57 You can learn more about the self-connected approach to eating in Aletha Solter's book *Cooperative and Connected*, and there is a chapter on this in my book *I'm Here and I'm Listening*.
58 I offer more ideas for *attachment play* in the next chapter.

You might be curious about that last point. If we offer *Loving Limits* in response to other *control patterns*, they will have the opportunity to release more of their healing-feelings, so they will be less likely to need *control patterns* with food.

However, as always, please listen to yourself here. If on occasion you feel really called to offer a *Loving Limit* with food, I invite you to trust yourself.

The difference with *Loving Limits* with screens

In Aware Parenting, we also don't recommend just offering random *Loving Limits* to children in relation to screens, including before sleep. This is because they might experience this as arbitrarily overpowering them.

> ### Self-Compassion Moment
> If you're feeling frustrated, powerless, incredulous or any other uncomfortable feeling when you read about refraining from initially offering Loving Limits *with relation to food or screens, I'm sending you so much love. This information can help us connect with painful feelings, and having regular opportunities to express those emotions with our empathy buddy and/or Aware Parenting instructor can make a huge difference.*

However, again, not offering random *Loving Limits* with screens doesn't mean not doing anything. Our child still needs our support. Yet, our options for how we might respond to their screen *control patterns* are slightly different to our responses with food.

We might:

- Have *conversations* with our child;
- Make *agreements* with them about their screen use;
- *Remind* them when the time (or other measure, such as game level) that we agreed is coming to an end;
- *Communicate* our *trust* in them and their capacity to stick to the agreement;

- Offer connection and *compassion* if they're finding it hard to stick to the agreement;

- Offer *attachment play*[59] to support them to get off the screen;

- If they still don't get off the screen, offer a *Loving Limit* along with the information, e.g. *"I'm not willing for you to watch any more/play any more, sweetheart, because I want us to stick to the agreement that we made, and I'm here and I'm listening."*[60]

Self-Compassion Moment

If you're tempted to pick up sticks because you've often offered Loving Limits *in relation to food or screens, I invite you to put those sticks down. I wonder if you find it helpful to know that I sometimes used* Loving Limits *with my son with screens in the evenings when he was in his early teens (and that it didn't go very well!) which you'll read about in the teens section. I didn't have this information back then. As always, I invite you to be compassionate with yourself, and trust what you feel called to do.*

Later childhood and trust

Once they move into later childhood, they might need our help if they are clearly tired but are dissociating from their tiredness (and possibly healing-feelings) through various *control patterns*.

Our aim is to trust them to listen to their bodies, but also to see when they are repeatedly not doing that, and to support them to reconnect with that inner listening in helpful and respectful ways.

We might:

- Have compassionate conversations in the daytime about whether they notice when they're tired.

- Ask them how they feel in the morning and respond with empathy.

- Lovingly help them see the connection between what time they went to bed and how they feel.

---

59 I offer more ideas in the next chapter.
60 There's a whole chapter on screens in *I'm Here and I'm Listening*.

- Ask if they want help to listen to their bodies.
- Experiment together with plans, e.g. everyone getting off screens or stopping reading at a certain time, and having a family alarm go off.
- Bring in *attachment play* or general humour in the evening.

> ### Self-Compassion Moment
> If you see your child staying up past when they're clearly tired, and you feel frustrated, powerless, or angry, I'm sending you so much love. If we feel concerned about their future, whether that's how they will feel tomorrow, or how they will be when they grow up, we can easily move into using power-over. I'm here to remind you that it's so important that we tend to whatever shows up in us first, so that we're more likely to be able to respond to them in loving and supportive ways.

Moving in with judgment or power-over is likely to lead to disconnection. However, if we're able to be calm and compassionate, because we've attended to whatever has shown up in us, we're much more likely to be able to respond to them in helpful ways.

Moving close with connection, compassion, warmth, fun, and support is way more likely to be helpful in supporting them to listen to themselves and trust what their bodies are telling them.

You might find it helpful to remind yourself that our long-term goal is to support them to respond to the three ingredients for restful sleep in themselves, through internalising our responses to them.

Our aim is to help them listen to when they are tired, to be willing for their own needs for safety and connection to be met, and to express feelings that arise in the evening in healing ways.

Focusing on helping them to know how to do these three things by how we talk with them and listen to them can be a helpful reminder when we are tempted to try to get them to go to sleep when and how *we* want them to!

Talking can be a *control pattern*

If they are wanting to talk about their day, you'll be able to tell whether the talking is helping them feel more relaxed, or whether it's the kind of talking that is actually distracting them from expressing deeper feelings.

How might you distinguish the difference? If while they're talking, you notice them becoming more relaxed, more connected, and making more eye contact, then it is meeting that need. In contrast, if you have a sense that they're talking 'at' you, that they're just as agitated after talking for some while, and you don't seem to be connected with each other, it could be that the talking is actually a *control pattern* that is distracting them from their healing-feelings.

Your loving presence can support them to release those feelings if they are trying to distract themselves. You might want to move in closer, offering eye contact, gentle touch, and letting them know that you're there with them. You might offer some *attachment play* related to talking, or offer a *Loving Limit* (although that can be hard with talking as a *control pattern*). As they move into later childhood, humour can increasingly replace *attachment play* as a way to bring about connection and laughter.

A *control pattern* related to our body can prevent them from timely independence

If a child has a *control pattern* related to our body, this can get in the way of them becoming independent in their own intrinsic timing. This can happen if we often breastfed them when they had healing-feelings to express, or if we rocked them to stop them from crying. They might need to be curled right up under our arm to go to sleep, or be glued to us, or pinch our skin or twirl our hair to suppress feelings. These *control patterns* can get in the way of their own timing of being ready and willing to sleep more independently. The innate next step for them might be still co-sleeping, but not needing to always have physical contact when sleeping, or that might be in their own bed in our room, or in their own room.

If this is the case, supporting them to express the feelings that these *control patterns* are preventing can help them not only sleep more restfully, and for us to sleep more restfully too, it can also support them to be free to sleep more independently at their innate timing and pace. Starting off with *attachment play* can be a helpful part of this process, and then you might want to offer *Loving Limits* and listen to the healing-feelings.

Restlessness and moving to their own room

I often hear from co-sleeping parents who want to move their child into their own bed because the child is so restless. If you're in that position, I'm sending you lots of love. However, the child is likely to be restless because of accumulated feelings, and putting them in their own bed while they are still in that state is likely to lead to more stress. Instead, supporting them to release those feelings so that they can sleep in a relaxed way will be much more helpful for them. Then, the child can move into their own bed when they are developmentally ready to not need that closeness anymore.

When can we trust a child to choose their own bedtime?

Once a child no longer needs closeness with us in order to go to sleep without dissociating, we can support them to take responsibility for when they go to bed. For most children, that will be sometime between six and twelve years of age.

The outcome of the attachment-style-parenting aspect of Aware Parenting is true independence at their own timing and pace.

When we support them and trust them to learn about going to sleep from their own experiences, that means that they continue to learn from listening to their own internal barometer. They learn about when they feel tired, and what happens if they don't go to bed when they're tired, and how they feel the next day.

However, if they have a *control pattern* that they're using regularly before bed, such as reading or screens, which is preventing them from being able to respond aptly to their own tiredness cues, we can support them with that, through conversations about *control patterns*, suggestions, such as to experiment in doing without that *control pattern* for a night or a week, and to see what happens, or joint agreements (which might be followed up by *Loving Limits*). We might offer plenty of *attachment play* to bring about warm connection and presence. This might require us to have lots of listening for our feelings first!

These are with the intention of supporting a child to be connected with their body, and their innate wisdom regarding sleep, rather than the aim of getting them to do what we want them to do. This is a vital difference.

What if we didn't practice Aware Parenting when they were younger, or we always fed them when they were tired?

In situations like this, we can help them reconnect with, and accurately read, their tiredness cues and sensations, while conveying trust in them and their bodies. We might offer repair for the times when we taught them to not accurately understand when they were tired, or if we used rewards, punishments, or harshness to get them to go to bed when we wanted them to. Putting down the guilt sticks can be an important part of this process!

Self-Compassion Moment

I'm sending you loving compassion if you are new to Aware Parenting and have done lots of things differently. As always, I invite you to put down any guilt sticks, to be deeply compassionate with yourself, and to remember that it is never too late to change things.

A note on language and 'not being a good sleeper'

You might find yourself saying that your child "isn't a good sleeper" or similar. How we think about and speak about our child affects how we feel and respond, and also affects their core beliefs about themselves.

Instead of thinking that their sleep is about who they are, I invite you to speak of their behaviour in the form of specific descriptions.

For example, *"My daughter woke up four times,"* or, *"My son took two hours to go to sleep last night."*

The more that we understand that our child's sleep is deeply affected by how much connection they experience, how safe they feel and how much stress, tension, and accumulated feelings they have, rather than being an innate trait of theirs, the more likely we will feel powerful in knowing that we can help them change.

We're also more likely to be compassionate with them, and to know that they don't want to be experiencing whatever it is that's going on that's challenging with their sleep. They want to sleep as much as we want them to sleep!

Note – this is unless there are really exciting things going on and they want to be a part of that, or they're really needing connection with us because they haven't experienced that during the day, so they're staying awake to connect.

Another note – however, being a night owl or an early bird does appear to be an innate trait, a chronotype!

I love this next story from Kylie (who is a Marion Method Mentor) and her son, Jake. Kylie shares a story from when Jake was a baby, and then another one from when he was seven years old. This is a lovely example of how the principles of crying with loving support before sleep remain the same between infancy and childhood, but look very different in practice:

"When my youngest child was somewhere between six and nine months old, I saw a post shared by my beautiful friend, Georgie, about Marion's work about Aware Parenting that was in relation to sleep. I was feeling desperate with my baby waking so frequently through the night at 45 minute intervals, and we were not getting quality sleep. Not knowing what else to do, I would breastfeed him back into another short stint of quiet. I looked up more about Marion and learned about crying in arms. I found enough information to help me understand the benefits and how to do it. That night, after we'd all gone to bed, and my baby woke for the first time, I got up and took him into the lounge room where I did crying

in arms with him. While he cried, I didn't try to stop or distract him, but instead was able to hold him lovingly and listen to his feelings while his perfectly designed body connected in, processed, and released what it needed to.

To my surprise and sheer delight, his feelings shifted, he became deeply relaxed in his body, and drifted off into the most peaceful, contented and lengthy sleep. It was a miracle! I remember sharing a post on social media at the time saying – there is a God and her name is Marion Rose! Haha!

Last year, when my same son was seven years old, he had a really big buildup of feelings at bedtime. I sat beside him while he raged, thrashing and kicking and hitting the bed and pillows. At times he would yell at me to go away. I continued to sit with him. Over the years Marion had offered me lots of information and support to help with the reassurance I needed to know that even though he was yelling at me to go away, he really wanted me to stay with him and didn't want to be alone with his feelings. At one stage, however, I lost my confidence and my faith wavered in what I was doing. I got up and walked towards the door to leave when he called out to me, 'Don't go, Mum!' Gosh... I am teary remembering it. What an incredibly beautiful, powerful moment for us both.

For me to have doubted myself and my ability to support him and then receive his confirmation that he did need me to continue being present with him in that way and for him to call me back and have the safe experience where I compassionately responded and continued to be there with him and all that he was feeling. I am so grateful that I had the awareness and understanding to be able to respond to him lovingly, without any judgement or shaming thoughts towards his seemingly contradicting requests that I likely would have had in earlier years of my parenting journey.

Soon after this, his raging shifted into a big sobbing cry where he shared the big challenging theme he was feeling really sad and powerless about. He cried and cried. I offered lots of love, empathy and reflection of what he was sharing with me including validation of his feelings. When his tears dried up and his sharing was complete, he drifted into the most relaxed, peaceful, rejuvenating sleep. I am often in awe of this incredible approach to supporting not only children but adults as well, including myself.

I so deeply value understanding and experiencing how life-changing the simplicity of:

- *meeting our needs;*
- *having adequate information; and*
- *the support we need to process and shift big feelings truly is.*

Lifetimes of love and gratitude to you, Marion, and Aletha Solter, from Kylie and Jake xoxox"

CHAPTER SUMMARY

There are three ingredients for restful sleep in children:

i. To feel tired (sleepy)

If we generally responded aptly to their sleepiness cues when they were younger, we can trust that they will listen to their own sensations of tiredness as a result. Through observing them, we'll see when they know how to take responsibility for going to bed themselves when they are tired. If we often distracted them from their healing-feelings when they were tired, we can support them to reconnect with the sensations of tiredness in their bodies.

ii. To feel connected (closeness creating a sense of safety)

It is normal for children to need to be close at bedtime. Our emotional state will also affect how safe they feel when we are close with them. Each child is unique in their timing of being able to go to sleep without closeness and without needing to dissociate. It can be helpful to see this process as a gradual movement towards independence and them knowing their strength and safety. Once they no longer need closeness with us to go to sleep without dissociating, we are invited us to trust their timing of when they want to go to sleep.

iii. To feel relaxed (by releasing any healing-feelings present)

Crying with our loving support, play and laughter, and talking are all ways that children release feelings before sleep, and we can follow their lead with whichever they choose. Our aim is to trust them to listen to their bodies, but also to see if they are dissociating from healing-feelings, and if they are, to support them in helpful and respectful ways. Our long-term goal is to help them respond to the three ingredients for restful sleep in themselves, through internalising our responses to them.

In Aware Parenting, we don't generally recommend using *Loving Limits* with food. We also don't recommend offering random *Loving Limits* to children in relation to screens before sleep. However, this doesn't mean not doing anything when we observe a *control pattern* with food or screens. There are lots of other options for us with both of these.

If a child has a *control pattern* related to our body, this can get in the way of them becoming more independent with sleep in their own innate timing. If this is the case, supporting them to express the feelings that these *control patterns* are preventing supports them to be free to sleep more independently at their innate timing and pace.

I so deeply trust that you can help your child grow up to have a healthy relationship with sleep.

24. Playing before sleep

Laughter and play, like crying and raging, are two of the key ways children heal from stress and trauma and release tension from their bodies so they can feel more deeply relaxed.

Big shifts can happen when we understand these natural relaxation processes, because we now can welcome rambunctious play before sleep.

Rather than trying to 'calm down' a child when they are being playful, we can trust that they are using their effective and innate healing process to become deeply relaxed.

When we understand that a rambunctious child is simply trying to use their intrinsic wisdom to feel deeply relaxed before sleep, how we feel and respond can change radically.

If we're telling ourselves that they're fighting sleep or 'being annoying', we're likely to feel frustrated.

If we're telling ourselves that they're trying to use their innate body wisdom to feel relaxed, we're more likely to feel calm and compassionate, and to be able to cooperate with those processes.

We can cooperate by:

- Joining in with their play utilising *attachment play* principles and practices.
- Offering *attachment play* if they're clearly agitated but not moving into crying.
- Listening to them crying or raging if it comes spontaneously during or after the play.
- Offering *Loving Limits* if they move into aggression during the play, or if they want to play for hours when they are clearly tired (to help them express the underlying healing-feelings).
- Offering humour and jokiness as they get older.

For play to be maximally powerful in helping a child feel both connected and relaxed, they need us to be present with them.

> ### Self-Compassion Moment
> *I'm sending you love if you're thinking, "Oh no, what, another thing for me to do!!" and I so deeply acknowledge all that you are already doing. I also want to offer the possibility that you actually might really enjoy this time. You might also find that you feel more connected with your child/ren. You may even feel more relaxed afterwards and sleep more peacefully too! However, I invite you to not coerce yourself to play with an "I should do some attachment play".*

Yet, if you are willing:

If they're running around the house, how about running around with them!

If they're jumping off the sofa, would you like to jump too?

If they're playing being a character, what about becoming a complementary character?

If they're using humour and laughing, how about joining in with the laughter?

Trusting that our child knows what to play to help them feel more relaxed, and joining in with them, brings more effectiveness to the play. Understanding *attachment play* and bringing in particular elements to the play can help a child feel even more connected, relaxed, and powerful, all of which are helpful for their restful sleep.

Attachment play is a core part of Aware Parenting, based on the book of the same name by Aletha Solter, which I highly recommend.

Attachment play:

- helps children *heal* from stress and trauma;
- supports them to *express* and *release* feelings such as fear and powerlessness; and
- equips them to both *prepare* for, and *process*, new experiences.

I'll always remember a really clear experience of the power of play and laughter, when my daughter was a tween. One afternoon, we were given tickets to see her favourite band the next day. That required us getting up very early the next morning to get on a plane. For several hours in the evening, she was literally jumping up and down with joy, dancing around the kitchen, expressing all her exuberant excitement. I was with her, reflecting back her excitement to her, and enjoying seeing her joy. I was excited too, but I forgot that joining in with her play would also be helpful for me, and so didn't join in with her loud exuberance. After all her releasing through rambunctiousness and laughter, she had a beautiful restful sleep and woke up bright-eyed and bushy-tailed at 4am, whereas I lay awake most of the night, full of excitement, and felt really tired the next morning. It was such a clear demonstration of the power of releasing feelings before sleep through exuberant play and laughter!

There are nine types of *attachment play*. I'll share a few examples of some of the types and specific games that you might find particularly helpful in the evenings to support your child/ren to feel more deeply relaxed.

However, most of all, I invite you to hold in mind the power of trusting that your child knows what they need, and that you can follow their lead with play.

As children get older, *attachment play* can morph into silly and humorous conversations with lots of laughter.

Before sharing the examples, here is a story from Helen, who shares how her perspective of play before sleep changed. She says:

"I used to think that high energy play was for something outside of the bedtime routine. But one night, my children both seemed playful and not ready for sleep. So we played the 'I'm the demanding baby' game, where I pretended to be the demanding baby who asked for ridiculous things such as 'bring me the cookie with diamonds on top' and if I didn't get what I asked for, I would throw it out and ask for more! This really hit a sweet spot for my daughter, so she had the most laughs out of this game. Then when I said, "Playtime is over, time to sleep," they cooperated and jumped into bed."

Self-Compassion Moment

I'm sending love to you however you feel when you read this. If you've tried to stop your child playing before sleep, and you're tempted to pick up those sticks, I invite you to put them down! You might feel sad instead, and I invite you to welcome the sadness. I'm here to remind you that it's never too late to bring more playfulness and laughter into parenting.

Power-reversal games

Power-reversal games can help children release feelings of powerlessness that are so common for them to experience in this culture at this time. This is where we play the less powerful or competent role, often in a mock-exaggerated way, or where we pretend to not be able to do something, along with pretending that we're suprised, frightened, or angry. If they're clearly enjoying it and are laughing, we can know that it's helping them.

When children go through stressful or traumatic experiences, they feel powerless. In day-to-day life in *The Disconnected Domination Culture*, it's common for children to feel powerless, even if we're doing everything we can to prevent that. The more they feel a sense of true power in their bodies as a result of power-reversal games, the more likely it is that they will feel safe and relaxed enough to be able to sleep.

We can add power-reversal to many of the games that children are already playing. This makes the play even more effective in releasing stress, especially feelings of powerlessness.

If they are laughing during the power-reversal games, that indicates that they are effectively releasing powerlessness.

If they're wanting to play chasing games, we can invite them to chase us, and keep on being over the top mock-surprised when they they catch us. If we jump up in the air with huge surprise, or fall over each time they catch us, or add in, *"You'll never catch me THIS time!"* with a big smile on our face, these can help them release their feelings of powerlessness.

If they're jumping off the sofa, you could pretend to keep getting in their way and being knocked over by them, again in a big, exaggerated way. You could say, *"You're not going to do that AGAIN, are you?"* – with a big smile on your face!

If they're playing one of their favourite characters, you could pretend to be the younger one, or the smaller one, or the one who doesn't get to do things. *"It's NOT FAIR! Why don't I get to the the one who...."* Again, ham it up, play the role, and watch their delight.

Note: not all games work for all children at all times. As always, observing your child is key. They will let you know whether to continue what you're doing, or to stop.

Another note: I invite you to focus on the balance of attention *here too. Remember that they need to feel physically and emotionally safe in the present, while also being connected to past experiences, for the play to help them heal from past stress or trauma.*

Leila shares about an incredible experience she had with her son when she invited a power-reversal game:

"I have been practising Aware Parenting to the best of my ability since my son was born eight years ago and I have to say that I often struggle with attachment play. *To be honest, I found it much easier when he was younger, for example the 0-4 age bracket felt easy for me in terms of* attachment play, *but I find the 5-8 age bracket really challenging. There are a few reasons for this, not the least of which is (and I feel guilty even saying it) that I just don't really enjoy it, and often after a long day I am tired and the last thing I feel like doing is playing and making things untidy at bedtime.*

However, I absolutely know the benefits of it, and I do put my whole heart into it as often as I can, with loving time limits. The other big reason that I struggle with it is that it is hard to come up with new ways that will work in the moment, and we often default to the old standard in our house, which is pillow fights. My son loves pillow fights, but I find that we end up standing around because he doesn't come after me with the pillow and if I try to get him started with what I call "the clapper" (two pillows clapping him in the middle) we get the laughter, but not the "power over" piece that is so key to the release for him.

So, the other night I had what I thought was a brilliant idea while I was listening to my son's feelings as he was having a rage. A BIG rage. Screaming, crying, banging on the floor, all of it. I had been contemplating this idea for a while, but I had to wait for a time that I was really comfortable with it, otherwise it would defeat the purpose because I would likely get angry. So, here's what I did: I let him completely mess up my bed while I did everything in my power to 'stop' him from doing it. If you knew me, you would likely gasp at hearing this because it's common knowledge among my friends and family that my bedroom is my sanctuary and that I am very particular about how my bed is made. I love fine linens and a well-made bed. More importantly, my son knows this. So, suffice to say my bed is usually off limits, except for falling asleep together. I also made sure to wait until laundry day; the day that I usually change the sheets. This made it so much easier for me to do it with a happy heart, but I still made sure to make the bed properly so that he was none-the-wiser.

After about 30 minutes of just being with him and listening to his feelings, he had stopped and was visibly calmer, but clearly not completely finished, so I said, "I have an idea, instead of a pillow fight, how about this one time you mess up my bed?" Well, all I can say is his whole face lit up and he could barely believe what I was saying. We then launched into a full-on attachment play *with me throwing myself onto the bed pretending to stop him, yelling, "No, no, no, I won't let you do it!" and "You'll never get the sheets off with me on the bed! It's not possible! I won't let you!" Followed by, "How did you do that? You are so strong, how did you get them out from under me?" It was fantastic, effective and I actually enjoyed it, too. He said it was the best day of his life. Hahahaha!"*

> *Self-Compassion Moment*
>
> *I'm sending love to you and how you feel when you read this. Does it inspire you to play something that you know is particularly relevant for your child/ren and you, and that will bring lots of healing laughter? Remember to not coerce yourself to do it, but to only do it when you're willing, and to make it as easy as possible for you, like Leila did, when she chose to play the game on laundry day.*

Note: Leila's story shows how effective *attachment play* can be after a cry, if there are still healing-feelings to be released and the release seems to be incomplete but they aren't crying. However, please remember that if a child is in the middle of crying, we would not recommend going in with play, because that would be distracting them from the healing process of the crying.

Nonsense play

Nonsense play is where we act silly and goofy, doing things that are obviously different to how they're meant to be done, or otherwise exaggerating feelings or challenges. It's particularly helpful to support children express and release feelings related to not being able to do things, or not knowing how to do things. Simply adding in silliness and goofiness to whatever they're playing will go a long way to adding more potency to the play.

Here are some suggestions:

- Put a hat on back to front and pretend that you don't know how hats go.
- Play chasing games but pretend to not know how to play, in silly ways, *"Oh, I thought chasing games meant that I cuddle you all the time!"*
- If they're jumping on the sofa, jump with them and make funny faces with each jump, or silly noises, or goofy words!

Again, I invite you to observe their response. They will probably take what you're doing and run with it, so that you end up co-creating new games together.

Nonsense play can be helpful when we're starting to feel frustrated, angry, or fed up. Megan shares her experience with this:

"I was lying next to my daughter, trying to help her fall asleep. She wasn't falling asleep and I could feel myself getting cranky, so I exaggerated the mood and made it into a funny game. I said, "Uh-oh, cranky Mummy's gonna come out! Raahhh, I'm cranky Mummy, I want you to close your eyes and go to sleep! I'm having a tantrum!" And she was laughing and laughing, and I pretended to have a tantrum, and she said, "No, I'm not going to!" And I said, "Oh but you HAVE to!" and was pretending to have a tantrum, and she was laughing and having a great time and then she fell asleep! I feel so joyful about these little parenting moments."

Separation games

You're likely to have already played separation games, even if you hadn't heard the term before. Right from infancy, most parents play peek-a-boo, and later on, hide and seek. These games support children to understand and heal from separations by including a short visual or spatial separation between our child and us.

Sleep is a form of separation, even if we co-sleep, because our consciousness shifts from being awake to being asleep.

For this reason, separation games can be particularly helpful before sleep, to help children release feelings from past separations, and feel more connected (remembering that a sense of connection is a vital ingredient for a sense of safety and restful sleep).

Children who have experienced traumatic separation, such as after birth, or going to daycare, preschool, or school if they didn't want to, will have feelings related to separation that can particularly show up at bedtime.

Playing separation games or adding separation elements to the play they're already doing can help them heal from those feelings and also feel more connected and safe, which results in more relaxed and sound sleep.

If you're playing chasing games, you might run behind the door while they can see you, and then jump out again, or they run and find you and you jump up in the air with surprise! Or if they're playing with throwing pillows, you could hide your head behind a pillow, and then move the pillow away and say, "Boo!"

Separation games include a small amount of separation that isn't scary for them, and the separation is short. If the separation is too long or too much, it won't be healing. They'll let you know if that's the case, because they won't laugh, and they might even show that they're scared.

Remember, we're always searching for the *balance of attention* with Aware Parenting. This is where they feel the safety in the present moment from our loving presence so that they can feel, express, and release painful feelings from the past. In this case, the emotions are from past experiences of separation, and the release is through laughter.

Contingency play

This is where children gain a sense of agency as well as power, and where their actions make things happen. In other words, our behaviour is contingent on their behaviour. These kinds of games can be particularly helpful if children have fears of monsters at night. A classic game to help with this is the magic wand game or the remote control game, where they wave the wand or remote control, and tell us to do things like jump in the air or bark like a dog.

Helen shared her experience of this:

"Sam had been having nightmares for a while, and was scared of monsters before bed, and I came for a few sessions with you, Marion. I remember feeling doubtful when you told me that the remote control

game might be helpful for him. I just thought that I'd have to help him directly with the fear of monsters. But I tried it anyway and went full on with playing it every evening. He laughed SO much! I was shocked to see that it really did help him, and the fear of the monsters disappeared. It came back temporarily when he watched a scary TV show, but I just used that play again and the fear went. It really worked!"

Activities with body contact

This kind of play is particularly helpful before bed as it offers both closeness and play, and thus attends to both the second and third ingredients for restful sleep.

Piggy back rides can be super fun, and you can add in other elements, such as them telling you which direction to go (which would then also become contingency play). You could pretend to be stuck together, you could hold hands as you go through the pre-sleep activities, you could roll around together on the floor and keep on bumping into each other and cuddling. Some children really enjoy having a massage at bedtime, which can help them feel safe and connected.

Attalia, a *Marion Method* Mentor, shares about the power of this kind of play. I love that she followed her daughter's lead with play and listening to crying, even before knowing about Aware Parenting. She says:

"Wrestling before bed is one of my daughter's most favourite things to do. Together, we experience more connection, closeness, and playfulness in these moments. My daughter is nine, and we started rambunctious play when she was five. There were times when my two daughters and I would wrestle and it would often end in tears. I was curious about this, and then I noticed that the wrestling became the conduit for tears that were being held back after a stressful day at school. My youngest daughter naturally brought this activity to me before I knew about its therapeutic and healing benefits. Her innate wisdom knew that this was what she needed to relax and release before sleeping. There are times when I don't have the capacity for physical play, and I can feel she is more restless when she sleeps next to me. My daughter often wants me to wrestle with her and help her laugh.

Helping her laugh is a recent addition and it has reminded me of the healing power of laughter and play."

Cooperative games and activities

Playing games where cooperation happens can bring such a lovely warm connection between parents and children. For example, perhaps your child/ren might like to take turns adding a sentence to a story you build together.

I remember when my children were about six and ten, they wanted to play on a new app all together one evening. I was reluctant at first, because it was a screen and I had some painful thoughts about them going on screens. However, we used the app and sang funny songs together and videoed ourselves and we all laughed so much. It was so fun! I realised that it was kind of like a cooperative game, because we were learning song words together and making up these little skits together where we needed to be in time with each other. We were so connected and relaxed afterwards. It helped me remember to trust that connection and release come in many forms, and to just keep on being willing for closeness and fun, even if it comes in surprising ways!

Regression play

Some children can benefit from regression play before going to sleep. They might want to pretend to be a baby, in which case you could join in and effusively tend to this beautiful little being. This can be particularly helpful for an older sibling who has a new baby brother or sister, or if a child is going through a developmental leap.

Sienna shared about this with her daughter:

"Abigail went through this phase where she always wanted to be a baby in the evenings before bed. Looking back, I was newly pregnant and she was clearly trying to process it all. At first, I tried to convince her that she was a big girl, but she kept on asking me and then I remembered about the regression games, and went with it. Every night for about two weeks, she wanted to be bundled in a blanket and rocked and sung to sleep, so I did

what she wanted. I actually leant into it even more after a bit when I saw how much she was obviously getting from it, and it helped me too, because I remembered those early days when she was a baby. I think it supported us both to process that there would be a new baby coming and that our relationship would change. And all of a sudden one night, she just didn't want that any more, announcing, "I'm a big four year old." I look back on that time with fondness now. In retrospect, it was very special."

Attachment play during pre-sleep activities

You can also bring in *attachment play* to the pre-sleep activities, such as having a shower or bath, brushing teeth, and putting on pyjamas.

In my *Attachment Play Course*, Jenny (who was the Editor of the first draft of this book) shared an example about how closeness can naturally seep into the things we do with our children before sleep:

"I have had some lovely moments with my youngest, who is nine, around bedtime. Quite organically (inspired by your attachment play *games), at toothbrushing time I now sit on the closed loo seat, and she sits astride me, facing me and brushes her teeth (there is a towel on my lap for frothy toothpaste spillages). She stays there quite a long time and we have plenty of eye contact, she strokes my hair, I stroke hers, we have eye contact, I study her face (and vice versa) and she nuzzles into my neck. It is soooooo lovely and feels like such a beautiful connection before bed (and she ends up brushing her teeth very well!). Thank you!"*

Bath games

Being in the bath together can bring about more connection and often more fun. You could pretend to be sea or river creatures together, or characters that are relevant to your child/ren. You might name the character, and chat with it about all the bathtime activities, and make them relevant to what that character does. If you're not in the bath with them, you could still play games in these ways, perhaps pretending that they're a seal and you're giving them toys to find in the water. Children may also enjoy games such as pretending to be a car at the car wash, and you aren't very competent at your job of cleaning the car (*"Oops, I missed another spot!"*) so you keep going back to clean them over and over again.

With older children, once you are no longer sharing bath time, there are still ways to make bath or shower time a fun and playful opportunity, perhaps (depending on your bathroom) taking turns at spraying each other and avoiding the spray. If you're washing their hair and they don't enjoy it, you could ask them to wash your hair first. You could turn it into nonsense play, e.g. by making funny noises each time they put water on your head, or power-reversal games, *"No, pleeease don't put any shampoo on my head!"*

From a child: Since you got into that Aware Parenting thing, you're always trying to get me to let out my feelings. But I don't want to let my feelings out tonight. I'm in the bath, and you said you'd come in with me. You come in the door, and what's this? You've got on the snorkel that we had for our holidays, and you've brought mine too. And you're wearing a swimming costume! Mum, that is so weird! You jump in our big spa bath, and the water goes all over the edges, and you don't even go on about it like you do when I make the water do that! You've bought my cozzie too, so I stand up and put it on. This is funny, wearing cozzies in the bath! Then you put on a funny voice and start pretending that we're looking for tropical fish. Mum! We are in the bath! There are no tropical fish here! But you insist that there are, and then somehow, these little plastic fish appear! You must have had them hidden in your hand! We pretend to be snorkelling like we did on holiday. I have a tickle of happiness in my tummy.

I'm so glad that you're not asking me if I have some feelings to tell you. I was getting bored of that. I'm loving having so much fun with you! After a while, we jump out of the bath, and we have patterned beach towels instead of our usual plain bathroom ones. After we've put our PJs on, we get two dry beach towels and you tell me that you know of a great beach nearby. We go to the bedroom, and lay out towels out on the bed. Then you pretend to sunbathe. "What a great beach this is!" you say. I laugh out loud. This was a fun evening, Mum! You are a bit crazy! I feel all warm and relaxed. We cuddle up together and we talk about the things we did on our holiday. My heart is like a happy little seahorse. Good night, Mum!

Brushing teeth games

There are lots of games you can play with teeth brushing. Yes, it really is possible to bring fun into this! If you are brushing their teeth, you could pretend to brush their hair, their ears, and their arms with the toothbrush, and be mock-surprised that their teeth are so hairy today! *"Oh THIS is where your teeth are! Oh no, THIS is your teeth! Oh, your teeth look so blue today!"* You may find they desperately ask you to brush their teeth with a smile on their face.

Or perhaps you could use their hair brush and pretend to keep on being surprised by how big toothbrushes are nowadays and why they won't fit in mouths anymore. Or you could pretend you're AMAZING at brushing teeth, and whilst you are going on about how amazing you are, you're looking away and you're brushing the air, and missing their teeth altogether.

If they brush their own teeth, you could sing silly songs whilst they're doing it, or pretend to inspect how much they've cleaned them but look in their ears and eyes instead, remarking, *"Oh your teeth are SO clean!"* You could brush your teeth at the same time, and take turns in trying to sing songs while brushing teeth. The more you play, the more likely they are to join in, and you'll both come up with new ideas.

Helena, an Aware Parenting instructor in the UK, shares some of her favourite toothbrushing games:

"The game that really worked with my kids was when I held a toothbrush and pretended not to know where it went. Under their arm? In their ear? They then took great delight in then showing me where the toothbrush is meant to go. The second game I loved was to pretend that the toothbrush is really scared of going into their mouth. I played the silly voice of the brush and again, my children took great delight in putting the brush in their mouth and chomping down in it."

Karenna shares her breakthrough with toothbrushing:

"After breastfeeding my three-year-old daughter to sleep most nights since birth, my husband and I had become a little slack on the teeth-brushing-before-bed front and we wanted to get into a healthier routine. At first she was quite resistant and we tried lots of approaches: making it fun, being silly, singing a 'brush your teeth' song, attachment play games *(pretending the brush was a toothbrush and the toothbrush was a hairbrush); pretending to brush elbows, knees, etc. and being confused about where our teeth were, giving choices (the big bathroom or the small bathroom? Sitting on the bench or standing on the stool?).*

Although there was much laughter and connection, there wasn't much tooth brushing going on. It was becoming frustrating and I noticed my own 'I'm already defeated' attitude creeping in before I even attempted to get her cooperation to brush her teeth each night. Around this time I was at the supermarket and on a whim bought her a few toothbrushes with a character that she enjoys on them (she occasionally watches the show with the character in it and absolutely loves it) and a mini herbal kids' toothpaste. When I gave them to her I made a big deal about it being her own special tooth-brushing kit that she was responsible for and that nobody else in the family could use. I also mentioned how she had to be the one to squeeze the toothpaste onto the brush while I was her 'assistant' and held the brush. I didn't have high expectations but I figured I had nothing to lose. She took to this straight away and seemed to love the independence of being the one to squeeze the toothpaste onto the brush (slightly more than I would squeeze, but I held my tongue). This was all it took to fall into a nightly teeth brushing rhythm quite quickly and now she even reminds me some nights and mornings as well!"

Putting on PJs games

For younger children, you could pretend that you're putting on their PJs yourself, and remark on how well they fit you, *"Look at my lovely new pyjamas! Do you love them? They fit me so well, don't they!?"* Or you could put the bottom part of the pyjamas on your head and pretend you have a new hat, *"No, don't take my hat! That's my hat, it's not your PJs!"*

As well as these games, which our family really enjoyed, another game I used to love playing with my lovelies before bed was that they would pick which PJs they wanted to wear, and we would run around the bedroom and I would try to throw the pyjamas and hit them with the nightwear (gently of course, and there were no buttons or zips!). When it touched them, they put that part of their pyjamas on.

You could also hide the pyjamas and pretend they are buried treasure and see if your child can find them. For older children, you could pretend that they are dressing up as particular characters off to an adventure, *"(Insert character's name), let's get ready for your nighttime adventure! Right, you'll need your special outfit, what else? Let's get into the (relevant) vehicle off for our adventure!"* The bed can be a significant place in the adventure! Again, you'll probably find that once you start games like this, they will not only run with it that time, but also ask for it again in the future.

Attachment play for if your child is trying to dissociate with food before sleep

If they are asking you to get them food, and you are really certain that they're not hungry, you might come back with a tray with a tea towel over it. You could pretend to be a waitperson and announce in a funny accent that you are bringing them the most delicious food! Then you could whisk away the tea towel to reveal something funny on their plate, like a sock. If they laugh, you could keep going with the game, pretending to be surprised: *"How did that get there? I will speak to the chef straight away!"* or *"What! Do you not like the special of the day, sock soup? It is soooo delicious!"* You might go back and get some other non-food item and continue the game, if they are laughing. If they're not laughing, then it's back to the drawing board!

Some games will bring about connection and laughter with some children on some evenings, others will not. If the game you choose clearly isn't supporting them to laugh and connect, I invite you to stop playing and move on to something else.

I used to have the following practice when my children were younger. If I was doing attachment play *or offering* Loving Limits *before bed and nothing much was moving, I would stop after about 10-15 minutes. I learnt to do this after several times where I just kept going and going, and felt really frustrated, which wasn't helpful for anyone.*

Another game might involve you pretending to be food. *"I'm a lovely salad, would you like to eat some of me?"* And then offer your hand, or a part of your clothing, pretending, for example, that your red shirt is a tomato. *"Oh, you don't like tomato, what about pineapple?"* and offer your yellow jumper.

Or you could say something like, *"Oh, would you like a sandwich? I know a really delicious sandwich!"* and then see if you and they can become a sandwich together by them lying on top of you and then putting covers over the top. You could offer silly ideas about what kinds of toppings are in the sandwich, using the sheet or blanket or duvet/doona, or whatever you have on your beds.

A game I used to play with my daughter, when she was about three, was that if she asked for food and I thought she might have feelings, I would say something like, "Are you hungry for food, or for love?" If she said "love", I would give her loads of hugs and affection.

Attachment play for if your child is trying to dissociate before bed with screens

If your child is watching something, you could sit next to them and watch it with them, and tap them on the shoulder from behind, and when they look at you, just keep watching the screen, pretending you haven't done anything.

You could pretend to be one of the characters, and talk to them about getting off the screen, offering to play out what they are watching on the screen.

I'd love to share a nonsense play game that I learnt from Chiara Rossetti, a dear friend who was an Aware Parenting instructor who is no longer with us. This game is to go away and draw an iPad on our stomach. Then come back into the room and pull up our top to reveal the iPad, and then invite them to play a game. We might then go through each of the apps that they enjoy playing, making the sounds or character voices.

A game shared by Belynda, an Aware Parenting instructor in Australia who is also the main Editor of this book, is to spend some time connecting with your child while they are on their screen and then to offer them eye contact and say in a delighted voice, '*Pick me! I'm waaaay more fun than* [the name of the game]'. Your child will often say, *'No way!'* and you can continue to beg and plead with them that they play with you instead of the screen, offering more and more outlandish 'features' – *'But I have a much more impressive range of volume, see?* [and then shriek!]' or *'But can a screen do THIS!* [and then give them a brief foot massage or some other thing you know they like]'.

Games from Vivian

Here are some ideas from Vivian, an Aware Parenting instructor in Europe.

Get tangled up!

Pretend that you need to fall asleep completely tangled up. Arms, legs – all tangled up! If you have more than one child, get tangled up all together!

Where did the bed go?

Play that you want to bring your child to bed but you think the bed is somewhere it is not, for example in the office or kitchen. Pretend to be surprised and confused: "Where did our bed go? It always used to be here, this is so strange!"

How would you like to go to bed?

Ask your child how she or he (and you) would like to go to bed. For example, as policemen, firefighters, airplanes, or does he/she want to be a prince/princess and be picked up by a horse? Everything in that bedtime routine is coloured by what you and your child are pretending to be. As firefighters, you might put out a fire whilst brushing teeth, or as airplanes the plane seats might be cleaned (teeth). You can take your child on your back or in your arms and fly or drive in a police car. You might even get a phone call to quickly put out a fire or rescue a cat from a tree before going to bed.

Bed on the ground or underneath the bed

In this game, you play that it is the most normal thing for you to sleep underneath the bed (if that is possible with your bed) or on the ground. Pretend to be surprised as to why the cushions and blankets are all on the bed and place them back on the ground again so that you can go to sleep with your child.

What animal would you like to be for bed tonight?

Ask your child what animal he or she would love to be for bed that night. For example: a dog, or a spider, or a lion. Your child can pretend to be that animal and you respond, or both of you might pretend to be that animal.

Catch

Play catch and the bed is the safe spot. When your child is on the bed you can playfully try to catch them. Crawl around the bed with your arms out wide, trying to catch them. Your child can choose how close he/she comes to the side. You can pretend to be a lion, a dog, a shark; anything your child has an association with, or requests as you try to grab them.

Lie down differently

Go and lie down in bed in a different way and pretend to be oblivious about you lying in bed in a way different to usual – for example, upside down.

What shape/number am I drawing on your back?

Draw an image, shape, letter or number on your child's back (or belly) and let him/her guess what you are drawing. (You can include oil or lotion.) Your child might enjoy taking turns.

Where is the go to sleep button?

Pretend to look for a button on your child's body. "Is this the go to sleep button?" If your child responds with something else you can include that. "No, that's not it, that is apparently the xyz button! Is this the go to sleep button?"

Magic wand / Remote control

Use your magic wand or remote control to make your child go to sleep; pretend to be surprised or frustrated when it doesn't work.

Silly bedtime stories

Make up a silly bedtime story. Include things your child is focussed on in their lives, or something about that day, but in a silly way.

Bedtime for the toys

Play with your child to bring her favourite toy(s) to bed. Your child might enjoy having a play bed for them too!

You will never be able to push me over!

In this game you sit on the bed, or on the ground, and you pretend that you are a tree and a house and a mountain, and your child will never be able to push you over. But every time she/he does, and you pretend to be surprised and/or upset that she/he pushes you over.

I want to bring him/her to bed!

In this game you play with your partner (or a grandparent, or even a stuffed toy) – and playfully fight over who is going to bring your child to bed. "I want to bring him/her to bed!" "No , I want to."

Are you sleeping?

In this game you pretend to be really impatient when you are lying in bed with your child, and ask him/her: Are you sleeping already? And now? You ask your child this when he/she is obviously not sleeping yet.

Hold your child and sing her/him a lullaby

In this game you play by holding your child to gently rock him/her and sing a calming lullaby, but instead of that you're rocking wildly and singing a loud song and pretending to be surprised that your child doesn't fall asleep.

Good morning!

In this game you yawn loudly and stretch, and get up to open the curtains because it is morning! "Good morning! Did you sleep well? Come let's go and start the day!"

Roll off the bed

In this game you pretend to not be able to stay on the bed, you roll off the bed no matter what you do.

I am so happy that it is bedtime!

Pretend to be so incredibly happy that you can finally go to bed – over-the-top happy: falling on your knees or doing a happy dance."Oh yes, finally, finally I can go to bed!" You can even start during the day by saying, "Are you tired already? Can we go to bed?" You might also enjoy asking at very random times during the day, in a very unknowing way, if it is bedtime already? "Is it bedtime already? Can I bring you to bed?"

I don't want to bring you to bed

Play that you don't want to bring your child to bed. You don't want to be separated from your child, you don't want to say good night. "No, I don't want to bring you to bed, I don't want to say good night."

Don't fall asleep!

When you are lying in bed, pretend to not want to fall asleep. Keep your eyes wide open! "I don't want us to fall asleep, let's lie here looking at each other. We can't close our eyes!"

We can't fall asleep

Pretend to be anxious about all the things that might happen when you fall asleep and come up with silly things. "I can't fall asleep, what if I fart! Or what if I kick you in my sleep?! Or what if I talk in my sleep! Or roll off the bed? We can't fall asleep!"

User manual

Pretend to have a user's manual and try to find what to do for your child to be able to fall asleep, and come up with all sorts of silly things: "I need to hold my left ear and put one finger in my nose. Hey, you are not sleeping! We need to turn around three times to the left and five times to the right.... then lay down make a fart noise and you will be asleep." Pretend to be upset or frustrated that it is not working. And your manual has all sorts of silly suggestions! If suggestion one doesn't work, try this, if suggestion two doesn't work, try this, etc.

Bed throw

In a mock frustrated way throw your child to bed: "I am going to throw you to bed this evening!" Pick up your child and throw him/her gently on the bed. I imagine they would like to be "thrown to bed" multiple times! "How did you get up? Now I need to throw you to bed again!"

I am so tired!

Pretend to randomly fall asleep yourself. If you are reading to your child, start nodding and pretend to fall asleep. You might include some snoring. If you are playing you can pretend to fall asleep as well. "I am so tired (big yawn), I think I am falling asleep zzzzzzz." Your child might enjoy waking you up. You can be silly about it: "Did I fall asleep again?!"

You can also pretend to be too tired to do anything, like brushing teeth/ washing/pyjamas and pretend to fall asleep then or to fight to not fall asleep while brushing teeth, etc. You can even pretend to not have control over it; "Oh I am falling asleep again! Keep me awake!" But you keep on falling asleep.

You can't lie down yet!

When your child wants to lie down, pretend that he/she can't lie down yet. "Oh, you can't lie down yet! You first need to do three somersaults!" When he/she then wants to lie down: "Oh, you can't lie down yet, we first need to tell the plants good night/run around the room/ give the wall a kiss, do a handstand etc." Come up with silly things your child or you both need to do before your child can lie down in bed.

Where are you?

When you lie down to go to bed with your child, pretend that you don't see him/her. "He/she was right here and now she is gone?! Where are you?" Look for your child underneath the sheets, behind the cushions, underneath the bed etc., until finally, miraculously 'seeing' her right in front of you.

What is bedtime?

Pretend to be completely oblivious about what to do at bedtime. "What is bedtime? What do we do? Do we go outside for bedtime?"

Where is our bed?

In this game you start searching for your bed in silly places. Is it in the fridge, outside, in the bathroom, underneath the table?

The fall asleep chair

Pretend that your arms are some kind of calming, fall asleep chair. Instead of this being a calming chair it moves in all sorts of ways!! Legs up, to the side, it shakes. You can also pretend to be surprised yourself too: " This is not a calming fall asleep chair!!"

Switch roles!

Let your child bring you to bed.

I can't lie still!

The parent pretends to not be able to lie still and moves from one weird and funny position to the next one., saying, "I can`t lie still!" The child might join in and lie in all sorts of strange positions too.

Vivian says

"I love to invite parents to welcome their own feelings into the play. This can create lots of emotional safety. We model that all feelings are welcomed and invited to move through us in connection and play. Children then receive a message that is congruent with what they are experiencing. Inviting our own feelings into play can be very refreshing and healing for both parent and child."

Attachment play in the morning /waking up games

Emily shared this game with me that her son created. It helped them both heal from experiences where he'd woken early in the morning.

The It's Still Night Game

"I just wanted to share a cool attachment play *game that my son (who is four) initiated himself this morning. Background: he gets up at 4-5am every day full of beans and wanting to play. I am in my own judgment NOT a morning person, and often resist getting up and ask him to go play alone/get a book to read in bed/stay in bed and give me cuddles. It's often a really challenging way to start the day (for us both) as we just have SUCH opposing needs and capacities at this time of day. He asked me to pretend I really, really wanted to get up, while he held me down, pulled me back, pushed me back into bed, chased me down the hall and brought me back, closed the curtains, turned off the light and pretended it was still nighttime.*

He then asked to reverse the game where I tried to make him get up even though it was still night and he didn't want to get up, he pretended to still sleep and crawl back into bed as I tried desperately to waken him and entice him to come and play with me. This was so healing for us both. We both laughed so hard. I absolutely adore that children just naturally GET this, that they truly do know EXACTLY what they need to heal and grow. We can learn so much from them. I wonder how tomorrow morning will look now?"

Play, crying, and *Loving Limits*

Attachment play is a really powerful and effective way of helping create a deep sense of connection, which helps create restful sleep. It also helps children release light fears, powerlessness, and other feelings, through the laughter and the play. It helps them heal from stress and trauma and helps them feel more relaxed in their bodies.

So you may well find that after playing, your child is happy to lie down, either with or without you, and drift off to sleep, because they feel tired, connected, safe, and relaxed after the play.

However, sometimes, *attachment play* is not enough to help them feel deeply relaxed, and a child still has accumulated feelings at the surface that are preventing them from sleeping.

They might want to keep playing and playing, even though they're clearly tired (and you are too!). Or they might lie down but they're wriggling around, or asking for lots of things. Or they might suddenly have a really big cry about a really small thing.

Attachment play also creates the conditions for deeper feelings to come up to be expressed. The connection is part of what brings emotional safety, which is a core element of what is required for tears and tantrums to be healing.

Those healing-feelings might come out without you needing to do much, via a **broken cookie moment**.

Perhaps you've been playing lots, and suddenly they start crying in response to something small, such as they don't like their new toothbrush, or the colour of the pyjamas, or the way that you did something.

If the feelings are big and loud and full-blown, you can trust that it's not really about any of those things, and it's simply the power of the play you've done together that has facilitated the feelings to bubble up. This is simply the emotional coat hanger that they are hanging the emotions on.

By expressing these big feelings and releasing the tension in their bodies, they will probably be able to sleep more easily and more restfully.

I invite you to simply be present with your child, offering them empathy and listening to their feelings. "*I really hear that you don't like the new toothbrush, sweetheart. I'm right here and I'm listening.*" Remember that the bigger and louder and more intense the feelings are, the more stress your child is releasing from their body and the more relaxed they will feel afterwards. Staying with them and their feelings is you supporting their natural relaxation-through-release process.

Or, your child might start pinching, biting, throwing, pushing, or hitting. That tells you that the connection and play has stirred up some deeper feelings but they're not quite safe enough to express them in healing-raging, and are in fight or flight. Here's where it's important to hold in mind that they are **trying** *to become more relaxed but they need more of your help so they can feel safe, and move out of the fight mode. This is where you can move in with a* **Loving Limit,** *which is where we say no to the behaviour, and a yes to the feelings that are causing the behaviour.*

That means moving in close and, first of all, doing the minimum possible to stop the behaviour. That might be holding their hand if they are pinching, throwing, pushing, or hitting. Or it might be putting your hand on their forehead if they are biting.

Then you can communicate to them in your posture, tone, voice and words that you are saying no to what they are doing, and you are compassionately willing to listen to the feelings that are causing that behaviour. I love phrases such as, *"I'm not willing for you to bite me, sweetheart, because I'm here to keep everyone safe, and I'm right here, and I'm listening."*

A note on language and *Loving Limits*[61]: I don't recommend saying, *"It's not okay to hit,"* because this is a judgment and is likely to lead to more painful feelings and is less likely to create a sense of emotional safety. Likewise, saying, *"Be gentle!"* is not likely to stop the hitting, nor to help them feel and express the feelings underlying the hitting. Thirdly, I also don't recommend, *"We don't hit in our family,"* because if they have, what does that mean for them?

---

61 Please note that all this language is specific to me and is not Aware Parenting. Please feel free to use whatever words deeply resonate with you!

Please note that there is no specific language in Aware Parenting for *Loving Limits*. I invite you to choose language that helps you feel safe, loving, and truly powerful, and which helps your child feel safe and loved.

I specifically choose, *"I'm not willing,"* because I find that it helps me connect deeply with my true power, which can help a child feel safe. The *"... and I'm listening,"* can help them feel our loving presence.

It's the combination of our loving presence and the clear grounded 'no' that helps them feel physically and emotionally safe, so that they can exit out of the fight or flight response, and resolve the experience through releasing the emotions.

The aim of the *Loving Limit* is not just to stop the behaviour. It's to help the child feel physically and emotionally safe, so that they no longer need to be in the fight response (and hitting or biting). The *Loving Limit* is also to help facilitate the feelings to be expressed in healing ways, through crying and raging, along with vigorous body movements.

This is what helps them move out of the fight or flight response and into a calm relaxed state, which will likely mean that they can have a lovely restful sleep. It's really normal and natural for children to have really big feelings when we offer that *Loving Limit*. They might cry and rage for a long time – and really loudly and intensely.

This is where it's so important for us to keep reminding ourselves that this is their natural and wise healing and relaxation process, and that they need our help to feel, express, and release these feelings from their bodies. If your child has been sleeping restlessly, you might find it helpful to remember that these are the feelings that have been sitting in their body, making it hard for them to feel relaxed while sleeping.

If you can stay present with your child right through to the end of the big feelings session, you are likely to see them in a very different physical and emotional state.

You'll see them move through the rage, often to sadness and crying, and then to presence. You'll probably feel how much more relaxed their muscles are. You might feel that beautiful calmness in their body. They might cuddle up with you in a beautifully soft and melting way. They might gaze into your eyes or tell you that they love you.

After they've had a big release like this, I invite you to stay with them as they drift off to sleep. That might mean carrying them to bed, or if they were already on the bed, lying down together and cuddling up.

Being close with them after they've expressed some of their deepest and most painful feelings can be a profoundly beautiful experience.

From a child: I know it's getting late, because I just want to run from one end of the house to the other. I get Simon to join in, and soon we are laughing and laughing. You come out of the kitchen, Mum and Dad, and I wonder what you'll do. Will you tell me to quiet down? I don't like that. I want to run and laugh! But what's this! Dad, you say, "We'll need to get the laughter police, you know there's no laughter in this house!" And you actually giggle! Well, that gets me and Simon laughing more, and when you run to the other side of the house, we chase you there and back again. And this time, Mum joins in! "Where are the laughter police! There's WAY too much laughter going on here!" That just makes me laugh more and more. We run up and down, up and down, and you both keep on saying funny things like that. I haven't laughed this much for ages. I love it! Simon and I run again, but this time I somehow trip over him. OUCH!

It's like my balloon has popped, and all the air comes out. I start to cry. You come over to me, Dad, and Mum goes over to Simon. I cry so loudly. I don't know why! It's like all the sunshine has turned into a big summer storm. I cry SO much. And you just stay with me, Dad, loving me. I cry and cry as if I had all the tears in the world inside me. I keep going and going. And going. And going.

Finally, it all comes to an end. I open my eyelids, and our eyes meet. I see the love in your eyes. You carry me to bed, even though I'm a big boy now. Simon's already asleep. And wow, I feel SO sleepy, Dad. Did you put magic dust on me? I snuggle up with you and I think I will be asleep so quickly. Nighty night, Dad, sleep tight.

This is the power of Aware Parenting, to transform bedtime struggles into lifetime memories of love.

All four of us in our family used to love playing The Laughter Police Game! I still remember running up and down the length of our house, pretending to be the laughter police, while our children giggled and laughed. And even though that was many years ago now, those memories are indelibly inked into my consciousness.

Alternatively, your child might enjoy *attachment play* games *after* crying and raging. For children, laughter/play and crying/raging are not as far apart as they generally are for us as adults. Remember Leila's experience of this, above!

However, please hold in mind that in Aware Parenting, if a child is already raging or crying, we would NOT ever recommend moving in with play at that moment, as that would be distracting them from their feelings – and the healing process.

Charlotte shares a story of how her nine-year-old daughter had a big cry before sleep, and later on they shared some lovely *attachment play* together. I love this story, because it really illustrates that it's never too late to start practicing Aware Parenting. Children stay connected with their innate healing wisdom, and can reconnect with that, however old they are when we first learn about it.

"I found Aware Parenting when my daughter turned nine years old and it resonated to my core. I grieved a lot that I hadn't found it earlier.

However, I am still finding it a game-changer for my daughter and me. It's supporting her – and me – to get in touch with our feelings, have them heard and validated and then enabling the stress/trauma to disperse. More recently, I have seen the profound impact this new lens and way of being is having on her sleep. She had always taken at least an hour to sleep and wriggled a lot in bed. It felt like she couldn't sleep unless she had a meditation on or something to (what I now know) mildly disassociate with. I have always stayed with her as she fell asleep.

I have been doing lots of work for myself and getting in touch with my own big feelings, having them heard, facilitated by Life and being mentored by Marion. My intentions around bedtime are now so different. Now I have integrated more of this understanding, I see my daughter beautifully setting things up for herself to discharge the emotion of the day – and some of the past – before sleep. Understanding that she just needs safe connection and to feel relaxed in her body makes total sense. I see it before my eyes.

Even this week, she came home from school, and wanted to go to an extra dance class that she'd been offered. But then she changed her mind and decided not to go. I suggested it might be best for her to wait as she had been unwell. A little later, she put on her dance stuff and I thought it was to play a game (she often does this). Then, after the dance lesson would have started, she said, 'Right, let's go'. When I said, 'It's already started, I'm not willing to go, sweetheart, as I don't think it's what you need right now,' she was upset. She was able to have a big cry and I could tell that it was a big discharge from the day.

Once that was done she was immediately fine again and said, 'Right, let's go upstairs,' and she got into her pyjamas and sat in bed. She said she still had some energy left and so she jumped up and said, 'Tell me what to do and I'll do it'. So she did star jumps and lots of yoga poses, and we ended up laughing together. We then had a long extended period of attachment play – starting with me saying, 'Let's get your covers on,' and then rolling her off the bed onto my knee. I then pretended she was squashing me so hard that I collapsed – with her laughing and laughing. After a long time, when I felt like I wanted to stop, she resisted a little, had a little cry, asked me to cuddle her, said she didn't want the usual meditation tape on, rolled over and went to sleep. It was like watching her doing what she naturally knew she needed to get to that place of readiness for sleep. Quite beautiful."

CHAPTER SUMMARY

Rather than trying to 'calm down' a child when they are being playful, we can trust that they are using their effective innate healing process to become deeply relaxed.

When children go through stressful or traumatic experiences, they often feel powerless. We can add power-reversal to many games to make the play even more effective in releasing powerlessness. If they are laughing during the power-reversal games, that indicates that they are effectively releasing powerlessness.

Not all games work for all children at all times. I invite you to focus on the *balance of attention:* they need to feel physically and emotionally safe in the present, while also being connected to past experiences, for the play to help them heal.

Separation games include a small amount of separation that isn't scary for them, and the separation is short. If the separation is too long or too much, it won't be healing. They'll let you know, because they won't laugh, and they might even show that they're scared.

Attachment play also creates the conditions for deeper feelings to come up to be expressed. During or after play, your child might start pinching, biting, throwing, pushing, or hitting. This is where you can move in with a *Loving Limit*, which is where we say no to the behaviour, and a yes to the feelings that are causing the behaviour.

I love the phrase, *"I'm not willing for you to hit me, sweetheart, because I'm here to keep everyone safe, and I'm right here, and I'm listening."* I don't recommend saying, *"It's not okay to hit"*, *"Be gentle!"* or, *"We don't hit in our family"*. There is no specific language in Aware Parenting for *Loving Limits*. I invite you to choose language that helps you feel safe, loving, and truly powerful, and which helps your child feel safe and loved.

It's normal and natural for children to have really big feelings when we offer a *Loving Limit*. They might cry and rage for a long time and really intensely. If you can stay present with your child right through to the end of the big feelings session, you are likely to see them in a very different physical and emotional state.

Being close with them after they've expressed some of their deepest and most painful feelings can be a profoundly beautiful experience. This is the power of Aware Parenting, to transform bedtime struggles into lifetime memories of love.

Alternatively, your child might enjoy *attachment play* games after crying and raging. However, if a child is still raging or crying, we would NOT ever recommend moving in with play at that moment, as that would be distracting them from their feelings and the healing process.

I'm here to support you to have even more joy, fun, and laughter in your family.

25. Dissociation and distraction from feelings when sleepy

There are three slightly different ways in which children can dissociate before sleep:

- *They* ask *us* to do things that will make them dissociate.
- *They* do things *themselves* to dissociate.
- *We* do things *to them* that make them dissociate.

If that sounds a bit complex, I'm here to explain! We might do things to them that make them dissociate, because we think we are meeting a need and don't realise that they are trying to express healing-feelings to us. Or, we don't understand that they have healing-feelings to us, or don't have the emotional spaciousness in ourselves to listen to their feelings, so they do things themselves to help them dissociate. Over time, they may then ask us to do things to help them dissociate, and/or they continue dissociating by themselves.

Asking us to do things that will make them dissociate

Does your child ever ask for lots of things before bed? Perhaps:

- to read them another book, and then another one;
- to play just one more game together; or
- to get them a soft toy, and then a different one.

You might keep doing what they ask, but they're just not satisfied. In fact, they might show all kinds of signs that they're frustrated and agitated.

Self-Compassion Moment

I'm sending you compassion if your child does these kinds of things often and you feel frustrated, overwhelmed, or angry. Perhaps you've responded in harsh ways, especially after doing what they ask over and over and they're not calm and still not willing to go to sleep. I'm here to remind you to put down any sticks that you might be tempted to pick up, and instead to be compassionate with yourself. Perhaps you might feel sad when you reflect on your responses. It's so common for us to feel tired and depleted at the end of the day, and to react in ways that we don't want to. I invite you to reach out for some loving listening, so you can express your feelings. The more you express your emotions to your empathy buddy, the less it will come out in ways that you don't want with your child.

As a form of attachment-style parenting, Aware Parenting advocates listening to your child's needs and meeting them promptly.

However, there's often a quality of asking for things, particularly when a child is sleepy, that shows us that they are trying to distract themselves from their healing-feelings. This is very different from them asking for a need to be met.

As you become more familiar with Aware Parenting, you'll be able to differentiate between the two more and more.

When they're asking for us to do lots of things, our aim is to discover whether they are expressing a need, or trying to distract themselves from their feelings. Then we can avoid distracting them from their feelings because we think we're meeting a need. Understanding the difference is likely to save us from frustration and powerlessness.

How can we differentiate between needs-feelings and healing-feelings here?

We can clearly see that they aren't expressing an unmet need if we observe the following. Our child asks for something, and we give it to them, and they're clearly still agitated and antsy. Then they ask for something else, and we give it to them, and they're still agitated and antsy. We can clearly see that they are trying to avoid feeling and expressing the uncomfortable feelings that are bubbling up inside them. Our responses aren't really working to distract them from their feelings, so even though we're doing what they ask, they're still feeling agitated.

***To support those underlying feelings being released, instead of saying yes to everything and the going to sleep process taking a very long time, we can offer a* Loving Limit.**

Because they are making requests of *us*, the *Loving Limit* in this case is *us* placing a limit on *our* response.

Loving Limits

We can offer a *Loving Limit* when we understand that a child is asking for something because they are trying to distract themselves from pent-up painful feelings. We are saying no to the request and yes to the underlying feelings.

In these kinds of situations, I love to express *Loving Limits* using phrases such as, *"I really hear that you want me to get you another toy, sweetheart, and I'm not willing to get another toy because I don't think that's most helpful for you right now, and I'm here and I'm listening."*[62]

Remember that when we offer *Loving Limits*, it's important that we include the information why we are doing that. In this case, I've used the phrase, *"...because I don't think that's most helpful for you right now."*

One of the many things I love about *Loving Limits* is that they really

---

62 Please note that this language is my preferred way to express a *Loving Limit*, but there are many other possible phrases to use. There is no set language for *Loving Limits* in Aware Parenting.

are loving! If your child keeps asking for that thing, or other things, you can keep on offering them empathy, while still saying no. You can show your willingness to listen to the feelings that are actually the real cause of all the requests.

What they really need is to express those feelings and release all the tension they're holding inside, and receive your loving support while they do that.

You might keep on repeating the *Loving Limit*, even keep asking for the distraction. *"I really hear that you want me to go and get you another toy, sweetheart, and I'm not willing to get any more toys tonight, because I don't think that's the most helpful thing for you right now. Ahh, and I really hear that you want me to get another toy, darling, and I'm not willing to do that. I so hear that you want another toy, and I'm not willing for more toys tonight."* Once you've given the information the first time around, you might not keep repeating the information part.

They might even move to then wanting to change their pyjamas, or go back to a different part of the house, or some other request. It's common that they will keep trying to avoid feeling and expressing their healing-feelings. In which case, you could offer a *Loving Limit* about the new request, since you are clear that it isn't to meet a need.

The aim is to help them feel, express, and release the feelings that are sitting inside their bodies, preventing them from being able to relax enough to sleep soundly.

Once you offer the *Loving Limit* and they are expressing the feelings through tantrumming or crying, your role is to keep being as present as you can with them, keep listening to the feelings, and to keep letting them know that you're still there with them and still listening.

It's normal for all children to have big, loud feelings. You might find it helpful to remember that these feelings have been sitting inside their body and making it harder for them to feel relaxed enough to sleep soundly. Remembering that might help you feel more willing to feel calm and keep supporting their crying, knowing that it will lead to more sleep for you both.

From a child: My body is like a whirlwind, and I'm being blown all over the place. I know you want me to go to bed, but how can I? I'm the wild wind, getting wilder and wilder. Oh look! What's this? I love this teddy. I haven't seen him for ages! Can you get him down from the shelf for me? Oh and look at this! My old painting smock from daycare. Can I put it on now, Dad? Will you help me? Oh actually, look at that old dinosaur toy I had. Where's the other one that went with it? I really want to find it! Can you help me? Dad, can we go back to the kitchen? I really want the dinosaur to play on the counter top! Oh look! Will you read this book to me? I love this book! Oh, and there's my blue truck. I was wondering where that had got to! Will you help me find the person that goes with it? Oh Dad, my wild whirlwind is getting faster and faster and it's like I can't get off. I need to keep going, faster and faster, but I don't really like it. Can you help me, Dad?

What's that? I see you come close and put your hand on my hand as I'm about to reach out for my new board game and ask you to play it with me. I feel the warmth of your hand on mine. My hand is the only place I can feel. My hand, your hand. You say some words to me. I hear that "not willing" thing that you like to say so much nowadays. My swirling whirlwind has something to centre around now. There's my hand, and there's your hand, and you are still and sure. I feel safe.

But also, the wind gets wilder, now it's not swirling everywhere, and I start to get so mad, Dad. "I WANT TO PLAY SOME MORE!" I shout at you. You say no in that warm way, and I can feel my hand, and your hand, and your voice, and my ears. "I WANT TO PLAYYYYYYYYY," I shout some more. The whirlwind goes out a funnel. I shout it out. I rage it out. I stamp my feet. You're there. Your hand, your voice, your eyes. I see you. You're here with me. I'm safe. The whirlwind has let me go.

I start to cry, and I fall into your arms. I cry and I cry, so loud, but so different to the whirlwind. I'm the wild wind all coming out in the rain and the storm. I already feel so much more relieved. The tension is melting away, the more that I cry in your arms.

You hold me and I can now feel my chest and my back, I'm cuddled up to you and your arms are around me. My body is here again. The whirlwind is dying down now. A few funny sighs come out of me, like the last of the *whirlwind needs to get out. Then I sink into you. I feel peaceful at last. We stay like that for ages.*

Then I look around, and I see my lovely room with all my things. But I don't need to go to them all. They are there for me and will be there for me tomorrow. You carry me to bed and we cuddle up together. I start to drift off to the sound of your heartbeat. I love you, Dad.

Distracting themselves with *control patterns*

Have you ever noticed that when your child is tired, they distract themselves from the feelings that naturally bubble up as part of their relaxation response? For example, perhaps they suck their thumb when they're tired, or if they can read, perhaps they want to read books, or watch a screen.

This is subtly different to when they are asking us to do things to distract them from their feelings – because they don't require us to do anything in order to dissociate. So, our response is different in nuanced ways, too.

When you understand that their innate healing process is to release feelings rather than hold them in, you might feel called to help them move from the suppression to the expression of the feelings. It's those accumulated feelings which is making it hard for them to sleep.

The first step, if we're wanting to support our child in this way, is to tend to ourselves, and receive regular and ongoing listening for our own painful feelings. This is particularly important if we used to do (or still do) what they do to dissociate – such as suck our thumb to go to sleep, or read books, or watch TV.

Then we are more likely to be able to move in to help them and they are more likely to be willing to express those feelings rather than suppress them.

With *control patterns*, I find it helpful to think of four steps:

1. Doing our own inner work so that we can offer our loving support.
2. Moving close with compassion, warmth, and presence.
3. Offering *attachment play* related to the *control pattern*.
4. Offering *Loving Limits* and *listening* to the healing-feelings.

Thumb-sucking before sleep

Let's go through these four steps with an example of how this might look.

Firstly, if your child has a thumb-sucking *control pattern*, you might start by receiving some loving listening from your empathy buddy or Aware Parenting instructor, or perhaps doing some journalling to explore your own feelings and experiences.

You might consider questions such as:

- Did you ever suck your thumb as a child?
- If so, how wasyour thumb-sucking perceived and/or responded to when you were young?
- What other *control patterns* did you use as a child and how were they responded to?
- How do you feel and what do you think when you see them sucking their thumb?
- What do you need so you can offer them unconditional love when they're doing it?

Secondly, when you see your child sucking their thumb, you might sit next to them and beam at them lovingly. You might feel the presence in your hand and put it on the centre of their back or on their arm, if they're willing. You might cuddle up with them, if they're willing. I invite you to do this and connect in with your sense of unconditional love for them.

Thirdly, you might experiment with *attachment play*. You could pretend that you want to taste their thumb, and ask them what flavour it is. *"Is it strawberry?"* And then you pretend to taste it, and say something like,

"Oh NO! That's not strawberry! That's poo flavour! You're not going to trick me again like that, are you? What flavour is it this time?" You might find yourself playing that again and again. Or you could pop your own thumb in your mouth and pull it out with a really loud POP, and do it again, but each time it makes another different funny sound.

Playing games like this has no element of shaming or teasing, rather, the play is designed to bring connection and warmth to where the child is in freeze, i.e. dissociating from healing-feelings.

You might find that they then use thumb-sucking less often, and will express their feelings more often. After some play like this, they might take their thumb out and start crying instead. That might happen with a pretext, such as they don't like the way the blanket is folded, or the way you looked at them. You can trust that after the *attachment play*, they're feeling the connection and safety to let out deeper feelings, and those feelings are likely to come out in the form of crying and raging.

Finally, with thumb-sucking, we don't recommend *Loving Limits* in Aware Parenting, because we don't want to override what our child is doing with their body and what they are communicating about the emotional safety available to express their painful feelings. However, with *other control patterns*, it may be that a *Loving Limit* is useful and helpful, depending on how the *attachment play* went.

From a child: *Whenever I'm tired, Daddy, my thumb just goes in my mouth without me even thinking about it. I don't know why. It just happens. Sometimes Aunty Gemma tells me to take it out, but when I do, I feel all funny. I don't like it. And I think I must be tired now, Daddy, because it's just happened. My thumb is in my mouth. Everything feels different when I do it. My world becomes a bit hazy, like I'm watching my favourite cartoon. It's like I'm in a dream world. You come over, and you're a bit fuzzy. I don't hear you like I do when I'm not sucking my thumb. I look away, and I go back to more sucking. I expect I will fall asleep like this. I create my own world with pink and fluffy clouds.*

What's this? I hear a funny noise. I look up at you. You're putting your thumb in your mouth and making a really loud sucking noise. And then all kinds of other funny noises. That's so strange, Daddy. Why are you doing that? You keep doing it, but this time your face is making weird expressions. I start laughing. My thumb comes out of my mouth, just a bit. I can see and hear you a bit more clearly, and there's a breeze of freshness drifting across my face. Oh.

But then I put my thumb back in my mouth again. That's it. I look away from you again, and the sucking gets stronger. Then I hear another noise. What is that? I look at you, and this time, you've popped your thumb out of your mouth, and you have a big smile on your face. Your thumb starts dancing around, and then your other thumb joins in. You start singing a funny song about thumbs. I smile again, a bubble of laughter coming out of me. I feel this warmth, and my thumb pops out of my own mouth. How funny is that, Daddy? We both have our thumbs out of our mouths. Your thumbs come over to mine and say hello. We do a little thumb dance. I'm smiling. Your thumbs sing a funny song about loving my thumb. Oh, now I'm laughing. And it's so strange, because my pink clouds are moving away. And there's a kind of freshness and clearness coming. We keep laughing together, Daddy.

Oh, but what happens? There's rain in this cloud. I can feel it. It's coming out. Ouch. This hurts. I can feel tears coming to my eyes. I look in your eyes, and you're there with me. You nod, and offer to hold my hand. I take your hand. I can feel your warmth. The rest of the pink clouds float away and the rain cloud is there, full to bursting. Some tears start to come. My laughter turns to tears. Oh Daddy, I feel so sad. So sad. I start to cry. You move closer, and gently put your arms around me. I can feel your warmth. I cry more. I cry a river. I cry a storm. I didn't know that this storm was hiding in my pink clouds. You are here with me, Daddy. I am safe here with you. I hear you saying warm words to me, and I know I am safe, even though I love my pink clouds. I keep crying and crying. My pink clouds have had such a lot of rain in them. I didn't know. My tears keep coming, and you keep on holding me. I cry even though I don't really know why I'm crying. I know that I feel very sad. You have been asking me whether I've been feeling sad lately, with all that's been going on, but I didn't know what you meant. Perhaps this is the sadness you've been talking about. My heart feels sore. I start to remember some of the sad things that have happened, and I stop crying to tell you about them. You nod, and listen. Somehow your love helps me feel more. I return to crying. Now I'm in your arms, and you just keep holding me. I cry and cry as if there was only crying in the world.

Oh, what's this, Daddy, my tears are coming to an end. I do this sighing thing, and I look up at you. I gaze into your eyes, and I can really see you. I can really see your eyes. I love you, Daddy. Instead of my heart hurting, now it feels all open and loving. I look around me and I see Benny the cat and I love him so much. It's like I'm a part of everything I see. I can see so clearly. I don't need my lovely pink clouds right now. I feel all soft, like Benny, sleeping on the mat. Ahhh, I yawn. I feel tired too. Can I go to bed now, Daddy? Will you stay cuddling me? I don't even think I will need my pink clouds and thumb to go to sleep tonight. Nighty night, Daddy.

Self-Compassion Moment
I'm sending love to however you feel after receiving this story.

Maru, an Aware Parenting instructor in the UK who is originally from Mexico shares about her two-year-old daughter's *control pattern*:

"I was practicing Aware Parenting and training to become an Aware Parenting instructor. Around the time that my daughter turned two, she started waking up after three hours and it took her a long time to go back to sleep and she was moving around a lot in her sleep.

It took me a while to see that she had some control patterns. *She liked stroking my arm to go to sleep. It was really subtle, and only became evident when she started to stroke my arm again once she woke up, and the need increased as the feelings accumulated. It was impossible for me to sleep and it took me many months to realise what was going on, and that she was stopping herself from expressing her feelings through this* control pattern, *which was why she kept on waking up. I love sharing this, because otherwise parents wonder why sleep isn't improving, when there's a subtle* control pattern *in play."*

Us distracting them from their healing-feelings

We're so often taught that we need to help children calm down before bed, and so it's very common to give children a dummy, or to read stories with that intention, and to generally do things to try to 'make them' feel more calm, which can actually help them mildly dissociate from their healing-feelings.

Giving a dummy when tired

A dummy is *control pattern* from an Aware Parenting perspective – a habitual way to mildly dissociate from feelings.

That's why, if your child has a dummy, they will probably ask for it when they're tired, because they're trying to suppress their feelings that are naturally arising to be expressed before sleep.

Your approach with the dummy will depend on how long they've been using it and how many feelings it's been holding in.

If they've had it for a long time, there will be a lot of feelings that they have sitting in their body, and thus it may take a longer time for them to gradually stop using the dummy. However, if you keep offering them a dummy, they might think that you don't welcome their feelings, so, as with all of Aware Parenting, I invite you to listen in to yourself, observe them, and experiment. You might decide to not give them the dummy any more and trust that when you're not there to listen, or they don't feel the *balance of attention*, they will find other ways to dissociate that *they choose* (unlike the dummy, which was *our choice*).

You can use the four steps again here!

In the *attachment play* phase, you might want to play silly games with dummies, or suck on one yourself and make funny noises and faces, and bring laughter and play into their relationship with the dummy.

Then, you could offer a *Loving Limit* when you are ready to listen to the underlying feelings before bed: "*I'm not willing for you to have your dummy now, sweetheart, because I don't think it's the most helpful thing for you, and I'm here to listen to your feelings."* You might choose other information to offer instead, such as, *"I'm here to help you go to sleep without needing it. "* I invite you to connect in with which information is *true for you* to express to them.

After the *Loving Limit,* the most helpful response is to listen, and keep on listening, and to keep on offering empathy.

It is normal and natural for them to have a lot of healing-feelings to express and a lot of crying and raging to do. You might want to reflect back on all the times that they have been using the dummy, recognising that those were times when they had healing-feelings that were bubbling up to be expressed.

After they've had a big cry or rage, they might then cuddle up with you, and you're likely to be able to feel a difference in their body in terms of how relaxed and present they are.

After the big cry they may still want to have the dummy afterwards, in which case you might give it to them if you aren't able to listen any more (and you've done what you can to support yourself to be able to listen more). There might be several crying sessions before they feel relaxed enough in their body to not want the dummy to suppress feelings anymore. Or, you might experiment with this. What happens if you still don't give them the dummy? This way, you are communicating that you are willing to listen to all of their feelings. If they need to dissociate, they will find another way. As with all of Aware Parenting, I invite you to listen in to which most resonates with you, and to experiment and observe what happens.

Self-Reflection Moment

If you've experimented with offering attachment play and Loving Limits in this way, afterwards do you notice that their muscles are more relaxed, that their face and mouth look more relaxed, and that they then sleep more peacefully?

Every time you do listen to their healing-feelings it will make a difference to them. They will be holding less feelings in their body. They will not need to be as tense. They'll feel more relaxed, and they will have released stress from their system. They'll have healed from trauma. They will know that they are loved however they feel, and that their feelings are welcome.

> *Self-Compassion Moment*
>
> *If your child uses a dummy, or used to, or you used to use one as a child, I'm sending lots of love to you and your feelings as you read this. You might feel called to share those emotions with a loving listener, or to do some journalling, or to connect with your Inner Loving Mother, if you're familiar with The Marion Method work.[63]*

Reading stories and singing songs before bed

It's interesting, isn't it, how common it is to read stories before bed? From an Aware Parenting perspective, we can see that this might their needs for connection and fun, but we can also see that it is possible that this can be a way to distract children from their feelings.

From an anthropological perspective, we can imagine that it has been common over millennia to tell stories, perhaps around a fire, to share about the ancestors and to pass down traditions and stories. Dancing and drumming are also likely to have been common. This is similar to lullabies; singing and chanting around campfires has probably been around as long as there were campfires and the capacity to sing!

However, the *way* we read stories today, from books, can bring about very different experiences for a child, depending on our intentions.

---

63   You can find out more on my website, www.marionrose.net, or on my Psychospiritual Podcast.

Stories and lullabies can be used for connection and healing, but they can also be used to distract children from their healing-feelings. Some children might actually become more alert after hearing particular stories before bed, when feelings or thoughts are stimulated.

How can we maximise the connection and healing power of stories and songs, and minimise the suppression factor?

Supporting yourself to be present in your body, and offering closeness when you're reading stories can help.

I also recommend avoiding stories if your child is antsy and agitated or starting to cry. At those times, moving in to listen to feelings will be way more helpful than books to help them feel truly relaxed.

In addition, making the books come alive can really help – reading in funny voices, or even bringing in *attachment play* – such as:

- pretending to fall asleep and snoring loudly each time you turn the page;
- jumping up in the air with surprise with each new page; or
- starting at the end of the book and being mock-shocked that the book begins at the end, "What a STRANGE book! It's starting at the end!"

Alternatively, if your child is quite relaxed already and doesn't need to play or cry, you might lie down together and make up gentle stories together, including tales about them and their lives.

Children can experience a deep sense of being cared about, loved, and mattering when we tell them 'once upon a time' stories about them.

Simply being aware that you don't want to suppress your child's feelings through reading can transform the experience, so that it can turn into times of deep connection, attachment play, or even healing crying if that's what they need.

For example, if they clearly have a lot of feelings and are urgently wanting you to read more and more books, you could let them know that this is the last book, and then offer a *Loving Limit*, *"I really hear that you want me to read you another story, sweetheart, and I'm not willing to read any more tonight, because I don't think that's the most helpful thing for you right now. And I'm right here and I'm listening to all of your feelings."* This *Loving Limit* can help them express the feelings that were causing the agitation, and will help them feel calmer and more relaxed, which is likely to affect their sleep in enjoyable ways.

Self-Reflection Moment

Do you remember being read stories before bed as a child?

Did you read before bed as a child or teenager?

Do you need to read before bed to feel relaxed as an adult?

How do you feel after reading?

How do you feel if you don't read before bed?

Have you had any 'aha!' moments?

Would you like to do anything differently with your child as a result?

CHAPTER SUMMARY

There are three slightly different ways in which children can dissociate before sleep:

- *They* ask *us* to do things that will make them dissociate.
- *They* do things *themselves* to dissociate.
- *We* do things *to them* that make them dissociate.

Asking us to do things that will make them dissociate

Our aim is to distinguish between needs-feelings and healing-feelings. We can clearly see that they aren't expressing an unmet need if they keep asking for things, and we respond, and they're still agitated and antsy. Then we can offer a *Loving Limit* when we understand that our child is asking for something because they are trying to distract themselves from pent-up painful feelings.

I love to express *Loving Limits* using phrases such as, "*I really hear that you want me to get you another toy, sweetheart, and I'm not willing to get another toy, because I don't think that's most helpful for you right now, and I'm here and I'm listening.*" However, there is no set language for *Loving Limits* in Aware Parenting.

Distracting themselves with control patterns

With *control patterns*, we can think of four steps:

1. Engaging with our own inner work so that we can offer our loving support.
2. Moving in with compassion, warmth, and presence.
3. Offering *attachment play* related to the *control pattern*.
4. Offering *Loving Limits* and *listening* to the healing-feelings.

Us distracting them

Dummies, reading to them, and singing songs are three of the ways that we can do this. Simply being aware that we don't want to suppress our child's feelings can transform the experience. It can turn into warm connection, *attachment play*, or even healing crying if that's what they need.

I'm here with you while you and your child/ren become even more present and relaxed.

26. Your own inner work

It is common for our own feelings to bubble up when we respond in these Aware Parenting ways. We might have always had a dummy to go to sleep, or we might have been left in a pram in the garden with a bottle for our naps. We might remember calling out in the night and no-one coming to us, or clutching on to a soft toy to go to sleep. We might have been told to go to bed at a certain time as an older child, and often been awake and alone, not feeling tired.

As we offer our child connection and the opportunity to talk, play, laugh, cry, and rage so that they can naturally feel relaxed enough to fall asleep and stay asleep, we might experience all kinds of our own feelings from the past bubbling up.

Self-Compassion Moment

I'm sending so much love and compassion to you if you experience this. I'm here to remind you that this is a normal part of our own healing process and is the way that our own psyche is inviting us to feel and express painful pent up feelings, and receive reparative experiences. Again, I will invite you to connect in with an empathy buddy (or three! I so recommend structuring in lots of this support for ourselves), or an Aware Parenting instructor if you're needing extra support. Journalling and connecting with your Inner Loving Presences (from The Marion Method) can also be really helpful here.

I had a soft toy rabbit that I had with me when I went to sleep. I had him from when I was a baby, and I even took him away to University with me! We can form very deep bonds with our bedtime control patterns!

Self-Reflection Moment

I invite you to contemplate the following. You might write the answers in a journal, or share them with an empathy buddy or Aware Parenting instructor. Please check in with yourself beforehand as to whether you are willing to do this, and that you have the emotional bandwidth to listen in to feelings from your past.

- What did you do before going to sleep as a young child?
- Did you have something to help you go to sleep, such as a dummy or a soft toy?
- How did that change as you got older?
- Do you remember how you felt going off to sleep as a child?
- Do you remember waking up in the night? If so, what did you do next?
- Did you have nightmares, night terrors, or did you sleepwalk?
- What would you have longed to have as a child before, during, and after sleep?
- Did you sleep in the same bed (or in the same room) with your parents, siblings, or other family members? Or did you sleep alone in your own room? Or a mixture? How was that for you?
- Did one of your parents stay with you until you fell asleep? Or did you usually fall asleep alone? Or did you fall asleep in a room that you shared with your sibling/s?
- If you did co-sleep or share your room with a sibling, how old were you when you first slept alone? Do you remember how that was for you?
- At what age did you start choosing when you went to sleep? How was that for you?

To your inner children:

I'm sorry for all the times you were alone before sleep or in the middle of the night, when you longed for closeness.

I'm here to listen to all of your feelings about that.

It's your birthright to have closeness at night when you need it.

There's nothing wrong with you for wanting closeness.

It's natural to want to be close.

I'm sorry for all the times you needed to dissociate to go to sleep.

I so celebrate all the ways you found to dissociate when your feelings weren't welcome.

There's nothing wrong with you for having big feelings.

Your big feelings are normal and natural and healthy and healing.

You were so wise to dissociate when you didn't feel safe to express your feelings.

I trust that you will know now when you feel safe to express those feelings.

I'm so sorry for any times you were judged, shamed, or punished for crying or raging before bed or in the middle of the night.

That wasn't your fault, sweetheart.

Your feelings are beautiful gifts.

It's your birthright to have your feelings heard.

I'm sending love to any times you were judged or shamed when you were being playful before bed.

Being playful before bed is actually really wise, did you know that, sweetheart?

You are so wise.

There is nothing wrong with you when you get rambunctious.

I welcome your play.

Your play and your laughter are so beautiful.

I'm here with you.

I will stay with you for as long as you need.

I love you.

CHAPTER SUMMARY

It is common for our own feelings to bubble up when we respond in these Aware Parenting ways. As we offer our child connection and the opportunity to talk, play, laugh, cry, and rage so that they can naturally feel relaxed enough to fall asleep and stay asleep, we might experience all kinds of our own feelings from the past bubbling up. I'm sending so much love and compassion to you if you find this happening.

I invite you to connect in with an empathy buddy or three, or an Aware Parenting instructor if you're needing extra support. Journalling and connecting with your *Inner Loving Presences* (from *The Marion Method*) can also be really helpful here.

I also invited you to contemplate your own childhood experiences with sleep.

I'm here with you. You're not alone with this. I so deeply acknowledge all of your feelings.

27. The steps of supporting your child to sleep

Whether your child is two or twelve, I'm sending you so much love as you start, or continue, your Aware Parenting sleep journey.

As I did in Part 1 on babies, I'm going to offer you some suggestions for steps as starting points. As you continue to develop your own Aware Parenting sleep practice, you'll discover what is most supportive for you and your family. You can always experiment, observe, and go back to the drawing board. Once you find ways that really resonate with you and work for your family, I imagine you'll find that they become easy and habitual.

I'm here to remind you that as our children get older, our aim in Aware Parenting is to gradually give over the responsibility for tuning in to each of the three ingredients to them – when we observe that they are ready for that.

Here are the steps:

1. Thinking: Hold the theory clearly in your mind

The three things needed for sound sleep:

- to feel tired (sleepy);
- to feel connected (*closeness creating a sense of safety*); and
- to feel relaxed (*by releasing any healing-feelings present*).

If they are clearly tired and connected and are not going to sleep, this is generally because they are not feeling relaxed enough, often because of accumulated feelings (but of course always check out other physiological reasons first).

The three ways children heal from stress and trauma:

- *attachment play*;

- crying/raging with vigorous movement and loving support; and
- talking (less effective for younger children, more helpful and important with older children).

Children have unexpressed feelings bubbling up when they are:

- playing rambunctiously;
- trying to distract themselves by asking for lots of things;
- wanting us to read to them or play with them more, even though they are clearly tired[64];
- suppressing feelings, e.g. with thumb-sucking or a dummy; and/or
- wriggling or antsy.

2. Feeling: Have your own feelings heard

The more you have your own feelings lovingly heard before supporting your child for a nap or sleep, the more spaciousness you will probably have to be loving and playful, and welcome your child's feelings, and the less likely you will react in ways that you don't want to towards them.

In addition, this will mean it's more likely that they will experience feeling safe, both to feel relaxed enough to sleep, and to release any feelings that are bubbling up to be expressed through laughter and play or crying and raging.

Your emotional state has a big effect on them and their ability to feel relaxed.

The wonderful thing is that a little listening can go a long way. So if your days are busy, that might even be just two or three minutes connecting in with your empathy buddy or Aware Parenting instructor on voice note

---

64 However, please hold in mind that if they haven't had much connection with you during the day, their need for connection might override their need for sleep.

in a voice-messaging app before you go in with some *attachment play* or *Loving Limits* with your child before a nap or bedtime. Knowing that someone else understands, welcomes your feelings, and supports you wholeheartedly, can make a huge difference to your own capacity to be present. This in turn affects the emotional safety you create for your child and the likelihood that they will experience connection and fun in play or the freedom to release any healing-feelings before sleep through talking or crying with you.

You will probably notice that if you've received less listening time for a day, few days, or weeks, that your capacity to be present with your child/ren's needs and feelings goes down, and you are less able to move in with *attachment play* or listen to their feelings. That's a really strong *indicator* and *invitation* to reach out for more empathy for yourself.

As your child becomes more independent and doesn't need closeness in order to go to sleep without dissociating, and starts choosing when they go to sleep, you might find big feelings showing up for you. Or perhaps they are wanting to choose when they go to sleep but are using reading or screens as a *control pattern*. Having your feelings heard is more likely to mean that you'll be able to stay connected with them and be truly supportive in whatever they most need, whether that's *attachment play* or *Loving Limits*, or listening to them share about their day.

If you really don't want to play or listen to feelings, you might leave a quick voice note with your empathy buddy to tell them that (out of earshot of your child, of course!).

3. Presence: Connecting in with yourself and helping yourself become present

The more connected with yourself and present you are, the more likely it is that your child will feel connected with you and safe.

This will aid them in feeling a sense of emotional safety to release feelings through *attachment play*, crying or raging, or talking with you.

Here are a few suggestions:

- Gazing at your child's face, or eyebrows, or irises, or skin.
- Stroking a dog or cat.
- Dancing around the kitchen when you're cooking dinner.
- Noticing the sensations of food when you're eating.
- If you share a bath with your child, noticing the sensations of the water on your skin.
- Stretching exercises or yoga with or without your child/ren.
- Connecting with your *Inner Loving Mother*, from *The Marion Method*.

4. Preparation: Preparing yourself physically and emotionally

If you know that your child generally wants to do *attachment play* before sleep, or if you sense *attachment play* is going to help them feel more connected and relaxed, preparation for this could include having comfortable clothes on so you can join in wholeheartedly. You might prepare for this in simple ways, such as putting on a funny hat and running back into the room where they are, ready to be goofy and silly. You could watch a few minutes of your favourite comedian, so that you are in a humorous mood. If you sense that you are going to need to offer them some *Loving Limits* to help them cry, that might be making sure you're feeling powerful in your body by doing some yoga poses or dancing around the kitchen in the evening.

5. Tired: Watching for tiredness signs

As they get older, you will probably have an approximate idea of what kind of time they tend to get tired. However, if they've had a day with lots of physical activity or new experiences, they might feel physically tired earlier on. If they've had a nap or woken up later, that might also affect when they tend to get tired.

As much as possible, I invite you to hold in mind that it's harder for them to both release feelings and go to sleep when they're not tired. Whereas, when they are tired, they will be more likely to move into those natural relaxation processes of playing, crying, or raging, and also, of course, to be able to fall asleep.

Remember that our aim is to support them to notice their own tiredness signs as they get older, so they can increasingly take responsibility for their own going to sleep process as part of their unique timing of becoming more independent.

6. Connected: Offer them closeness and connection

I invite you to focus on connection with yourself, and from that place, offer connection to your child.

There are many ways we can bring deep closeness and connection into *all* the activities that happen before sleep. You might do that as much as you can throughout the late afternoon or evening if you are together (and if they still have naps, for the hour or so before that, if possible). That might include inviting them to join in with preparing the dinner, or being close with them and chatting or singing together whilst making dinner. That might mean offering eye contact whilst eating, and touching them gently (for example as you put their plate on the table, you might gently touch their back). You might offer endearments and sing little songs. You might pretend to be a chef and offer funny pretend dishes to them, or ask them to be the waiter or waitress and pretend to work in a restaurant together.

For younger children, you might have a bath or shower with them, or you might wrap them in a towel when they get out of the bath or shower and give them a big cuddle, perhaps pretending that you're a big bear hugging your little bear. If you're brushing their teeth for them, you might get down to their level and talk warmly to them. If they brush their own teeth, they could do that sitting on your lap, or with you cuddling them from behind. If they are older, you might sit down next to them on the sofa or on their bed, and be curious about their day, if you weren't together. You might sing songs together, play board games together, or do little family rituals, such as family bed gymnastics.

For older children, once they no longer need us to be with us while going to sleep, offering warmth and closeness during the evening will still help contribute to a sense of ongoing connection and safety in their bodies.

7. Relaxed

1a. Notice where you might be inadvertently distracting them from their innate relaxation processes (this is more likely to be for younger children)

They might be trying to be playful and you might be trying to 'calm them down'. They might be trying to distract themselves by asking for one more snack, one more drink, one more toy, one more game, and you're doing all the things they are asking for, but they are still clearly antsy and agitated and keep asking for different and more things, and you keep giving them those. They might be asking you to distract them from their feelings, such as by asking for you to read them more stories, and you keep on reading and reading.

However, please hold in mind that they might be trying to meet their need for connection with you, especially if you've been separated from each other during the day.

Or,they might be trying to find a pretext – an *emotional coat hanger* – to hang their feelings on – to have a big cry over a small thing. Perhaps the dinner isn't quite right, or the towel, or the PJs – and you keep trying to 'fix' it. But then realise that they are still agitated and keep trying to find another pretext. You might be offering them a snack, or a dummy, or a screen, or a story, when they are trying to move into having a big cry.

You might be distracting them in other ways, such as changing the subject, offering a story, or lessening their feelings through your words, for example: *"It doesn't matter,"* or, *"There's nothing to be upset about."*

1b. Notice when they are distracting themselves with *control patterns*

If they are clearly distracting themselves from their healing-feelings through *control patterns* such as: thumb-sucking, a dummy, being busy, moving from one thing to the next, reading, watching screens, the most helpful initial response will generally be *attachment play*.

In the last chapter, I shared a four-step process:

1. Our own ongoing inner work (e.g. sharing our feelings and thoughts about their *control pattern* to our empathy buddy, or perhaps journalling).
2. Moving in with warmth and compassion (thinking about the warmth melting the freeze).
3. Offering *attachment play* that's related to the *control pattern* in some way.
4. Offering a *Loving Limit* and *listening* to their healing-feelings.

2. Instead of distracting them, follow their lead. If they're trying to distract themselves, move in with *attachment play* or *Loving Limits*

If they invite play, join in with them. Do what they're doing, or add in *attachment play*, such as:

- *power-reversal play* (by being less powerful and mock-surprised about how much bigger, faster or more powerful they are); or
- *nonsense play* (by being silly and goofy and incompetent); or
- *separation games* (by bringing in elements such as peek-a-boo or hide and seek).

The more they laugh (as long as there's no tickling), the more they are releasing stress and tension.

I invite you to trust them and to be mindful that they know what they need to release, heal, and feel relaxed enough to sleep.

If they are trying to distract themselves with one more toy, and you clearly see that this isn't about here and now needs (because they're not happy with anything), you could offer a *Loving Limit*. "*I hear that you want to get another toy from the living room, and I'm not willing for you to do that, sweetheart, because I don't think that's the most helpful thing for you right now. And I'm right here and I'm listening,*" and then listen to the feelings that they've been trying to distract themselves from.

If they are wanting you to distract them from their feelings such as by asking you to read them more stories, you could also offer a *Loving Limit*, "*I hear that you want me to read you more stories, and I'm not willing to read you any more, sweetheart, because I don't think that's the most helpful thing for you right now, and I'm right here and I'm listening,*" and then listen to those feelings that they were trying to distract themselves from.

If they're trying to find a pretext – an **emotional coat hanger** *to find a reason to have a big cry or rage*, once you realise that that's what they're doing, you could simply offer them empathy and stay with their feelings, "*Oh sweetheart, I really hear that those pyjamas aren't the ones you wanted tonight, and the other ones are all wet in the washing machine. I hear you. I'm listening. I'm right here with you.*"

If they're using a **control pattern** *to dissociate,* offer *attachment play*, followed by a *Loving Limit* if necessary.

If they start trying to cry, simply be with them and their feelings. Move in close, offer warmth and eye contact and a loving tone, "*I'm here with you, sweetheart. I love you. I'm listening.*"

As they get older, talking will increasingly replace crying as a way to release feelings.

This might involve them wanting to share about their day, or about things that interest them.

You listening lovingly to their sharing through talking is as important as your loving presence with their tears and tantrums at younger ages.

3. Keep following their lead or doing what they really need to feel truly relaxed

If your child is immersed in play with you and you're both laughing and enjoying the play, keep going for as long as you can.

If you start getting tired or just don't want to play any more, you can offer them a *Limit*[65], *"I've so enjoyed playing with you, and I'm going to put a timer on for five minutes, and I'm not willing to play any more after that, because I'm tired. Then, I'm going to help you go to bed.*[66]*"* And when the timer goes off, *"I'm not willing to play any more sweetheart. Let's go to the bedroom now."* You might want to do some *attachment play* to get into bed – *"Let's pretend we're sloths and we're moving reallllllllyyyy slooooowwwwwly to the bed."* If they have feelings in response, we can listen lovingly to those. *"I hear that you wanted to play more, sweetheart. I understand. I'm listening."*

If they're wanting to play for hours and you sense that there are deeper feelings underneath that are preventing them from feeling relaxed enough to be able to go to sleep, or if you think a cry is bubbling, you might offer a *Loving Limit*, *"I'm going to put a timer on for five minutes, and I'm not willing to play any more after that, because I don't think it's the most helpful thing for you."* And when the timer goes off, *"I'm not willing to play any more sweetheart, and I'm right here and listening."* If this brings forth tears, listen lovingly, offering empathy. If the crying intensifies when you offer warmth or empathy, that tells you that you're helping them express the feelings that have been sitting inside them.

65 It's a *Limit*, not a *Loving Limit*, because it's from your own unwillingness to play for longer, rather than to support them to express feelings that are causing them to want to keep playing.
66 This is for younger children who are still needing our support to go to sleep. Once they are older and no longer need that support, we wouldn't recommend a *Loving Limit* in relation to when to go to sleep.

"You really wanted to play more, sweetheart. I hear you. I understand. I'm listening."

If they keep asking for things, or trying to distract themselves, or focusing on the pretext, and they're crying, keep offering the limit and listening lovingly to their feelings, *"Oh sweetheart, I really hear how much you want me to play for longer, and I'm not willing to play any more any more, because I don't think it's the most helpful thing for you right now. I'm here with you and all of your feelings. I love you."*

If they start getting rough in the play, you can also offer a *Loving Limit,* starting with doing the minimum to stop the roughness, and then something like, *"I'm not willing for you to do that, sweetheart, because I'm here to keep everyone safe. And I'm right here and I'm listening."*

If they continue to cry, I invite you to remember that it's normal and natural for all children to have a lot of big feelings sitting inside them.

The crying might get louder and more intense if you offer empathy, come closer, or offer warm touch.

I invite you to listen in deeply to yourself and to them and to play with the *balance of attention*, seeing what is most helpful for them. You might find that during the most intense crying, they're sweating and moving their arms and legs around a lot.

I invite you to remember that the fight or flight response mobilises energy in their arms and legs, and that during this crying, they are releasing this tension, so that instead of being wriggly, they will feel more relaxed and more able to sleep restfully and restoratively.

You might find it helpful to think about how much energy it takes to hold in these feelings, and to see clearly how these feelings, when held inside, lead to them finding it hard to go to sleep and stay asleep for as long as they need.

If you're able to stay with the whole process, they are likely to let out a whole chunk of feelings, and then come out the other side, completing the whole crying cycle.

If you stop them, it's possible that they will wake up later to continue crying, to try to complete the process.

Remember to focus on keeping connected with yourself, staying present if you can, through:

- *connecting* in with your *breathing*;
- *noticing* the *details* about their face or hair; and
- *feeling* the *sensations* of your sitting bones on the chair or floor.

It's very common for our own feelings to bubble up from the past, as well as conditioned thoughts.

If you do feel concerned that they have an unmet need, you can always stop and offer them what you think will meet that need, and then observe them afterwards.

They will tell you what was really going on when you know what to look for. If, when you meet the apparent need, they're still agitated, tense, or avoiding eye contact, it's likely that it wasn't an unmet need after all.

If you keep listening to the end of the release process, the crying will eventually taper off and come to a natural completion.

You might find they then fall asleep, or there might be some awake time before that. I invite you to keep offering warm connection as you hold them in your arms or lie with them. You might notice they are particularly cuddly, and you might also feel deeply connected with them after hearing their biggest feelings.

4. Notice whether they're becoming more relaxed and present

You might notice that their muscles become more relaxed, their face softens, and they are more present after the playing, raging, or crying.

Noticing things like this is important in terms of you receiving reassurance that attachment play *or expressing these big feelings has been helpful for them. Remember, this is the research process, and you are the researcher!*

8. Keep connected: Stay close with them as they fall asleep

If they're in your arms, you might want to keep holding them as they fall asleep, or you might want to put them in bed and lie next to them. I invite you to choose and experiment and see what happens for both of you, while staying close with them.

As children get older, they will naturally come to a time where they don't need closeness to be able to sleep without dissociating. I invite you to follow their lead on this. This is part of trusting their own individual timing of increasing independence.

9. If they wake up soon after

If they wake up soon after, it's likely that they have more feelings to express.

I invite you to move close and not say much. Saying, "*I'm here with you,*" and offering a soft touch might be enough to help them feel connected, and they might express some more feelings.

10. Your feelings

During the play, laughter, crying or raging, or talking, you might have experienced your own feelings bubbling up – it's so normal and natural if you did. You might also feel drained, exhausted, overwhelmed, frustrated, sad, or numb afterwards. These responses may tell you that being with your child as they expressed their emotions helped you to connect with your own feelings. Often these feelings are from our childhood.

If we are going to be able to consistently offer presence, playfulness, and listen to our child's feelings, it's vital to have our emotions that bubble up when we do that lovingly heard.

If you have a partner, that might mean sharing with them. If you have an empathy buddy, you might leave them a message or connect on a phone or video call.

I invite you to connect with a supportive listener before you're tempted to go and sit in front of a screen, go to the fridge, or drink a glass of wine. And of course, I send you unconditional love if you do go and do those things!

And I want to lovingly remind you that if you do, those feelings will sit inside you and might be ready to come up the next time your child is crying (or some other event)!

11. Observation

Notice any differences after listening to their feelings, before, during and after sleep, and when they are awake too. Increased relaxation can be seen in the following ways:

During sleep:

- Relaxed muscles
- Melting into your body
- Relaxed and open hands
- Moving around less whilst sleeping
- Able to stay asleep without being in one particular position, e.g. under our arm.

When awake:

- More eye contact
- More smiling
- Face more open and luminous
- Concentrates for longer periods
- More happy
- Less whining
- Less agitation

The more of a difference you see, the more it will give you reassurance that what you are doing is helpful for them. That can also help you acknowledge and appreciate all that you're doing and the difference it's making to how they feel.

CHAPTER SUMMARY

To support your child to sleep, you can focus on thinking (holding the theory clearly in your mind), feeling (having your feelings heard), presence (connecting in with yourself), preparing yourself physically and emotionally, watching for tired signs, offering closeness and connection, and supporting them to feel relaxed through *attachment play, Loving Limits,* and listening to them sharing about their experiences.

I so deeply acknowledge
all that you're doing.

28. Specific suggestions for particular situations

Your child won't nap

It could be that your child is ready to drop their nap because they are no longer tired during the day. However, they might still be tired enough to need a nap but not relaxed enough to nap. This is very common if a child has quite a few accumulated feelings sitting at the surface. They're not as tired as they are at nighttime, and so it's easier for them to suppress the healing-feelings which might be preventing them from feeling relaxed, and so it's harder for them to nap.

One option is to forgo the nap, then when they get more tired in the evening, they'll be more able to express the feelings that are preventing them from falling asleep for a nap (because it's harder to suppress feelings when they're more tired). After supporting them to express the feelings for a few evenings, you might notice that they are generally feeling both more relaxed in their body and also more able to access their feelings. They might then be able to go back to having a nap, or they might not really need one any more after all.

However, it's also possible that a child who doesn't have a nap could be so sleepy in the evening that they fall asleep before doing any of the crying they need to do, or without completing a whole crying cycle.

When toddlers stop having regular daytime naps, bedtime can be unpredictable and a little chaotic for a while until their body fully adjusts to no naps.

You might want to avoid late afternoon car rides or other activities which might lead to a late nap and them going to bed later.

Your child expresses their feelings at other times, but not before sleep

As children get older, the effect of tiredness making it harder to suppress their painful feelings lessens. You might find that they cry or tantrum at other times of the day rather than when they are tired. If so, I invite you to follow their lead as much as possible, and welcome the healing-feelings when they do come. It's likely to mean that they then feel relaxed enough to sleep when they are tired, and don't have any feelings to express then, because they've already expressed any healing-feelings that they need to for that day, earlier on.

Your child always wants to play wild games before sleep

From an Aware Parenting perspective, this is their natural relaxation-through-release response in operation. Rather than trying to 'calm them down', I invite you to follow their lead. That will probably mean joining in with the play and bringing in elements of *attachment play* where relevant – such as power-reversal games, nonsense play, and separation games. If they're laughing (as long as you're not tickling them), they are releasing tension through the play, which is likely to help them relax. You playing with them in these special ways is likely to have a more powerful relaxing effect than if they just play on their own or even with a sibling.

Your child sucks their thumb to go to sleep

They are likely to be sucking their thumb to suppress the healing-feelings that are naturally bubbling up when they feel tired. If you're wanting to help them feel the emotional safety to express those emotions, one of the first things I recommend is to share your feelings about them sucking their thumb with your empathy buddy or an Aware Parenting instructor. That might include any feelings from your own childhood, if you used to suck your thumb too. Then, if they do suck their thumb before bed, you could offer them lots of warmth, and then *attachment play* related to the thumb-sucking. For example, being mock-curious about what they have in their mouth. Do they have a tiger in there? They might take their thumb out and you act surprised that it's not a tiger. And then if they put it in again, you might be curious about whether it's a toothbrush, and again show mock-surprise when they show you that it's their thumb. And then repeat it! As they laugh and laugh, they are releasing some of the lighter feelings that the thumb-sucking has been holding in. That in itself might be enough for them to now feel relaxed enough to fall asleep. Or, it might be that the connection and laughter have loosened up some deeper healing-feelings and they might suddenly start crying in response to a small pretext. The more of these feelings they express, the more relaxed they will feel, and the more easily they'll sleep.

Please note that we don't recommend taking a child's thumb out of their mouth or offering *Loving Limits* with thumb-sucking.

Your child wriggles around in bed, talks a lot, fidgets, etc.

Wriggling, talking, fidgeting, and agitated talking (as long as you've checked out that there's nothing going on for them physiologically) is generally a sign that your child has accumulated feelings that are sitting close to the surface. They're feeling agitated as a result, and that's causing all the wriggly-type behaviour. Knowing this in itself can make a huge difference for us as parents.

Instead of thinking that they're doing it deliberately, you might want to keep in mind one of my favourite parenting mantras – "They're not doing it deliberately, they're not enjoying it, they need my help."

And they do need our help, because they have these innate relaxation processes which often we have inadvertently worked against, and so they are left with the healing-feelings that haven't been released. They need our support for their relaxation-through-release processes to work effectively, whether that is *attachment play,* where our child releases feelings of powerlessness, fear and frustration, or crying and raging along with vigorous movement and our loving presence, or sharing about their day with us. The more they do of those, the more they release those feelings. Our children want to feel relaxed, just as we do. We don't enjoy feeling agitated and antsy, and neither do our children.

Deep relaxation is so enjoyable, and you do have the power to support your child to feel that more of the time.

Your child is scared of monsters or has other fears during the night

There are various contributing factors to these kinds of fears, such as a lack of information, or a developmental awareness of death that can happen for many children at around the age of three years. Giving children accurate information is an important part of Aware Parenting.

However, if these fears are caused by scary, stressful, or traumatic experiences, you can help them heal from these. Information may still be an important part of that, such as if they watched a movie with monsters, and we give them accurate information that monsters don't exist.

The *first* thing I would do is to check out whether there's anything going on in their daytime life which is frightening for them. And if there is, to do whatever you can to stop that. *Next*, I would increase the amount of closeness and connection they are experiencing before bed and whilst asleep. After that, I would recommend lots of *attachment play,* which can help release and resolve fears. You could pretend that your child has a magic wand or a remote control that they point at you, and when they do, they choose what you do – jump in the air, pick your nose, fall over. If you can do this in a goofy, exaggerated or mock-surprise way, it will probably increase their sense of power. If they're laughing, enjoying the game, and wanting to keep playing, you can trust that it is helping them release fears and giving them more of a sense of agency. Giving them more choice in their day-to-day life can also help. Then there are approach-avoidance games. For example, we might hold hands, and run towards something that might be scary for them, such as their bed, or the cupboard, or the dark shapes on the walls, and turn round together and run back again to hide. Doing that over and over again, getting closer with joint laughter, can also help children feel deeply supported, and the laughter can release powerlessness and fear. Finding opportunities to support them to express pent-up feelings through crying and raging, and lovingly staying with them whilst they do so, will also reduce and even eliminate the fear. Your confidence and calmness will also support them in knowing that they are safe. However, if you're doing all of these and nothing seems to shift after a while, I would recommend having a consultation with an Aware Parenting instructor.

Your child has nightmares or night terrors

From an Aware Parenting perspective, nightmares are often a sign that a child has accumulated feelings that aren't being expressed in the day, so their system is trying to process the feelings in a different way.

In working with parents over nearly two decades, I've found that the higher percentage of a child's healing-feelings are listened to in the day or evening, the less likely they are to have nightmares at night.

It makes such sense that the body has multiple systems to process painful feelings. If those feelings aren't being expressed and heard during the day, the body has a back-up system to bring about healing, and that seems to be through nightmares.

Some people believe that nightmares can be caused by certain foods or by EMF, so as always, please check out physiological factors if you feel called to. Once you've done that, I invite you to be an emotional detective.

The *first* task is to see if there's anything that they are experiencing during the day that is scary or traumatic for them, and to stop that thing happening wherever possible. For example, some parents have shared that their child has nightmares after watching TV. With Aware Parenting, we invite you to reduce the sources of stress in your child's life wherever possible. Perhaps they're experiencing harsh treatment at school: going into the school and advocating for them, or taking them out of that school, might be the first step. The *second* step is to create the emotional safety needed for them to express their feelings at home. Being able to do this often depends on you receiving some emotional support to express your feelings. *Third*, laughter and play are powerful ways to release fear. I recommend lots of *attachment play*, particularly games that bring about laugher (as long as there's no tickling).

Then, when your child is clearly indicating that they have painful feelings bubbling (e.g. they're crying or raging, they're suppressing their feelings, they're hitting, biting, throwing or taking, they're asking for lots of things and aren't happy with any of them, they're whining, etc.), move in with your loving warmth and presence and support them to express those feelings in tears and raging, and stay with them throughout the process. You'll see throughout the book there are ways to respond to each of these behaviours in ways which support their natural healing response.

I loved receiving this from Majule about night terrors:

"My son had some accumulated feelings building up for a while. One night, when I took him to the toilet, he started to cry and rage, and I realised he was still asleep. I recognised how incredible his innate body wisdom is. I just knew that it was exactly what he needed to do and I held space quietly, ensuring he was safe and speaking some words of reassurance over him in the same way I would if he were awake and raging/crying. This lasted about 20 minutes, with lots and lots of tears. When he briefly 'woke up', he said, "I want to go back to bed now, Mummy". I put him in bed and he went back to sleep. The next day he was so much more himself than I'd seen him for a while; he was more relaxed and loving and present in his body. This experience completely changed the way I understand night terrors."

Your child is wetting the bed

My first invitation would be to check out whether there's anything going on physiologically. Next, I'd recommend ascertaining whether there is anything stressful in their life that you can protect them from. The bedwetting could be caused by accumulated feelings from stress and trauma. Then you might want to offer the things I have suggested in the book to help them heal from stress and trauma, particularly plenty of *attachment play* and crying with your loving support before bed. One of these forms of play could be to offer them dolls or soft toys and a toy bed, and invite your child to play with these. Then you could support them in whatever they decide to play, trusting their innate wisdom for healing through the play.

Your child always wants 'more' before bed – more games, more stories, etc.

The *first* step I recommend here is to listen in to whether this is the expression of an immediate need, or accumulated painful feelings. If your child hasn't had enough connection with you during the day, they may want lots of it at bedtime. Doing extra non-directive child-centred play during the day can really help with this. Alternatively, if the requests for more are caused by accumulated feelings, you will notice that they have an *urgent* quality to them. This is one of the core signs that something is a *control pattern* (a way to mildly dissociate from feelings) rather than a here and now need. That means that although the requests are urgent, those are not the real needs. The real need is to express the feelings that they are trying to suppress. When you're confident that this is what's going on, you can very lovingly offer them a *Loving Limit*: "*I hear that you'd really like more games/stories, sweetheart, and I'm not willing to play (or read) any more because I don't think that's the most helpful thing for you right now. And I'm here, and I'm listening.*"

Remember that a *Loving Limit* is not just about stopping the behaviour. It is designed to elicit the feelings that are the cause of that behaviour, so we're expecting protesting, leading to crying or raging.

Our role is to stay calm, not take anything personally, and just keep on listening and offering the limit if necessary. "*Oh sweetheart, you really wanted more, and Mummy says no, because I don't think that's the most helpful thing for you right now. And I'm here with you, listening to all of your feelings."* When they can cry and rage with us, they are doing what their natural relaxation response is designed to do. That is to feel, express, and release the feelings that were underneath all those urgent requests. Then they will be much more likely to feel calm and relaxed and to be able to go to sleep.

Your child wakes up a lot at night

There are physiological reasons that may possibly cause children to wake up a lot, so please check these (see the Appendix).

And remember that connection is one of the core requirements for restful sleep for younger children, so I invite you to offer them closeness, if you're not already.

If they're already close and are waking up a lot and there's nothing else going on, the waking is most likely from accumulated feelings that are bubbling up to the surface when they're in lighter sleep. Some parents are willing to listen to those feelings in the middle of the night, and if that's you, I so celebrate you. Many parents prefer to listen to those feelings during the day or in the evening. If your child is already crying and they're safe and you're there with them, supporting them to cry loudly until they've finished will help them release a whole load of pent-up tension that wakes them up at night. I invite you to notice ways you might be distracting them from their feelings, either through trying to distract them from rambunctious play or distracting them from crying before bed. Instead, I invite you to join in with the play and listen to their healing-feelings. Children really do know how to feel deeply relaxed at night, and once we understand our own conditioning that often prevents that, their sleep can change markedly and quickly.

Please remember though, that sleep is the ultimate emotional barometer, so sometimes it may take a bit of time (that can be weeks or even months) for them to catch up on expressing those pent-up feelings. You'll receive reassurance that healing is happening by noticing any changes in other areas since you've been listening to more of their healing-feelings, such as them making more eye contact, smiling more, concentrating for longer periods, being more cooperative, naturally gentle, and cuddling up more.

You really can help your child sleep more restfully and restoratively!

Understanding why a child wakes up at night and what we can do to help can often make a huge difference to how we feel.

Linde, an Aware Parenting instructor in Europe, shares her journey of coming to Aware Parenting, and the difference it made not only to her children's sleep, but also to her thoughts and feelings when they weren't sleeping so restfully:

"When I first became a mother in 2016, I did not know of Aware Parenting (I have a Masters degree in psychology. However, that was not very helpful in my parenting journey). We did offer him lots of closeness the first few weeks. I was able to rest a lot and be very present with him. The first few weeks, my son slept 'fine' and did not cry much. He did sometimes cry and tense up, arching his back and tilting his head back like a banana. I thought that was his way of saying he was hungry but now I can see that might have been him trying to heal from his birth trauma, since his birth was very quick and I was very stressed.

It was only a few weeks later that he suddenly started crying more and more, often at the end of the day around the time my partner came home from work. Because I knew that my partner felt very overstimulated and overwhelmed by noise, I tried to put our son down for the day before he came home. I did not know then that babies accumulate feelings throughout the day and thus have a need to release, often in the afternoon or evening. So of course he started waking up a lot in the evenings and during the night. I tried everything to get him to sleep. I jiggled, sang, tried a pacifier, went on walks, and used white noise. When we were at our wits' end, we left him to cry in his bed hoping he would fall asleep. He did not! It broke my heart! It felt horrible but we did what people told us to do.

I also consulted with an osteopath who told me not to pick him up when he cried intensely so we would not 'reinforce this behaviour'. We 'could' pick him up when the intensity went down a little as to reinforce 'that behaviour'. It breaks my heart that this belief of babies manipulating us – and that we can and need to control their behaviour – is still widespread. But at this moment this sounded like what I've learned in school about conditioning behaviour, so we tried this. The midwife that came to check up on us also had her opinion and said that he had reflux, so not to feed him as much, and she told us to let him sleep on his belly. The doctor just said, "Babies cry, that's normal". My mom told me not to pick him up much as I might spoil him. (She's now on board with Aware Parenting and is learning all about emotional needs of babies and children!) There were a lot of different opinions and that made it very confusing and made me doubt myself even more than I already did!

The main thread throughout the advice we got was: let him cry on his own and he will fall asleep. And he did, after 15-20 minutes of tantrums in his bed, on his own, with tears streaming down his little red sweat-covered face. We watched him on the camera but switched off the 'noise'. My heart could not take it, but I was told, "This is normal, this is how they learn." It seemed to work, he slept 'fine'. He woke up sometimes, we gave him a bottle and he fell asleep again. During the day we did everything to keep him from crying. However, when he needed to sleep, we often let him cry himself to sleep. That was what I was taught, I thought that was what he needed. We believed he was fighting sleep and that he had to learn to surrender, and we did not want to make him dependent on us.

He did cry every time I dropped him off at daycare, and they had to pull him off me. It devastated me, but I thought this was normal. By the age of two, he had become very hyperactive and had a lot of tantrums and night terrors. All these symptoms I see now as signs of accumulated feelings and unmet needs. When he was two and a half, I gave birth to his brother. I remember my youngest waking up almost every hour on his first night. I was alone at hospital because my partner was at home with my eldest. I was miserable. My youngest cried a lot from birth, and it's that which made me reach out to other friends with kids for support and tips.

A friend then recommended Tears and Tantrums *[by Aletha Solter]. I remember thinking 'this makes so much sense' but also struggling with it, because at that time I had not cried in a long time. I started listening to his tears, however I don't think I had the capacity to really hold space for them. I did not read any other Aware Parenting books until a year later, when we went into lockdown. At that point when we went into lockdown, my youngest son was having difficulty falling asleep at night and was waking up every day between 3am and 5am and did not fall asleep again until 9am! We tried everything, a bottle, a sleep timer, darkness, coming to lie in our bed, anything. My eldest son was also waking up a lot during the nights again and was taking much longer to fall asleep.*

This in combination with daily struggles around not listening, not cooperating, aggression and hyperactivity, made me very motivated and willing to start reading ALL of Aletha's books on Aware Parenting. I could finally see that so much of what I was doing was working against their natural release mechanisms! Because I had only read Tears and Tantrums, *and was exhausted, I was not able to listen to as many feelings as I would have liked or they needed. My youngest son also started sucking his thumb (he seemed fearless and did not display anger, what I can see now is part of the freeze response) – a* control pattern *he still has now.*

I started with attachment play, *listening to tears, and figuring out my own needs. When my youngest woke up during the early mornings, I listened to tears, we got playful before bed, we offered more connection when they went to sleep, and soon enough they started falling asleep more easily and sleeping through the night. We had a period of them sleeping in our room again, because that met their needs for closeness and our needs for sleep. After a while we tried putting them back in their own rooms without success. They now sleep together in a room to have some closeness, and still fall asleep with us next to them in our bed and then we transfer them to their own beds. This works for us now.*

I can now see when they are moving a lot or talking a lot before bed, that there is something that wants to come out. When they wake up during the night and I'm exhausted I have my Inner Loving Mother [*from* The Marion Method] *there to listen to how I feel and that I do not want to get up and remind me that I do want them to feel safe, and have their needs met! I also can see so much of their behaviour through an Aware Parenting lens which helps a lot with staying calm and connected. When they wake up early, I no longer feel powerless, because I understand the reason for their behaviour and know what to do. I trust myself and them so much more. I am very happy with their sleep during the night now, I know they sleep around 11 hours per night, no matter at what time they go to sleep. We are still experimenting with different ways of bringing them to bed, because that is still something not going completely as we would like. We would like to have some more time to ourselves in the evening and meet their need for closeness and help them release before bed.*

Sometimes my kids wake up during the night, and they come to our bed. At times I let them sleep with us, and other times I guide them back to their bed and stay there for a while. But what is most important is not that it does not ever happen, it's that I can now see what is causing this, that I understand what is happening, and that I know how I can help them. I can see their innate healing processes as a beautiful thing instead of something annoying that needs to be avoided at all costs."

> ### Self-Compassion Moment
> I wonder how you feel when you read Linde's story? Perhaps you might recognise some of these elements in your own sleep journey? If you're feeling painful feelings, I'm sending you so much love and invite you to have those feelings lovingly heard.

Your child wakes up really early

From an Aware Parenting perspective, there are three possible reasons for this. One: they are alone and need closeness. Two: your child is inherently an early riser and has the early bird chronotype. Three: they have accumulated healing-feelings in their body which are waking them up. How can you tell the difference between the latter two?

If your child wakes up early but is clearly present and relaxed in their body, calm and willing to make eye contact, they are likely to simply be an early bird.

However, if they wake up clearly upset, or in hyperarousal (agitation) or dissociation (tense and avoiding eye contact, sucking their thumb or a dummy), it's likely that accumulated feelings are making it hard for them to sleep as long as they need to. If this latter is the case, you have plenty of choice about when you can help this change. You might want to listen to their healing-feelings when they wake up in the morning. However, you might prefer to do that in the daytime, and particularly in the evening. The more they get to express those uncomfortable emotions, the more relaxed they will feel in their body. They will be more able to sleep until they've had enough sleep, and to wake up feeling refreshed and relaxed.

You want to help your child move to their own bed in their own room

First of all, I invite you to receive some empathy and listening for your feelings and thoughts and whatever is going on for you that you're wanting them to move to their own room. You might discover that it is cultural conditioning, or it might be unmet needs of yours for sleep. You might need to receive some empathy for how hard things have been. Perhaps you've been being judged for co-sleeping.

If you want your child to move out because they're wriggling around and you're not getting much sleep, I recommend supporting them to be less wriggly through doing *attachment play* and listening to more of their healing-feelings *before* reassessing whether you want them to move. After they are feeling more relaxed while still co-sleeping, I invite you to reassess whether you still want to help them move into their own room. If you still do, it will be more supportive for them to do that after catching up with the crying, because they'll be carrying fewer painful feelings in their system.

If you still want them to move into their own room, and they don't want to, I invite you to reconnect with Aware Parenting theory. How do you feel and what do you think when you imagine that they might still be inherently needing closeness with you before going to sleep, or during the night? If you still feel called to move them, I invite you to make this a slow process. You might want to give them the information, and help them choose things for their room that will help them feel a sense of connection with the space. If they have naps, you might want to support them by starting off with naps in there.

I recommend letting your child know that they can always come to you in the night if they want to, and to make that possible for them physically, e.g. the door is left open if they are not able to open it themselves.

I also recommend doing things that support them to feel safe, e.g. a red night light in their room and in the coridoor to your room.

Most of all, I recommend lots of *attachment play* in their own room. That might be games such as:

- Pretending that you are sleeping in their bed and they are sleeping in yours, and be surprised when they say it's not how things are.
- Playing hide and seek in their bedroom.
- Offering *attachment play* with putting on PJs in their room.
- Playing games such as being lions looking for other creatures in their room.

I invite you to follow their lead with the play they instigate and trust that they will bring up their fears and concerns through play.

You might also listen to healing-feelings – perhaps they start crying when you tell them that you will be gradually supporting them to sleep in their own bed in their own room, and you can simply *stay with them* and listen to their big emotions. Over time, you are likely to find that they are more willing to be in their own bed.

Please also hold in mind that it is biologically normal for humans to sleep in close proximity to each other, and this is what still happens in many, if not most, Indigenous cultures. If your child wants to come and sleep with you, that is so normal.

In general, the bigger the percentage of their healing-feelings you've listened to through crying and raging, and the less accumulated feelings they have, the more relaxed they will feel. This might mean they are more willing to sleep alone.

However, children who are deeply connected with themselves because they've been brought up with Aware Parenting can also be very clear about what they need.

You might find that without many accumulated feelings, they still want to be with you. Closeness is a core need for children. Throughout this process, having lots of empathy for your feelings, as well as being willing for everyone to get their needs met – can really help.

From a child: I don't know why, Mummy, but I'm always like a wriggly worm when I go to bed. I heard you telling Dad last night that you don't want me to sleep in with you two any more, because of all the wriggling. You said that you can't sleep. I'm a bit scared, Mummy, because I don't know how to stop wriggling. And I think that if I slept on my own, I would be so wriggly that I wouldn't be able to sleep at all. Please don't put me in my own bed yet.

Oh, you've come to me! I was just playing with my bears on the bed. You come in with a smile on your face. You look happy. I don't think you will make me sleep on my own tonight. You go to the cupboard and get out two sleeping bags that we slept in when we went camping. You ask me if I want to play wriggly worms with you! That sounds fun, Mummy. We haven't done that before! I get in my yellow one that has butterflies on it, and you get in your boring brown one. Then you start being a wriggly worm who just can't stop wriggling. You keep wriggling into me and bumping into me! We keep laughing! I keep wriggling into you. We are wriggly worms together, Mummy. We pretend that we just can't stop wriggling. We wriggle all over the bedroom floor. I love laughing with you.

Gosh, I'm starting to feel a bit tired. I yawn. I'm tired, Mummy. I snuggle up with you. We are wriggly worms together. Funnily enough, I'm actually not wriggling now. My body feels all relaxed. Isn't that funny? One day I will be able to sleep on my own, but I'm so glad that I'm still here with you tonight. Nighty night, Mummy!

You're a daycare provider and wonder how to apply the Aware Parenting approach to naps there

If you're wondering whether it's possible to apply this understanding of sleep within a daycare situation, Steph, a Level 2 Aware Parenting instructor and Early Childhood Educator who runs a Family Day Care based on Aware Parenting principles in Australia, says:

"Many of the children who have attended our Family Day Care over the past 9+ years have experienced the benefits of an Aware Parenting approach to sleep. Firstly, we have never forced a child to sleep, or even to lie down. It is always very important to us to follow what Marion so beautifully presents with the three ingredients of sleep; tiredness, connection, and relaxation. From the moment children enter our care, we connect with them through play and listening to big feelings. We develop trust and safety, while learning each child's individual cues and methods of communication. We do not have one set sleep time, as every child is uniquely different and works on their own rhythms. We support children to be in alignment with their body's needs, whether that be thirst, hunger, sleep, toileting, or feelings. When we notice a child is tired, we connect in with them. Some children, especially the younger children, like us to cradle them in our arms. Some children like to lie on their bed with us sitting next to them.

When children first start with us, many have accumulated feelings, and we provide the connection and safety for them to release their feelings. For some children, this can be a process that takes weeks, for others, only a time or two, as their parents practice Aware Parenting. Then we have some children who have come from centres and other daycares, where they were forced to sleep. We learnt to recognise that, while on the outside it seemed like these children were easy sleepers, they were often in a dissociative state while they fell asleep. You can see this if a child avoids or is uncomfortable when making eye contact; their fists may be clenched; tummy tight; and they can often look like they are sucking as imaginary dummy, breast, or bottle. We provide a gentle voice, and perhaps a hand on their upper back, upper abdomen or resting just next to their side. This allows them to know they are safe, while bringing them back into the present moment. When this happens we often hear big sighs, a child will comfortably look us in the eyes, sometimes smile and hold our hand, and then fall to sleep.

We often have parents tell us how transformative it is for their child, even at home.

Children have gone from uncooperative, aggressive, withdrawn, lacking in confidence, with poor sleep, separation anxiety, etc., to embody the opposite of all of this. We always take more time and care around sleep, as it is a vulnerable time; children have no control over what happens while they are asleep. Sleep is also another form of separation. Our intention is for children to feel safe and connected; to have their needs met, either through their direct communication with us, or our observations of their nonverbal communication; and to feel relaxed through releasing any accumulated feelings with laughter, raging or crying."

Self-Compassion Moment

I'm sending you lots of love if you are feeling painful feelings reading this, especially if your child has experienced something different. As always, I invite you to remember that whatever has happened in the past, you can support your child to heal from stress and trauma with Aware Parenting. I invite you to reach out to share these feelings with a loving listener.

To your inner children:

I'm sending love to you every time you were made to go to sleep when you weren't tired.

I'm so sorry for all the times your own tiredness cues weren't trusted.

I trust your own timing.

I trust your timing for when you can go to sleep without closeness.

I'm sorry if you were made to sleep alone before you were ready.

I trust your timing for when you can choose when you go to sleep.

I'm sorry if your timing for choosing that yourself wasn't trusted.

I trust your timing for when you are ready for sleepovers.

I'm sorry if you went on sleepovers too early for you, or weren't supported to go on them when you wanted to.

I trust your timing in all things with sleep.

Your body is so wise.

Your body knows when you are tired.

Your body knows when you've had enough sleep.

Your body knows if you need closeness to go to sleep.

Your body knows when you're ready to sleep alone.

I trust you.

I trust your body.

I'm here to listen to all of your feelings, so you can sleep restfully.

I'm here to play fun games before bed if you want to.

I welcome your tears and tantrums.

I welcome your joy and rambunctiousness before bed.

I'll be here with you if you're scared before sleep.

I won't ever make you sleep alone if you're scared.

I will offer you closeness for as long as you need.

And I won't ever hold you back from being independent.

You know when you are ready for each new level of sleep independence.

I trust you.

I love you.

I so deeply acknowledge you
and all that you are doing.

29. Common sleep questions and answers for parents of children (ages 2–12)

In this next section, I respond to common questions about sleep. Even if they're not relevant for your family, you might want to read them to understand more about the nuances of Aware Parenting and sleep. Or, you might choose to only read whichever is relevant to your family situation.

I'm also here to remind you that these are generic responses, and may not apply to all children. Each child is unique. For the most accurate answers about your own family, I recommend consultations with an Aware Parenting instructor.

The questions are in categories, starting with naps.

Naps

Two-year-old has stopped napping and becomes wild

Q ~ My two-year-old has stopped napping. I know he's not ready to drop his nap because he's absolutely wild without it. It progressively gets worse throughout the day and he expresses it through destruction and defiance and then falls asleep at 5pm.

A ~ Hi lovely, I'm sending you and him lots of love. From an Aware Parenting perspective, we wouldn't see destruction and defiance as signs of tiredness. Rather, the tiredness is making it harder for him to suppress his unexpressed healing-feelings and they are coming out in those destructive ways – rather than through crying and tantrums. There are a number of things you could do here to help him release the emotions that are causing those behaviours. One is to see if he is showing signs of sleepiness in the middle of the day, and follow his lead with either *attachment play*, listening to healing-feelings, or offering *Loving Limits* to help him express those healing-feelings. Then to see whether he is then able to nap. Another option would be to respond to the destruction or defiance with *attachment play* or *Loving Limits* so that he can release the feelings causing it through laughter or crying. As a result, after catching up on releasing some feelings that day or for more days, he will be more relaxed in his body and then might then be able to go to sleep for a nap. The more healing-feelings he expresses, the more relaxed he will be, which will affect both his behaviour and his ability to sleep when he's tired. I wonder if any of these resonate with you?

I keep missing the window of tiredness with my two-and-a-half-year-old before her naps

Q ~ I'm trying so hard, but I keep missing the window of tiredness with my two-and-a-half-year-old daughter, and then she moves into an overtired delirium. I don't know what to do when she is giggling, not able to lie still, and rolling around. I find it so hard to be playful and to join in with the silliness, because my brain is thinking that she is overtired and needs to go to sleep ASAP. I start getting really frustrated, and she takes forever to fall asleep.

A ~ I'm sending so much love to you and to the frustration you've been feeling. I wonder if you find it helpful to know that in Aware Parenting, we don't have the concepts of sleep windows or overtiredness. Instead, we see that when a child is being playful or is crying, that is exactly what they need to do in order to feel more relaxed. She's rolling around because she has some accumulated feelings to express. I hear that when you tell yourself that she is overtired and needs to sleep ASAP, you feel frustrated.

I wonder if you would like to tell yourself that her body is so wise and knows what to do to feel relaxed? I imagine you might then feel calmer, and more able to cooperate with her innate biological wisdom.

The next step would be to follow her lead and join in with the play. If she's rolling around the bed, you could join in with rolling games, perhaps turning them into a nonsense play game where she rolls over you and you pretend to be surprised by the big creature that's rolling over you. Or you could make a big "eek" noise every time she rolls into you. If any of the games bring laughter and giggling, keep going! That is part of her releasing stress and tension from her body. You might find that with some full-on play for a while, she's then able to lie down and fall asleep. Or you might find that she suddenly starts biting or hitting you, or wants to keep on playing for hours even though she is clearly tired. In which case you could offer her a *Loving Limit* and listen to her feelings. Or she might bump into the edge of the bed and have a big cry. If you tell yourself that this is her innate wisdom, and it's how her body will feel more relaxed, you're likely to feel more calm and able to lovingly listen to her tears. I wonder how you feel when you imagine this?

Giving up on naps (two-and-a-half-year-old)

Q ~ Should I give up on naps? My two-and-a-half-year-old still naps with his grandma two to three times a week but never with me and almost never with my husband. I keep trying to encourage him to nap and stressing myself out about it. With my older child it was also hard but I didn't fully give up until he was four-and-a-half-years-old.

A ~ Oh sweetheart, I so hear that you keep trying and stressing yourself out about it. If you're stressed and the naps aren't happening, I wonder if you'd like to focus on listening to his healing-feelings in the evening instead. Without a nap, he's likely to be feeling more tired in the early evening, which means that he will find it easier to let out his feelings and have some lovely big cries. That way, he'll have more restful sleep, and you won't need to stress about the daytime naps. You might even find that once he's let out some big healing-feelings, he might feel more relaxed during the day and might sometimes be able to nap then. Does that resonate with you? If it does, I invite you to play with it for a while and see what happens. You can always go back to what you were doing before. Alternatively, you may find that when he doesn't have a nap, he is so tired in the evening that he falls asleep without expressing healing-feelings. At these times, you might find that he wakes up later on, to cry with you then. I so trust that you'll find the way that is most helpful for you both.

Before sleep

Child hates sleep

Q ~ How can I assist my two-and-a-half-year-old son to not hate going to sleep?

A ~ Hello lovely! From an Aware Parenting perspective, if a child is tired and connected but isn't going to sleep, rather than perceiving that they hate going to sleep, we would generally think that they don't feel relaxed enough to go to sleep. Does that resonate with you? Does your son have closeness while going to sleep? Is he getting to let out big healing-feelings before sleep? That's one of the most common reasons for children not being able to sleep – because they haven't got to implement their natural relaxation-through-release process of crying with our loving support. Laughter and play are another natural relaxation response. I wonder if this resonates?

Alternatively, it is possible that some children feel scared to go to sleep because they fear that they won't wake up again.

This can happen if they have heard expressions like "putting the dog to sleep" and are equating that with you talking about putting your child to sleep. If you think that might be the case, giving him correct information about sleep would be important.

Another alternative is that children who have experienced early trauma – including medical interventions – can sometimes feel fear or terror in relation to the experience of 'losing consciousness' that happens when going to sleep, because it reminds them of the past trauma.

In this case, they might need to do plenty of *attachment play*, perhaps separation games and power-reversal play in particular, as well as crying and raging, to heal from the earlier trauma. In this way, the shift in consciousness at bedtime will no longer help him connect with unexpressed fear. I would recommend one to one support from an Aware Parenting instructor if you think that this is what's going on and you're needing extra help with this.

Bedtime routine suggestions for two-and-a-half-year-old

Q ~ I would love a bit of an outline of what a bedtime routine looks like from an Aware Parenting perspective. I really struggle to get my two-and-a-half-year-old relaxed and ready for sleeping – so some strategies around that?

A ~ Hi lovely! I hear that you're looking for a regular routine. With Aware Parenting, bedtime might be different each evening. It will also be different for each family, so I invite you to connect in with what you would like to include.

After you've listened in to yourself, I invite you to be an emotional detective, observing when she might be trying to feel more relaxed though inviting play or expressing healing-feelings through crying and raging. Then, I invite you to follow her lead wherever you can.

If she's getting playful, I invite you to join in and add in some power-reversal games, nonsense play, or separation games wherever possible. If she's inviting a cry, rather than trying to rush through to get her to bed, stay with those feelings and listen to them. If she's clearly got feelings and needs help letting them out (for example if she's asking for lots of things and isn't happy with any of them), you could offer a *Loving Limit*, *"I hear that you want xyz, sweetheart, and I'm not willing to get you any of those right now, because I don't think that's the most helpful thing for you, and I'm here and I'm listening."* You could also add *attachment play* into bath time, toothbrushing, putting on pyjamas, and any other routines. If after all those, there hasn't been any play or crying, I would observe to see whether she seems ready to play and laugh or cry, and follow that. This may look like her chasing you around the house and you getting caught and being surprised. If she clearly needs to cry, you could move in close and offer her connection, and if the feelings have an *emotional coat hanger* (e.g. she wants you to read her a lot of books), you could offer a *Loving Limit* there and then listen to her feelings. *"I really hear that you want me to read you another book, sweetheart, and I'm not willing to read you any more, because I don't think that's the most helpful thing right now, and I'm here and I'm listening."* Play around with the order of doing things, and see what makes a difference to her sleep. I trust that between the two of you, you will find what works and will create your own unique bedtime routine if you still want one.

Helping two-and-a-half-year-old have a consistent way of falling asleep which also leaves time for one-on-one with older son

Q ~ My two-and-a-half-year-old has a bedtime and nap routine but no consistent way of falling asleep – sometimes we cuddle on an armchair under a weighted blanket, and those are my favourite. Other times he can't fall asleep with me in the room, so I sometimes tell him I'm going to the bathroom and will be back later. I tell myself it's not a lie because I always do come back to check on him before I go to bed! If I just set a limit and leave the room against his wishes he'll stand by the door and call and cry. If he does that when he's really tired, he'll fall asleep by the door. I don't like doing this. But if I stay with him in the room, especially for his nap, he won't sleep at all and it's a huge waste of my time and patience, and not fair to my older son who stays by himself (and the older one has even bigger issues with being by himself). I need to establish some consistency but I'm not sure how. Part of me would be sad to miss out on those perfect days when I can cuddle him to sleep under the blanket. But another part would be willing if it led to more consistent sleep and more efficient bedtimes (his bedtime has been taking two hours on average, sometimes more).

A ~ Hi lovely, I'm sending you so much love in all of this. Children need to feel tired, connected, and relaxed to be able to sleep restfully. The first thing I invite you to do is to check as to whether he is actually tired. He may not be, especially if he has had a long daytime nap. It will be very hard for him to go to sleep if he's not tired. Next is connection, and I'll suggest some ideas for this, below. The third ingredient is relaxation. From an Aware Parenting perspective, if we've tended to those first two things and our child is still not relaxed, it's probably because they have some healing-feelings sitting close to the surface that are preventing them from going to sleep.

If he can't fall asleep with you just sitting there in the room, and he's clearly tired and connected, and if it's taking two hours, it's most likely to be that he needs more help with releasing those feelings so he can feel relaxed enough to sleep.

I wonder if you are open to a different way of doing things, including the part about asking your older son to stay by himself? I trust that there are ways to meet both or their needs, and your own. Could you rethink sleep times to meet these needs? For example, one idea for more connection could be doing lots of *attachment play* with both of your sons before sleep, so that they are both getting lots of closeness, and lots of release through laughter. You could invite them both to chase you through the house and keep being surprised about them catching you. You could invite them to gently knock you off the bed over and over, falling onto cushions below. If they're both laughing, they are releasing feelings such as fear and powerlessness, as well as physical tension. This will help your younger son, but is also likely to help your older son with all the times you've asked him to be by himself. Then, you might find one or both of them might also need to cry, and you can then simply listen if the crying comes out naturally. If they start getting rough or start wanting lots of things, you can offer a *Loving Limit*, *"I hear that you want me to read another story, sweetheart, and I'm not willing to read any more, because I don't think that's the most helpful thing for you, and I'm here and I'm listening,"* or if there's roughness, *"I'm not willing for you to do that, sweetheart, because I'm here to keep everyone safe, and I'm here and I'm listening."*

As for naps, if you lie down with your son and he falls asleep quickly, you could do that, but with your older son there too. If he clearly isn't going to sleep, how about just not trying to get him to nap, and you will probably find that he'll be more tired in the evening and then will be able to let out his big feelings more easily. I wonder if the answer is not about routine at all, but rather with playing with ways for you to all get your needs met? I am so willing for you to all get your needs met in beautiful ways.

Letting off steam before bed (two-and-a-half-year-old)

Q ~ Hi, are there any resources/exercises you would recommend for letting off steam before bed? Our little one thrashes around and the only thing that seems to help is endless bouncing on her bed before listening to audiobooks snuggled up. I'm wondering if there's anything else we can try as it tends to take over an hour for her to settle. However, audiobooks seem to help her settle.

A ~ Hello lovely, I wonder if it resonates with you that her thrashing around is caused by accumulated feelings and that when she's bouncing, she's trying to release the energy of those feelings from her body. However, it sounds like that isn't helping her feel fully relaxed, because she's then needing the audiobooks to bypass the feelings and mildly dissociate. If you join in with her bouncing and play, bringing in elements of *attachment play*, it's likely to maximise the releasing effect of the play. For example, you could do some contingency play, and whenever she bounces, you jump up in the air next to her and make a funny noise. Or you could do some power-reversal play, and every time she bounces, pretend that her bounce knocks you over, and be mock-surprised each time it happens! Or maybe you've tried joining in with her bouncing? If she is laughing, she's releasing feelings.

You might find that then some crying bubbles up – perhaps nothing you do is 'right', or she starts crying over something apparently small.

You can trust that she is letting out some healing-feelings through crying. Simply be there with her, listening to her emotions. I imagine that you find that the more *attachment play* and listening to healing-feelings you do, the more relaxed she will feel, and she probably won't need the audiobooks to feel relaxed enough to sleep.

Two and three-year-olds need an hour of cuddles after nighttime routine

Q ~ Any advice please for my two and three-year-olds who both need more than an hour of cuddles and connection before they fall asleep? This is AFTER nighttime routine including reading books. It's been three years without me closing the door on them and walking out for more than one minute or so. Tonight, I gave it five minutes and ended up back lying down with them. But there has to be another way to help speed things up so that it's just half an hour maximum for our average. I am a single mother and I need my time back!

A ~ Oh sweetheart, I'm sending you so much love. I really hear how hard these long evenings are and so support you in making this process quicker.

I wonder if it resonates with you that if they're tired and connected but not relaxed enough to fall asleep for more than an hour, this tells you that there are probably some painful feelings sitting in their bodies, preventing them from feeling relaxed enough to sleep?

If that resonates, you might want to notice where they are trying to release those feelings, either through *attachment play* or crying. That's going to be a lot for you with two small children, *and* I trust that you can do it. Perhaps they're being silly and goofy and running around a lot whilst you're helping them get changed for bed. Could you join in with the play and get them to chase you and keep on being surprised that they catch you, or could you lie on the edge of the bed with pillows underneath and they keep pushing you off the edge? Or do you notice them inviting play in other ways? When you bring in these *attachment play* elements, it increases the power of the play to bring about relaxation, particularly if there's laughter (as long as there's no tickling).

You might also notice opportunities where they are trying to cry. Again, you can trust them and their innate body wisdom to release stress through crying with you. If you've been trying to distract them from the feelings, you could experiment with not distracting them, and listening instead.

I'm here to remind you that they want to sleep when they're tired as much as you want them to, and they really are trying to use their natural relaxation processes so that they can go to sleep. I wonder if reminding yourself of that might also help you feel less frustrated?

Finally, it's vital for all of us to get listening time and empathy for our feelings. Parenting is big and hard, and having our own feelings heard is vital if we're wanting to listen to our child's feelings. I wonder if you have much listening for your own beautiful feelings?

Lying down with our kids before sleep?

Q ~ Does Aware Parenting always encourage us to lay with our kids while they are going to sleep? My son wants me to lay with him but it can take hours for him to fall asleep.

A ~ Hi lovely, I'm sending you lots of love. In response to your first question, Aware Parenting encourages parents to offer physical closeness at bedtime for as long as the child requests this. However, that doesn't mean you need to be lying down with the child. It could be sitting on the child's bed or on a chair next to the bed, for example.

To respond to the second part of your question, if he is tired and has closeness with you and he's taking hours to fall asleep, that tells you that he's not feeling relaxed enough to sleep.

Tiredness and a sense of safety are *necessary* but *not sufficient* for restful sleep.

Children also need to feel relaxed, and they have natural relaxation processes before sleep, which are laughter and play, and crying and raging. Does this resonate with you? If so, I wonder if you would like to observe him in the couple of hours before bed to see where he might be inviting play and laughter, or crying and raging. Do you notice where you might be inadvertently distracting him? It really is possible to help him go to sleep more quickly.

Nearly three-year-old sings, talks and fidgets before sleep

Q ~ Hi, please could you give me some examples of *Loving Limits* I could give our daughter (who will be three soon), who resists bedtime by singing, talking, whispering, and fidgeting for at least an hour. I am finding it really difficult as I am exhausted (we have a two-week-old baby also).

A ~ Oh sweetheart, I really hear how exhausted you are, especially with a baby too. I'm sending you so much love.

Rather than thinking that she is resisting bedtime, I wonder if you resonate with the idea that it's likely that she is either trying to have more connection with you, and/or she has painful feelings bubbling in her body that are causing her to behave like this?

If it's the first reason, and she's trying to do everything she can to engage with you to meet her need for connection, you might add in daily non-directive child-centred play with her so that she doesn't have such a strong craving for connection with you in the evening when she's tired. It's also to be expected that she has a lot of big painful feelings, such as fear, confusion, frustration, jealousy, and powerlessness, having recently become an older sibling. Supporting her to release those feelings will help her go to sleep. I love that you understand that *Loving Limits* will help, since *Loving Limits* are what we can offer in response to behaviours caused by accumulated feelings.

However, offering* Loving Limits *in response to singing, talking, whispering, and fidgeting can be quite tricky, so I would recommend exploring other ways to support her to release the tension in her body.

One idea would be to offer her *attachment play* in response to these behaviours. *Attachment play* is powerful because it helps children feel deeply connected with us. This is important at this time in her life, as it helps children know that they are deeply loved. One example would be offering her contingency play, where you do different things in response to her singing; or nonsense play, where you pretend you don't hear what she's whispering, and respond in a surprised tone, changing the words, *"What! There's a poo in your shoe!"* You can see if that will bring laugher. If she's laughing (as long as there's no tickling), she's releasing feelings that are preventing her from sleeping, so keep on going!

In terms of *Loving Limits*, I imagine there are times, perhaps before she gets into bed, where there will be some tears bubbling below the surface and a *Loving Limit* will help. Perhaps she's asking for lots of things but not happy with any of them, and you could offer a *Loving Limit*, or perhaps you read her books and she wants more. In both of these cases you could say something like, *"I really hear that you want me to read you another book, and I'm not willing to read any more stories, because I don't think that's most helpful for you right now, and I'm right here and I'm listening,"* and you might find the tears come then. I so acknowledge what a huge amount you are doing, caring for a small child and a baby, and I'm sending you lots of love.

Three-year-old thumb-sucking to sleep

Q ~ My youngest son goes to bed very easily. He puts his thumb in his mouth and he is out. Sometimes he asks us to stay until he is asleep, but that's only five to ten minutes maximum. However, I'm not so sure the thumb-sucking is all that healthy. Is it?

A ~ Hi lovely, I hear that you aren't so sure that the thumb-sucking is all that healthy and I invite you to trust your sense of things here. From an Aware Parenting perspective, thumb-sucking is what's called a *control pattern*, which is a way that children mildly dissociate from their painful feelings. He's telling you that emotions are bubbling up when he's tired, which is normal and natural, because his body is trying to release those feelings so he can sleep more peacefully. Does this resonate with you? If it does, and you're willing to listen to those healing-feelings instead, I would start with *attachment play* with the thumb-sucking. There are lots of different games you can play. One might be to suck your thumb too, and pull your thumb out of your mouth and keep being surprised that it's your thumb, because you thought it was going to be your foot/your ear/your nose, etc. If he's laughing, keep repeating the game. You're likely to find that he starts creating games and you will find new ones too.

You might find that the laughter is enough to release his tension, or you might find that tears bubble up afterwards, because you've created the environment for him to feel safe enough to cry to let those feelings out.

Then you can simply stay with him: "*I'm here with you. I'm listening. You're letting it all out.*" It may take some while for him to catch up on expressing the painful feelings that his thumb-sucking has been holding in. You might notice his behaviour changing in the day too. For example, he might make more eye contact, smile more, be more present, and generally be happier and more relaxed.

Giving relaxing tea to four-year-old before sleep

Q ~ I'm curious about using relaxing tea for relaxation and sleep. I've used things like this a bit in the past with my four-year-old but I wonder if it could do damage in the future with a possible addiction to having something outside of yourself for support. Any suggestions?

A ~ Hi lovely! I hear your curiosity about whether using relaxing tea to help children go to sleep might lead to it becoming a *control pattern*.

Anything that is used regularly to help children suppress feelings that naturally bubble up in the evening could become a* control pattern. *Almost anything can become a* control pattern!

However, it generally would need to be a regular occurrence rather than an occasional event, for it to become a way to suppress feelings. Supporting them with their own innate relaxation response (which is to cry and rage, laugh and play, or talk), is generally the most powerful and effective way to help them feel deeply relaxed so they can sleep restfully and restoratively. You might choose to do external things occasionally when you don't have the emotional spaciousness to support your child with their innate relaxation responses, and I invite you to be compassionate with yourself whenever you do. That might be a signal for you to reach out for more support for yourself. Each of us has our own unique journey and I invite you to deeply listen in to yourself and make choices from that perspective.

Partner leaving three-year-old for short periods before sleep

Q ~ I have a son who is nearly three and I have just had my second boy six months ago. I was the primary night singer/settler/reader/comforter for our toddler until the bub came along. As I can't be in two places at once, I had to relinquish my bedtimes with him to his father. Since he was two, night settling and sleep in general had been difficult (his father used to just give him a bottle and say "night" and "love you" then leave, and he was happy and content and would drift off). He is a great dad but thinks spending an hour reading and cuddling is ludicrous, so he worked out tricks to get away sooner. He spends maybe 15-20 minutes supervising some play and bottle drinking then tells our son he is going for a shower or going to the toilet or just doing something quickly and will be back in five minutes but then just sits in another room on his phone until he hears silence. I can hear our son begging him to cuddle him or read to him, but no. In my opinion that's no better than 'cry it out' methods of abandonment, except without the crying. It breaks my heart. I've tried to tell him this but he doesn't believe me, and says our son is fine. It still takes up to an hour total for him to fall asleep and I just worry that his little cortisol is spiking and he is stressed and sad knowing that Daddy doesn't come back – and then he just gives up asking. Is this causing emotional damage?? Opinion please?

A ~ Oh, I so hear how heartbroken you are and I'm sending you so much love. And yes, I wouldn't recommend being willing for your son to be left alone when he is calling out to be cuddled or read to. If Aware Parenting resonates with you, remember that if a child is tired and connected and isn't relaxed enough to fall asleep, it's likely they have feelings sitting at the surface that they need help with releasing, through play/laughter or crying and raging.

With a new sibling, it's normal for children to have even more painful feelings to express to us before they feel relaxed enough to be able to go to sleep without dissociating.

If that still resonates, there are a few options you have. You could ask your husband to be with the baby whilst you help your son with *attachment play* and then *Loving Limits* and listening to his feelings which will show up through crying and tantrums. It is so normal for him to have a lot of big feelings now that he has a new sibling. Another option is that you could be with both of your boys, perhaps with your baby in a carrier on your back, so you can play some power-reversal games with your older son, or simply follow his lead with play. After some play you might find that he will indicate to you how to help him let out some healing-feelings through crying and raging. Perhaps he gets rough and you can offer a *Loving Limit, "I'm not willing for you to do that, because I'm here to keep everyone safe, and I'm here and I'm listening."* Perhaps he wants you to read him 10 more stories, *"I hear that you want me to read more stories, sweetheart, and I'm not willing to read any more, because I don't think that's the most helpful thing for you, and I'm here and I'm listening.*" Or perhaps he keeps asking for another toy or something else, and again you can offer a *Loving Limit*. The aim is to support him to express the painful feelings that have been making it hard for him to feel relaxed enough to go to sleep.

You may also find that your baby and older son both start crying together, and you can hold your baby, and keep offering them both loving compassion.

"*I'm here with you, sweetheart, I'm here and I'm listening. You're letting it all out.*" I invite you to keep experimenting until you find something that works for you all and is sustainable for you. Most of all, I invite you to be willing to receive as much physical and emotional support as you can. Expressing your feelings to an empathy buddy or Aware Parenting instructor, for example, can make a huge difference. I'm so willing for a beautiful shift for you all.

Five-year-old keeps talking before bed

Q ~ My oldest son just keeps talking and talking; another game, another question – no matter how I try to add a loving boundary it takes so much time – often 30 minutes up to an hour. He says he cannot fall asleep alone. So, I wonder, should I go away after the bedtime routine or wait until he is asleep every day?

A ~ Oh, I hear how much time it takes and I'm sending you so much love. As for your question, I wouldn't go away after the bedtime routine. He needs more help from you, rather than less. I invite you to go through the list of three ingredients needed for restful sleep to discover what he might need. If you're sure he's feeling tired, the next thing is to see whether he needs more connection to feel safe enough to sleep.

Having a younger sibling or siblings might mean that he is talking in this way to try to meet his need for connection with you. If you want to support this need in the daytime so it's easier and quicker for him to fall asleep, you might offer him short bursts of daily non-directive child-centred play during the day.

Finally, in terms of relaxation, there could be two different things going on here. At this age, talking can be a healthy emotional release process. I wonder if you've experimented with deeply listening to him, answering his questions, and seeing if he begins to talk about things that have happened that were upsetting for him. His questions might give a clue to his concerns or fears. Listening to his feelings and reflecting them back will help him experience being heard and feeling more relaxed and able to sleep.

There is also a possibility that his talking, wanting to play, and wanting to ask another question may be symptoms of him distracting himself from unexpressed feelings. If, after long conversations, he doesn't seem to be more connected or more relaxed, this might be possible. Experimenting will help you discover what is really going on for him and what he really needs. There are a few things you can do. One is to see if during the bedtime routine you might be inadvertently distracting him – either from being playful and silly, or from crying and raging – these are all part of children's natural relaxation processes. Instead of distracting him, I invite you to support those processes.

If he gets playful, join in with the play. If he starts crying over something small, listen to the feelings.

If he is still talking and talking, those are likely to be ways that he is trying to distract himself from feelings that are sitting in his body. Helping him release those feelings will help him feel more relaxed and mean that it takes less time for him to go to sleep. You could experiment with both *attachment play* and *Loving Limits*. *Attachment play* might mean you respond to the questions with silly answers and see if he starts laughing. If he does, that is him releasing some of the lighter feelings. *Loving Limits* might be offered in response to the request for more games: "*I really hear that you want to play another game, sweetheart, and I'm not willing to play any more games, because I don't think it's the most helpful thing for you* (or you might say it's because you're tired now yourself, which would be a *Limit* rather than a *Loving Limit*) *and I'm here and I'm listening.*" As we get more experienced in offering *Loving Limits*, we will often find that tears or raging flow afterwards. *Loving Limits* are different from what I think you are talking about with a loving boundary, because we're saying no to the behaviour, and a really big yes to the feelings that are causing the behaviour. Lots of love.

Attachment play for light sleepers (six-year-old and mum) who take a long time to fall asleep

Q ~ I'm interested in recommendations for sleep-related *attachment play* for a six-year-old and her mum (both of us 'light sleepers' who take a long time to fall asleep).

A ~ I'm sending you both so much love. Have you experimented with activities with body contact, such as a back massage or a foot massage, or cooperative games, such as creating a cooperative story or song together? I also wonder if you might like to play games where each of you pretends to fall asleep and then the other one makes a funny noise and the 'sleeping' one pretends to wake up with a really big jump into the air? Or perhaps you could pretend to be mice together, trying to find a comfy and quiet place to sleep?

If she is taking a long time to sleep and easily wakes up, it could be that there are some feelings that are sitting close to the surface that are making it hard for her to feel relaxed enough to go to sleep and stay asleep.

Something similar might be going on for you. I wonder if you have an empathy buddy or Aware Parenting instructor with whom you could share your feelings? You might find it helpful to explore your own childhood experiences in relation to sleep, too. As for your daughter, encouraging her to talk about her day might help, perhaps with prompts such as: *"What did you really love about what happened today? What was the most unenjoyable thing that happened? Was someone friendly to you? Was someone harsh to you?"* This is not *attachment play*, but it's a way of helping a child process events and emotions verbally, and it could lead to tears if they are needed.

Six-year-old bedtime anxiety

Q ~ What would you suggest for bedtime anxiety for a six-year-old? It's happening maybe once a week where she describes it as feeling scared and worried but she can't articulate a specific thing. I've suggested deep slow breathing, thinking of nice memories (I give examples), keeping eyes closed, or asking her body what it needs. I've given her a flower remedy sleep spray, offered sleep meditations, etc. Our nightly routine is PJs/toilet/teeth, then into bed for a story. Then we have cuddles, sometimes tickles and then it's time for sleep. We have two beds in the room, one I'm in with her nine-month-old baby sister, and she's on a separate bed but right next to us (although on floor level). I stay in the room until both are asleep. I've got a small amount of (red) light in the room as requested from the six-year-old.

A ~ I so acknowledge all that you're doing to try to help her feel more relaxed. I would recommend adding in *attachment play* before getting into bed, particularly games where she can laugh uproariously. Laughter is an incredibly powerful way for children to release fear from their bodies.

However, I recommend caution with tickling, because it can actually lead to overstimulation, even if a child is laughing and asking to be tickled.

You might find after the *attachment play,* that she either dissolves into tears, or wants to talk more about something that is bothering her. She innately knows how to release the fear, and you have everything you need to help her with that.

Seven-year-old needs cuddling, stroking or holding hands to get to sleep

Q ~ Can you offer tips for encouraging a seven-year-old to go to sleep by himself? He currently needs mum or dad to cuddle, stroke, or hold hands to get to sleep.

A ~ I'm sending you lots of love. I wonder if you're needing more ease at bedtime? I wonder how this is for you, being with him in this way? First of all, I would recommend some listening for you so you can have your feelings heard about supporting your son to sleep in this way. There are two possibilities here. Firstly, this cuddling, stroking, or holding his hand might be meeting his real need for physical contact before sleep. I wonder if you find it reassuring to know that it's very normal that a seven-year-old might still need this kind of closeness at bedtime. This is particularly the case for a Highly Sensitive Child (*Elaine Aron*) or one who has experienced many changes or traumas in his life. If you want to help him fall asleep alone (after exploring why you want to do this, and where it might be coming from in you), you could try to gradually offer him less physical contact, perhaps by touching his hand a bit less and then moving slightly further away each evening, and listen to him.

The second alternative is that the stroking or holding hands might be suppressing healing-feelings that are close to the surface. If you think that's the case, the first step would be to help him release those feelings, perhaps initially through *attachment play*, and then *Loving Limits*. For example, you might play *attachment play* games by pretending that your hand is an animal and his hand is an animal and you're playing little games together. The little animals might then start playing peek a boo or hide and seek. Bringing in separation games could also help him release any feelings he might have in relation to being separate from you.

You might then move on to offering *Loving Limits* with holding his hand, but only if you're sure that this is a *control pattern* rather than meeting a true need. If you're sure, you might say, *"I hear that you want me to hold your hand, and I'm not willing to hold your hand, sweetheart, because I don't think it's the most helpful thing for you right now. And I'm here and I'm listening."*

The core ingredient for healing to happen is that you are staying there with him and listening to those feelings that he's been holding in.

If, after he cries with you, he's more relaxed and connected, you might find that he finds it easier to go to sleep at night and needs less support. However, you might find that actually it was a need after all, and he does still need that for now. Only you will be able to tell what's really going on for him through observing him. Once he's expressed some more of those feelings and can go to sleep with just a cuddle, you might find that he is then willing to go to sleep on his own.

Eight-year-old avoiding going to bed

Q ~ My eight-year-old will do everything in her will not to go to bed, or find something 'very important' to do just before bed, to put bed off.

A ~ I'm sending love to you both. Your daughter might be wanting to put bed off because she wants some connection with you, or going to bed might be helping her connect with unexpressed painful feelings. She might want some connection with you and to share what's going on for her through conversation. Finding ways to connect together, such as cuddling up in a bean bag together, or playing pillow fights, might also help her feel connected and relaxed so that she can go to sleep. If she has some unexpressed painful feelings, I wonder if you've experimented with *attachment play* about this, perhaps nonsense play. You might make up games that are really over the top about not going to bed. *"Going to bed is TERRIBLE! I never want to go to bed. Let's stay up all night and avoid going anywhere near the bedroom!"* Perhaps you could play exaggerated nonsense play games like, *"If we go to bed now, perhaps our house will turn into a rocket ship, and we would fly to the moon, and the stars will be too bright for us."*

Nine-year-old expressed sudden ailments before bed

Q ~ My nine-year-old often complains of growing pains or a sudden ailment before bed (we have checked her nutrition and physiological needs).

A ~ I wonder if you think that she is wanting more connection, care, laughter, or crying at this time? Perhaps you might experiment with different responses to discover what it is she needs. Could you offer either lots of over the top exaggerated care for her, or some nonsense play about the ailments? How about pretending to fight over who can care for her sudden ailment? Has she been through anything stressful or traumatic lately? Does she seem to be trying to cry? If so, could you play with finding the *balance of attention* so that she could have a cry with you? Offering her loving connection and your presence, I trust that you'll discover what's going on for her and what she really needs. If things don't shift, I recommend working with an Aware Parenting instructor.

Waking in the night / night terrors / nightmares

26-month-old waking in the middle of the night screaming

Q ~ My 26-month-old son has been waking in the middle of the night a few times in the last week or so, absolutely livid and screaming. He's physically tense and almost seems angry and upset at the same time. He struggles and cries worse if he's being held or touched. He asks about going downstairs and turning on the lights. It seems like almost a really intense tantrum. Sometimes this lasts 20 minutes, sometimes almost an hour. Eventually he will calm down as I sit with him, and he will want to snuggle and go back to sleep, and then he is absolutely FINE in the morning. Is this developmental? Is there anything else I can be doing to help, other than by letting him know I hear and see how upset he is (about the light being off and not going downstairs)? At this point, he still needs someone with him to be able to go to sleep, but he's falling asleep calm and connected with no *control patterns*.

A ~ Hi lovely, I'm sending you and him lots of love. In response to your question, no, I wouldn't see this as developmental, and would trust that he has some big healing-feelings to express that aren't getting to come out in the daytime. It sounds like it could be night terrors, which are common at this age (when sleepwalking can also occur). Has he experienced a recent trauma? If so, I would recommend supporting him to heal from that during the day or the evening before sleep so that he isn't needing to try to process it in the middle of the night. I wonder if you find it helpful to know that the louder and more intense the crying, and the more vigorous the movement, the more feelings are being expressed, and the more quickly those feelings will get to be released.

Does it resonate with you that when you move towards more closeness with him, the feelings might be intensifying because he's feeling more emotional safety to feel those really big feelings?

And I hear you about falling asleep – I wonder if there are times in the evening where he might be inviting you to support him with some crying or *attachment play* that you might be unwittingly distracting him from? If he can let these feelings out in the evening, they won't then wake him up at night. *Control patterns* can be very subtle, such as needing to sleep in a particular position or clutching a toy. I invite you to observe whether he may be dissociating in very subtle ways before sleep. As for what you can do to help – yes, staying close with him, and letting him know you hear and see him. I would recommend a low-level red light so that he can see you when he's crying. And he's fine in the morning because his body knows what to do, and he's healing and releasing feelings. That's so natural! Big love to you both.

Two-and-a-half-year-old has rarely slept through the night

Q ~ I have a two-and-a-half-year-old who has very rarely slept through the night. He is in a particularly bad habit of being awake for long periods at the moment, and is needing a big cry even though there have been multiple cries throughout the day. We know he's overtired as he refuses to nap, so I am trying different strategies including going to bed at six pm (when possible). We have lovely play and connection before bed, but the nighttimes are disasters. The whole family is suffering, as he wakes our four-year-old in the same room. Any advice would be lovely.

A ~ Oh, my heart goes out to you. I so hear what a challenging time you are having. And I deeply acknowledge all the listening to feelings you're already doing and all the lovely play and connection you are sharing.

It's very common for small children to have a lot of big feelings, and so often much more than we would expect.

I'm going to offer some different ways of thinking of what's going on to see if those are helpful for you. You talk about him being awake for long periods as a bad habit. I wonder if it resonates with you that rather than it being a habit, he's probably telling you he has still some more big healing-feelings that are making it hard for him to go back to sleep. The same for the concept of 'overtired' – which we don't have in Aware Parenting. If you are taking him to bed before he actually feels sleepy, that's also going to make it hard for him to sleep. Remember the three ingredients for restful sleep – tiredness, connection, and relaxation.

I wonder if you would like to experiment? For example, you could see what happens if you don't try to help him have a nap. You could then wait until the big feelings bubble up when he gets tired in the evening – when he's tired, he's likely to be able to be able to express more and bigger healing-feelings, which you're likely to then see makes a difference to how relaxed he is at night. If you don't see him as overtired and then don't take him to bed so early, does he then let out more healing-feelings in the evening and then sleep more at night? The way we perceive what is going on makes a big difference to the actions we take, and changing the perceptions can change how we feel and how we act. I'm so willing for the subtle shifts you make to lead to more sleep for all of you.

Three-year-old waking up every hour

Q ~ We have a three-year-old and have practiced Aware Parenting since he was six weeks old. And I wanted to ask if there are any other healthy ways to help your child sleep. He will sleep from bedtime until 12am then wake up EVERY HOUR until morning. My husband and I can no longer support the lack of sleep and can't be the parents we want to be with lack of sleep. We really want to find a healthy way for our son to sleep through the night. He's in his own room but wakes up and I have to settle him more than five times a night. I'm currently expecting another, so the sleep deprivation is on a whole different level. How can we help our son put himself back down. We are trying to talk about it with him and see if there's anything we can help him with, but we can't seem to find a solution.

A ~ Hello lovely, oh I'm sending you both so much love. I can only imagine how you're feeling with that much sleep deprivation.

I wonder if you find it helpful to remember that as a form of attachment-style parenting, Aware Parenting advocates being close with your child at nighttime for as long as they need that.

The second ingredient for restful sleep is closeness. Since he sleeps alone in a room, I would suggest moving him into your room if you're willing to co-sleep. At three years, children can have a new awareness of death and typically develop new fears because of that. If he is aware of your pregnancy, he may also have fear, sadness, or confusion in response to that, which would further contribute to his need to be near you both at night. At three, talking with him about sleep is not likely to be very helpful, because it's probably needs-feelings or healing-feelings that are waking him up, which he can't think his way out of.

I so deeply honour all the listening to feelings you've already done. And, babies and children have so many more feelings than we often realise. First time around, we may listen to what we think are all of their healing-feelings, only to realise later on that we've only listened to half of them, or some other percentage, and that's why we're seeing the effects of their accumulated feelings.

If a child is waking up every hour, it often indicates that they have more unexpressed feelings bubbling in their body that are waking them up. Does that resonate with you? I wonder if your son is getting to do *attachment play*, particularly separation games, because he's been in his own room, as well as crying during the day and before sleep? The more you focus on big laughter and play, and loud crying and raging, the more you are likely to see a difference in his sleep. He wants to sleep as much as you do! I'm sending you all well wishes and am so willing for him to get to express lots more before the new baby comes, which will not only help him with his sleep, but also support him be more naturally gentle and loving with his new sibling.

Three-year-old waking at night

Q ~ My three-year-old (never been a great sleeper) is having frequent night wakings and wants me to sleep with her. Sometimes I lay with her but as soon as I try and leave, she wakes again. Or she doesn't want me to sleep in her bed but I'm not allowed to go back to mine either! This could happen three to four times per night. Help!

A ~ I'm sending you lots of love. Closeness is such an essential need in relation to sleep at this age still, and so I wonder if you are willing to play around with rearranging the bed situation. Can you have a single mattress or bed in your room and start with her having that closeness throughout the night? Then observe what happens next. If she sleeps, she's probably telling you that she was needing that closeness. If she is still waking, it tells you that it's probably healing-feelings that were waking her up, and then you can help her through listening to those feelings. Does this resonate with you?

If she has never slept very restfully, it suggests that perhaps she has healing-feelings from her birth or early days that she hasn't yet had the opportunity to express to you.

I wonder how her birth was? Does she get to regularly cry with you, especially during the evenings? It really is possible for her to sleep restfully, and for you to, too! I'm so willing for you to both experience beautiful restful sleep.

Three-year-old coming into my bed and I'm resentful

Q ~ I'm currently struggling with co-sleeping with my three-year-old. She used to sleep the whole night through in her own room, but when her sister was born eight months ago she started coming through to my bed (which I share with her sister) in the middle of the night. She snuggles right up to me and I find I don't have enough space. By the time it gets to morning I'm totally touched out, with a sore back from contorting, and feeling really resentful of her. I know it's coming from a place of needing me so I feel really guilty resenting her, and I don't want to do or say anything to her about it that she experiences as a rejection, so I'm at a bit of a loss.

A ~ I'm sending so much love to you and all the feelings and sensations you're experiencing whilst your daughter is snuggling right up to you. Ouch about your sore back, and my heart goes out to you, hearing how resentful you're feeling. I imagine you're longing for some restful sleep and a comfortable body. I also hear that you're feeling guilty, and I wonder if you might be willing to put that guilt stick down. I also have a few ideas; I wonder if any of them resonate with you. Do you have an empathy buddy who you can regularly share your feelings with? Having a dedicated space where you can express all your pain and resentment and any feelings you have is a huge part of Aware Parenting. The more we get to express our feelings, the more clear we can be about the steps we can take. After that, could you offer her some dedicated one-to-one time each day whilst your baby is sleeping or being looked after? Even five minutes of non-directive child-centred play can really help fill up a child's connection cup. Playing other kinds of *attachment play* like the 'she's mine' game, where you and another adult (or even a stuffed toy!) 'fight' over her, can also help too. In general, throughout the day, offering her warm affection and hugs wherever possible might fill up her connection cup a bit so that she doesn't need to snuggle up as much at night.

Is she getting to do much crying and raging? The more feelings she gets to release, the more relaxed she'll be in her body whilst sleeping and then she will be able to sleep in your bed without being right up close with you; she will feel the connection whilst co-sleeping without needing to be in that particular position. If the snuggling has a quality of dissociation, it might be that the particular position is helping her dissociate.

If that's the case, you could offer her a *Loving Limit* in relation to that position: *"I see that you want to cuddle in under my shoulder, sweetheart, and I'm not willing for you to cuddle right in like that tonight, because I don't think it's the most helpful thing for you, and I'm here and I'm listening."* If she can have a big cry in response, you might find that she still wants closeness with you, but not in order to create dissociation. She will be more relaxed and less desperate, and you're likely to be able to sleep more comfortably yourself. In addition, on a practical level, have you also thought of adding another mattress to your bed to make it a super big bed so that there's plenty of room for restful sleep for everyone? I'm so willing for you all to get your needs met.

How to help my three-year-old go to sleep independently

Q ~ Looking for resources/advice/stories about how to help my three years and four months old girl go to sleep independently. We co-sleep and she's always had help (company) to fall asleep. Once she's asleep she pretty much sleeps through. But getting her to sleep (for me) is impossible. Normally her dad does it and they have their way that works – stories and a cuddle and she will just go off in ten minutes. For me it never works like that, I think the *balance of attention* is off, she says she can't sleep because she's scared to leave me. She says she likes daddy bedtimes best of all. I am also sick of bedtimes and really want her to be able to go to sleep herself. What would be the Aware Parenting approach to this? My mum used to just give me a kiss and leave and I'd fall asleep but I'm not sure how she achieved that.... I want it though!! How is it done?! I know that more connection, play around separation, listening to feelings, etc., would help. Whilst I try to do as much of this as I can sometimes we have a stressful day, I can't put aside time and energy for a whole drawn-out routine every night. She is highly sensitive and had a traumatic first three years in one way or another and we are working on healing but that is a long process. I need a solution sooner than that last night she was still wriggling around at 11pm even though she was exhausted and I just needed to go to sleep myself. I have a couple of weeks of the summer coming up where I won't have my husband and I need to be able to get my own child to sleep. I will talk the ear off my Listening Partner as well of course but I also just need practical suggestions please!!!

A ~ My heart goes out to you, being awake at 11pm still, and also to your daughter, wriggling around and awake until then. I acknowledge all that you're doing with connection, separation games, and listening to feelings, and I understand that after a stressful day, you don't have the time and energy for a whole drawn out routine in the evening. I love that you have a *Listening Partner*, because that was the main thing I would suggest – lots of sharing about how you're feeling, with her not being able to sleep because she's scared to leave you, and you wanting her to go to sleep alone. And most of all, you being really heard about how sick you are of bedtimes. You also mentioned that your Mum used to just give you a kiss and leave and you'd fall asleep, and I trust that is relevant here. I hear that you want that. Do you sense what you needed to do within yourself to fall asleep without her? Do you remember how you felt when she left you? I trust your sense that there's something going on here which means there isn't quite the *balance of attention* for your daughter to express the feelings related to being scared to leave you.

I also hear that you are wanting practical suggestions. My first suggestion would be more listening for you. If a child has feelings related to past separations, and we're feeling frustrated and are wanting to leave them, it's likely that this might be getting in the way of the *balance of attention*. I imagine that bedtime is helping her connect with feelings in relation to a past experience with you, which is perhaps why she can fall asleep easily with her dad. I'd be curious about whether the traumatic experiences she's had are related to separation from you, and again, for you to receive lots of listening and support for all of that. The more calm and relaxed you feel, the more she will feel that, and will be more likely to experience the *balance of attention* so she can heal from whatever is coming up for her around sleeping time.

Being aware of what you are telling yourself might also help too, for example, to remind yourself that she wants to go to sleep as much as you do and has some frightening feelings that are preventing her from feeling relaxed enough to sleep.

Then, on a practical level, for the time before bed, I would focus on separation games for a length of time that you're willing for (perhaps putting a timer on), and then when the timer goes off, you might offer a *Limit* (or a *Loving Limit*, if you think she wants to continue playing to distract herself from painful feelings) which might help her connect with and express tears and crying. Also, watch out for opportunities for connection, play, and *Loving Limits* in the whole run up to bedtime, e.g. during dinner, bath, PJs, teeth brushing, etc. I wonder how you feel and what you think when you read this?

Six-year-old in our bed most nights

Q ~ I saw one of your posts about toddlers waking up in the night to express emotions they didn't express during the day and I can totally relate. But at the moment, my six-year-old is the one who spends most of the night in our bed, vs our four and one-year-old. Would you suggest it's for similar reasons?

A ~ Hi lovely, it could be, but it might be that this is a way for them to feel connected with you, especially since they are sharing connection with you with their siblings during the day. I wonder if this resonates with you?

Nine-year-old having nightmares

Q ~ My nine-year-old daughter has awful nightmares, not every night but most nights she will come running into our room. We don't watch TV during the week and watch suitable movies on the weekend. We read and I try and have a peaceful bedtime routine which doesn't always work. She shares a room with her seven-year-old brother which she is still happy with and knows she can move to her own room when ready. She has had broken sleep for years; a bad dream, thirsty, toilet, can't sleep. She falls asleep easily. She sleepwalks sometimes. I also get increasingly stressed the longer it takes to get to bed, knowing the harder it will be to get up for breakfast/school, etc., which doesn't help.

A ~ Hello lovely, oh I'm sending you lots of loving compassion, particularly at the times when you get stressed, while it's taking her longer to get to bed.

The fact that she has had broken sleep for years suggests to me (as long as there's nothing going on physiologically) that she has had some big healing-feelings bubbling in her system for a while.

I'm curious about what she does before falling asleep and whether any of those things might be suppressing those feelings which then wake her up at night or cause nightmares. I would recommend watching out for opportunities where she is suppressing feelings during the evening, and then moving in with *attachment play* or *Loving Limits* to support her to express more healing-feelings during the day and evening so that they don't wake her up at night. Love to you both.

Thinking of moving your child into their own bed?

Three-year-old going into his own bed

Q ~ My three-year-old has just gone into a bed. He's doing well with it, I'm trying to allow enough connection time with him prior to sleep, but I'm wondering if this is one of those 'big' transitions and would like to know ways to make sure he's well supported?

A ~ It is a really big transition, and here are a few things I suggest. I wonder if any of them resonate with you? Lots of connection, particularly separation games and body contact games. These will help him with any feelings related to separation from you. Staying with him until he goes to sleep, unless he tells you otherwise. And letting him know that if he wants to come to you in the night, that he is welcome any time. How do you feel and what do you think when you read this?

Three-year-old crying to lullaby

Q ~ I was listening to episode 126 of your beautiful *Aware Parenting Podcast*, as a specific word you mentioned made me want to have a bit more clarity on that subject. I'd just watched the brilliant video 'getting bedtime right' on YouTube (Dr Gordon Neufeld), where he explains the power of the lullaby. He says it can put your child to rest to hear your voice, when facing separation. In your episode on sleep, you mention that 'singing lullabies' can interfere with the 'letting go of feelings'. Is there a nuance to this 'lullaby' singing? What happens is that if I start singing a sad song to my three beautiful daughters (twins of age three, and one of age two), they start crying immediately (and it is not sadness I witness in their tears – it feels more like anxiousness or sometimes even madness) and they start yelling, *'Mommy, stop singing!'* My youngest daughter even turns away from me, and refuses my closeness, and if I then continue to sing our lullaby, it feels unnatural, like I'm forcing it. I hope you can help me clarify what is happening here, and how I could interpret the singing of a lullaby.

A ~ Hello lovely! Lullabies can have different effects on each individual child. For some, it is a lovely way to connect together when they're already happy. For others, if they have painful feelings to express, it may distract them from those feelings. For yet others, it may help them connect with unexpressed feelings – like when we listen to a beautiful song and have a lovely cry, or feel other painful feelings bubbling up to be expressed. I wonder if they get to regularly express their crying and tantrums with you? Did the twins experience separation that the singing is helping them connect with? Did you sing that song to them in utero or when they were babies? What is your sense of what is going on here? I trust that you will work out what's really happening for them.

Wriggly four-year-old

Q ~ I have a nearly five-year-old. We have co-slept since birth but I would love for him to sleep on his own. I'd be willing to share a bed with him but he is so wriggly, climbs on me, needs to hold me, etc., which then really disrupts my own sleep. I would love some new ideas!

A ~ Hello lovely, I'm sending love to you, hearing about all the disrupted sleep.

If you've checked out possible physical causes, it's likely that his wriggling, climbing on you, and needing to be held are caused by accumulated painful feelings that he's not getting to express during the day or in the evening. These feelings create a sense of agitation.

I hear that you'd be willing to share a bed with him if he was more relaxed so you could get your needs for restful sleep met. You really can continue to co-sleep and have sound sleep, and the first step would be to see if you are inadvertently suppressing his natural relaxation responses of laughter and play, or crying and raging before sleep, and instead, to cooperate with those processes. Does this resonate with you?

I would generally always recommend supporting a child to be able to sleep in a relaxed way while still co-sleeping – before thinking of moving them into their own room. Often parents are happy to continue co-sleeping when their child is relaxed.

Does this resonate with you? Love to you both.

Transitioning scared four-year-old into her own room

Q ~ I need some wisdom for our sleeping situation. Our four-year-old girl has been sleeping with us all this time in our bedroom, but I need to sleep. So, if you know some tips to help this transition to her own room, please share. She has a lot of fears – of darkness, monsters, nightmares, and needs to feel safe as she is highly sensitive.

A ~ Hi lovely, first of all, I hear that you need to sleep, and that you aren't sleeping well with her in the bed. I'm sending you so much love. Is that because there isn't enough room? If so, can you get another bed to put beside yours to make a bigger bed? Or is it because she's moving around in her sleep? If that's the case, it's likely to be because she has healing-feelings sitting in her body that are causing the wriggling.

Rather than moving her to her own room, the most helpful way to help her feel more relaxed, and for you to get more sleep, as well as for her to heal from the fears, would be to increase how many healing-feelings you're listening to, through **attachment play** *and her crying and raging, particularly before bed.*

With *attachment play,* that could be power-reversal games where she becomes the more powerful one, and contingency play, where what she does affects you. For example, she has a magic wand or remote control and gets to choose what you do, and you do it in silly and goofy ways. If she's laughing, she's healing from the fears. Laughter is an incredibly powerful way to release fear, as long as there's no tickling.

I would not recommend moving her to her own room whilst she has all of those fears, and instead, I invite you to help her heal from them whilst she is still in your own room.

This will mean that you get more sleep too! You really can both get your needs met, sweetheart!

Mum and dad and four-year-old all getting sleep?

Q ~ How do you set *Loving Limits* around your child staying in their own bed when you actually like them coming in to sleep with you? My four-year-old runs into our bedroom every night – perhaps there's fear there – and whilst I don't mind this, my husband finds it hard to sleep with him there as he always ends up getting pushed out of bed!

A ~ Hi lovely, oh I'm so willing for you to all get your needs met here! First of all, I'd love to respond to your question about *Loving Limits*. *Loving Limits* are for when a child has painful accumulated feelings which are causing behaviours such as suppression or aggression. With a *Loving Limit*, we say no to the behaviour and yes to the feelings causing the behaviour. This is different to what you are talking about here.

I would not ever recommend telling a child to stay in their own bed when they are wanting closeness in the night. Closeness is a core need for young children, especially at night. It brings a sense of safety.

I trust that there will be a way for you to all get your needs met. And it seems like you're wanting to find a way for your husband to get his need for restful sleep met, as well as your son's for closeness, and yours for connection with your son at night. Am I guessing that accurately? If your son pushes your husband out of bed, is it because the bed isn't big enough for all three of you, or because your son is agitated and moving around in bed? If it's because of the size of the bed, could you bring a single bed in next to your big bed and all sleep together that way? If it's agitation, I would recommend doing more *attachment play* before bed and listening to more healing-feelings before sleep, since the agitation is likely to be from accumulated unexpressed feelings. Does any of this resonate? I'm so willing for you all to get your needs met.

Can my four and a half-year-old go to sleep alone?

Q ~ We still put my four-and-a-half-year-old to bed and stay with him until he is asleep. I would love to transition him to being able to go to sleep without us, but I am not sure if he is too young still, and I am wondering what age people transition their children and how to do it?

A ~ Hello lovely, I hear that you'd love for him to be able to go to sleep without you, and my first invitation is to receive some listening in relation to this. I wonder what you need and why you want him to go to sleep alone? The more you have your feelings heard and get clear about your needs, the more that will help you in this process.

First of all, to answer your question about what age children are ready to fall asleep without closeness, every child is different. Some might be ready to fall asleep without their parents nearby at age three, others not until age 10. It depends on many factors other than the amount of emotional release at bedtime.

For example, the child's sensitivity level, whether there is a sibling sleeping in the same room, how far away their room is from the parents' room, the number of recent changes in their life, as well as stimulation levels and developmental factors. Next, is he taking a long time to go to sleep and would you like that to be quicker? If he's taking a long time to go to sleep with you, are you doing *attachment play* and/or listening to healing-feelings before sleep? If he's tired and connected but not falling asleep, that suggests he's not relaxed enough because he has unexpressed healing-feelings in his body. I would recommend supporting your child with his own timing and when he's ready to go to sleep without closeness, whilst also holding in mind that the more connected he feels in the evening, such as lots of affection, cuddles and *attachment play*, the more likely he will feel safe enough to go to sleep without you. Additionally, the more he gets to express his feelings through crying and raging, the quicker and easier he will be able to go to sleep without you. Letting him know that he can come to you if he needs you can also help. As can playing separation games, such as hide and seek in his bedroom. I'm so willing for you to find a way for you all to get your needs met!

From co-sleeping with five-year-old to sleeping in their own bed

Q ~ I'd love to know your thoughts on how and when to move from co-sleeping, to the child moving into their own bed. My son is five and we've been co-sleeping since birth. I get caught between letting the process be completely child-led and possibly aiming towards a bit more separation. He has done the odd evening in his own bed and then come back with me later in the night, when he wants to carry on co-sleeping. I wonder if I need to set a limit and let him cry and release or let him carry on co-sleeping. He sometimes also wants to be in my bed but have no contact with me. I wonder what this is?

A ~ Hello lovely, it's such a big journey, isn't it – and I so hear that you get caught between letting the process be completely child-led and at other times aiming towards more separation.

I'm here to remind you that Aware Parenting is about you both getting your needs met.

I wonder what you need here? Is there anything you're not enjoying about co-sleeping? Are there any other ways you can get that need met? As for your son, do you sense that his wanting to co-sleep is simply about a need for closeness, or do you think there are other feelings sitting in his body affecting that choice? When you connect in with both of your needs, what would help you both get your needs met? As for the times where he's in your bed but doesn't want contact, at five years old, I would imagine that is telling you he has some healing-feelings to express. What happens if you do some *attachment play*, perhaps pretending that a little rabbit (your hand), and then a little squirrel (your other hand) wants to come close to him, and see whether he joins in with the play. That might also help you gain clarity about whether what's going on for him is about needs for closeness, or accumulated feelings, or both. Does this resonate?

Seven-year-old still co-sleeping and doesn't want to go on sleepovers

Q ~ My seven-year-old daughter still loves co-sleeping and doesn't want to go into her own room, and I've always thought I would trust her timing for when she doesn't want to any more. However, recently, I've had some comments from other parents, because she doesn't want to go to sleepovers. Can I really trust her timing? Or can there be a *control pattern* at play here? Would it be helpful for me to encourage her to sleep in her own room?

A ~ I love that you really trust your daughter's own journey and timing with independence. Aware Parenting is so much about trusting children's innate wisdom in terms of their journey of attachment and individuation. Each child is unique, and Aware Parenting is all about supporting that uniqueness.

I wonder if you would see her as Highly Sensitive (as described by Elaine Aron)? I ask this, because Highly Sensitive Children often want to co-sleep for longer. They also want to go on sleepovers later than their peers too. This makes so much sense, doesn't it, because they are taking in so much more information.

However, if you think there might be some *control patterns* that are preventing her from becoming more independent in her own natural timing, I also trust you in listening to that hunch. This could be the case if breastfeeding was a *control pattern*, and if you regularly fed her to sleep, and if that then spread to her mildly dissociating when she was cuddled up with you in bed.

One way you can ascertain that that might be happening is if she needs to be in a particular position in bed, and if she starts crying if she's not in that position.

If you notice something like this, *attachment play* in relation to this will probably help loosen up those feelings. After the *attachment play,* you might also find that some crying and raging is loosened up and she has some cries before bed. You might then offer a *Loving Limit* in relation to her being in that position. You could also ramp up the separation games in the evening, such as playing some hide and seek, if she has accumulated feelings related to separation that are getting in the way of her own timing. I trust your timing and hers.

11-year-old missing out on sleepovers

Q ~ I co-slept with our now 11-year-old boy. He now finds it very distressing to go to sleep without either myself or my husband laying with him. He misses out on sleepovers with friends and is missing out on his year six camp as we can't be there with him overnight. The anxiety and distress he goes through each night if we can't lay with him (e.g. hubby works away on night shift and most nights I have to study) is very distressing and debilitating for all of us. Any suggestions please would be so greatly appreciated.

A ~ I'm sending love to you all. I don't know how long you've known about Aware Parenting and how much opportunity he had to express his healing-feelings through crying, raging, laughter, and play when he was a baby and younger child. If you didn't know about these, it's likely that he has quite a few accumulated painful feelings in his body that are preventing him from feeling relaxed at bedtime. This is particularly the case if he experienced traumatic separations, e.g. directly after birth, or related to daycare or school. It's possible that the idea of separation when going to sleep might be helping him connect with those unexpressed feelings from earlier. To start with, I'd recommend lots of fun and laughter before bed, to help loosen up the feelings, and to listen to any crying that naturally arises. I'd recommend working 1:1 with an Aware Parenting instructor to dive in deeper to what might be going on for him.

Mornings

Q ~ My 9-year-old has a *control pattern* with her alarm clock and wants to get up very early each morning (to feel in control of her day) but is exhausted and judges herself harshly if she oversleeps.

A ~ I'm sending her and you so much love. I imagine you might find it painful to see her judging herself in this way. I have a few suggestions. I invite you to listen in to whether any of them resonate with you. I wonder if on weekends and holidays when she doesn't need to get up for anything specific, playing around with ideas of alarm clocks and times for getting up in an *attachment play* way might help. Perhaps you could do nonsense type play around getting up, or not being able to do things. I would also explore more about where this might be coming from. Is she experiencing harshness at school? Are you or her other parent judging yourselves harshly? Discovering the root of this and creating change there is also likely to be helpful for her. I'm so willing for you to get clear about what she most needs.

Self-Compassion Moment

I wonder how that was for you, reading the questions and answers? Learning that other parents have similar experiences can be reassuring. Or perhaps you've remembered some past experiences and are feeling painful feelings. My heart goes out to you if that is the case. As always, I invite you to reach out for loving listening in the Aware Parenting community.

Your feelings are beautiful gifts.

SECTION 3 SUMMARY

How are you feeling, having read this section? There's a lot of information here, so if what you've read resonates with you, I invite you to re-read it! Most of all, I want to acknowledge what a big process this is, not only changing our beliefs and conditioning about children and sleep, and listening to our own feelings, but also, being with our children and their needs and feelings with deep presence. I so deeply acknowledge and appreciate you for all that you are doing.

I'm here to remind you that although sleep is possibly what called you to Aware Parenting and to read this book, that since sleep is the ultimate emotional barometer, when you address a child's sleep you are attending to all parts of their emotional wellbeing.

Responding in an empathic and attuned way, offering plenty of closeness, joining in with their play and listening to their big, loud, and intense feelings, means you are not only making it much more likely that they will feel the kind of deep *relaxation* that brings sound sleep. You're also helping them *heal* from stress and trauma, meaning that they have less painful feelings sitting in their bodies.

They're less likely to need to suppress and dissociate from feelings, which will affect many more aspects of their lives than just their sleep. They will probably feel much more comfortable with the full range of their feelings, which will be important for their whole lives.

And most of all, they are likely to experience a sense of being unconditionally loved and supported, which will create belief systems which affect their future relationships and life.

I so deeply acknowledge all that you're doing.

29. Common sleep questions and answers for parents of children (ages 2-12)

PART 4

Teens and Sleep

30. The three ingredients for restful sleep – and what you can do to help your teen sleep restfully

Because of our teens' ever-increasing independence, we now have a different relationship with them and the three ingredients for their restful sleep.

I'll remind you of the three ingredients:

i.   to feel tired (sleepy);

ii. to feel connected (*closeness creating a sense of safety*); and

iii. to feel relaxed (*by releasing any healing-feelings present*).

Our long-term aim with Aware Parenting is to help them stay deeply connected with their sensations, needs, and feelings, so that they:

- *know* when they are tired and listen to their needs for rest and sleep;

- *understand* if they need closeness when they're tired, and are willing to ask for it; and

- are *connected with* their innate relaxation-through-release responses to cry, laugh, and share feelings through talking.

Why our role is now different

Our role is to give them responsibility to take action when they are tired, so that they feel relaxed and can sleep restfully.

We can observe whether they are connected with their own sensations of tiredness, their needs for connection, and their innate relaxation-through-release response. If they are, we can trust them to take responsibility for each of the ingredients.

However, if we observe on an ongoing basis that they are not connected with one or more of these, we are invited to support them in reconnecting with that, in a way that respectfully trusts that they still have that innate wisdom within them.

If there have been ruptures between us, or we're new to Aware Parenting, or they either have other needs or *control patterns* that regularly interfere with them listening to their bodies regarding sleep, our role now is to connect with our teen to see if they are willing to receive our support with these issues.

In Aware Parenting, if we want our teen to go to bed earlier than when they want to go to bed, and their sleep habits don't interfere with us getting our needs met, that is seen as a conflict of values rather than a conflict of needs. In other words, our needs are not being directly affected by their choice to stay up later than we would want.

This is why we wouldn't recommend offering them a *Limit* to go to bed because we want them to go to bed at a particular time.[67] We also *don't* recommend *Loving Limits* with bedtimes.

However, if they are not connected with one or more of the three ingredients, we still have an important role in our teen's relationship with sleep, and can contribute to them reconnecting with their innate wisdom for restful sleep.

Our aim is to:

- Stay *connected* with our teen
- Help them *release painful feelings*
- Give them *information* about sleep
- *Role model* the sleep behaviour we value
- *Encourage* them to tune in to what their body tells them
- *Support* and *trust* them to connect more with their needs for sleep

---

67 A *Limit* is a no based on our own needs or unwillingness. A *Loving Limit* is a no in response to behaviour, followed by listening to their feelings.

I wonder if the role modelling jumped out at you? If we always go on a screen before bed, or read, or often stay up late and feel tired, we are modelling that to them.

If we want our teen to listen to their body, we are also invited to listen to our own!

Self-Compassion Moment

If you're tempted to pick up the guilt stick, I invite you to put it down. This is a loving invitation, rather than judgment and coercion.

Trust and independence

You'll remember in the early chapters I shared that the first aspect of Aware Parenting is attachment-style parenting, which includes supporting and trusting a child's own timing and pace of increasing independence regarding sleep.

Our aim is to support and trust our children's inherent biological wisdom about when to go to sleep. This helps them to remain deeply connected with it, or reconnect with it.

So, we can hold this balance of trusting their innate body wisdom, while also seeing where past experiences (including with us) may be getting in the way of them being connected with that intrinsic intelligence.

As referenced earlier in this book, Aletha Solter says in *Attachment Play* (p.111), that children can learn to take responsibility for when to go to bed sometime between six and twelve years of age. She suggests that once a child no longer needs us to stay with them until they fall asleep (the age at which this happens varies immensely between different children), we may then choose to stop suggesting or telling them when they go to sleep.

We can support teens to learn about what, when, and how much sleep they need through inviting them to listen to their body's responses.

For example, if they need to get up early for school on weekdays, they will learn through experience about how much more enjoyable it is for them to go to sleep at an earlier time (often after experimenting with staying up late a few times and being tired the following day). The most powerful learning is through direct experience, and our role is to support that embodied learning, for example, by offering them compassion when they express that they're tired, and asking them if they want to share more with us about how they feel (even if we're tempted to move into judgment or lecturing them!).

In section 1 of the book, I shared about the freedom given to children and teens in many Indigenous cultures. To support our teen, we are invited to question our cultural conditioning, as well as lovingly listen to the painful feelings that this might help us connect with from our own teenage years.

> ### Self-Compassion Moment
> I'm sending love to whatever feelings you feel when you read this. You might feel shocked, imagining not telling your teen when to go to bed. If so, I'm sending love to the shock. Or you might feel scared, imagining how late they might go to bed. If so, I'm sending love to the parts of you that feel scared. You might feel incredulous, doubting that your teen would ever listen to their tiredness cues. If so, I really hear that incredulity. You might feel sad, knowing that there have been ruptures between you, and that your teen would not ask your perspective if you didn't try to foist it on them. My heart goes out to you if this is the case.

This journey of staying connected, or reconnecting with our teens, trusting them, supporting them to be independent, and offering support if required with sleep, is massive, particularly in this culture, where teens are not trusted. It's so natural that so many of our own feelings will show up to be lovingly listened to.

Joss Goulden, a Level 2 Aware Parenting instructor in Australia, shares:

"Aware Parenting in the teenage years became so much about offering connection, especially when they invited it, and continuing to prioritise our close safe relationship so they still shared their feelings with me. It required

me to keep coming back to trusting their own knowing, having conversations (without nagging or lecturing) about sleep, listening to their thoughts, observing when they were using control patterns *and moving in with extra warmth, compassion and connection and lots of* attachment play. *I got really skilled at repair, at finding so many different ways to offer connection and to ensure I was regularly getting my own feelings heard, in order to be able to support my teens with sleep. Any time I noticed myself having strong feelings of fear, frustration, or worry about them and their sleep, if I started to try to have conversations with my teens without supporting myself first, it was never helpful. On the other hand, when I got to share my feelings and speak out loud whatever was coming up for me first, I was able to have really helpful and supportive conversations with my teens."*

From a teen: *Mum, you keep telling me that I'm going to bed too late, and I'm starting to feel really pissed off. You're like a broken record. It's got to the point that I don't want to tell you when I go to bed any more, because it just leads to an argument every time. The thing is, the more you say it, the more I want to go to bed even later, just because I can do that. I just wish that you'd trust me and treat me a bit more how you want me to treat you – with respect.*

Oh, what's happening here? You're knocking on my door. You come in and smile a kind of weird smile. What strangeness is going on here? You start talking about wanting me to go to bed at 4pm, and tell me that 5pm is too late. Oh, I get it, you're doing some of that joking stuff you've started to do recently. I roll my eyes a bit, but you keep on going. You tell me that when you were a teenager, you went to bed before you got up. Oh, I get that one, it's like that really old TV show we watched together a while back. You've lost that serious face that you usually have when you talk about what time I go to sleep. Phew, I feel relieved. You keep going with the jokes, and I can't help it, I smile a bit too!

Then you tell me that you're sorry that you've been trying to tell me when to go to bed and you're going to change how you do things. I'd like to trust you, but I don't know if I can yet. I wonder whether you will do what you say. You say you want to trust me to listen to my body. Well, that would make a change!

I feel a bit warmer towards you. It's like your jokes have warmed the air between us. I ask if you want to watch that clip from the 'going to bed before getting up' show, and you say yes and come and sit on my bed. We watch it together and start laughing. That leads to us watching another couple of funny videos together, and chatting about them. It's weird, but after that I actually feel more relaxed and I kind of want to go to bed soon. I don't tell you yet, but how strange is that? Let's see how this goes....

i. To feel tired (sleepy)

Tiredness is still the first ingredient for restful sleep. However, with teens, our role is no longer about taking actions once we notice their tiredness. Rather, we are invited to trust *them* to be connected with their sleepiness sensations, and for *them* to take action as a result. They are likely to be connected with their body and to listen to themselves if we helped them stay connected with the sensations of sleepiness in their bodies when they were younger.

> ### Self-Compassion Moment
> I'm sending love to you if you feel painful emotions when you read this. I'm here to remind you that if we didn't have the knowledge or presence to help them with this when they were younger, we can still help them now – in the ways outlined in this chapter.

If we repeatedly see them overriding their sensations of sleepiness, this doesn't mean not doing anything. We can still have an influence without coercing, judging, or threatening them, and without using Loving Limits.

What this means in practical terms

Conversation

Being connected with them through conversation is likely to help them to be more connected with their bodies and their sensations of sleepiness.

If they talk to us about feeling tired, we can offer them compassion, *"Oh, I hear that you're feeling tired, lovely,"* rather than telling them *"Well, that's because you went to bed so late last night,"* or, *"I told you that you'd feel tired if you stayed up late,"* or even a slightly more subtle but still unenjoyable for them, *"I'm not surprised."*

We can ask about their plans for their evening, and express our interest and curiosity in what they're doing, and tell them about what we plan to do for the evening. If we've only recently stopped telling them when to go to bed, we might want to wait a few weeks before doing this, so they can trust that we're asking because we're interested in them and their lives, rather than because we're wanting them to go to bed when *we* think is the most helpful.

We might also model what we value in terms of listening to our body's cues. For example, sharing about when we are tired and want an early night, or when we're planning to stay up late to do something we enjoy or a thing that we really want to get done by the next morning. With these topics of conversation just a part of family life, we can avoid trying to get them to do what we want them to do regarding sleep. Instead, we can simply and lovingly model our own relationship with sleep, and show them our care for them. We can clearly communicate to them *when we* are tired, *how we* know that we are, and *what we* do in response.

Modelling listening to and acting upon our own sensations of sleepiness is a powerful communication to them.

Talking to them with compassion and respect will mean they are more likely to talk to us about their sensations of sleepiness, be influenced by us to act upon those cues, and ask for help if they need it.

Self-Compassion Moment

I'm sending so much love to you if you are feeling painful feelings having read this, if there have been things you did that helped them disconnect from their sensations of sleepiness. It's so common that these things have happened by the time they become teens. If you coerced them to go to bed when you wanted them to, or used punishments or rewards, or distracted them from their painful feelings when they were tired and were trying to share their painful feelings, my heart goes out to you. You might have known about Aware Parenting and regularly offered Loving Limits about going to bed at a certain time, and if you're feeling uncomfortable feelings hearing that we don't recommend doing that, I'm also sending lots of compassion to you.

I'm here to remind you that the more you are willing to put down any sticks, and have your painful feelings about this heard, the more likely you will be able to keep offering them the kind of loving connection that will help them reconnect with, trust, and act upon, their sensations of sleepiness. The more your own feelings are heard, the more you will be able to respond to them in calm and compassionate ways. Change really is possible, and you have so much power to create that change.

If we can still see ways in which our responses to their tiredness earlier on in their lives is affecting how they perceive and respond to their own tiredness, we might give them information about that. For example, if they tend to always want to eat when they are tired, and we think that's because we always fed them to sleep as babies and toddlers, we might tell them about that. We might explain that babies can learn to think that their sensations of tiredness are actually hunger if they were often fed when they were tired. We might have conversations about how we learnt to differentiate between our own sensations of hunger and tiredness ourselves as adults, and how we came to listen to what our bodies are communicating to us about sleep.

You might find it helpful to know that for the first three months of my daughter's life, I always fed her to sleep. Once I started to realise that it wasn't the most helpful thing for her, her dad and I started to listen to her healing-feelings every evening before sleep when she was three months old. However, even after this, she would still often fall asleep at the breast during the daytime. I was still learning about her healing-feelings when she was tired and would often feed her when she was tired or had healing-feelings to express during the day.

However, as I understood more about Aware Parenting, I helped her disentangle tiredness from hunger. Despite how I had responded to her when she was a baby and a toddler, she became deeply connected with what her body was telling her in regard to tiredness, hunger, and feelings by the time she was three years old.

As a result, when she was a teen, I found it easy to trust her self-connection in relation to sleepiness. I didn't ask or tell her when to go to bed as a teen or even as an older child, and I loved observing how connected she was with her body and her needs for sleep. She would sometimes stay up later, such as if she suddenly got into a project that she was loving, or was enjoying reading a particular book. However, she was, and still is as a young adult, deeply connected with her body and when she feels tired.

So, from personal experience, I can offer that whatever we do when they are younger in relation to sleep, it is possible to help them regain their accurate understanding of what their sensations are communicating to them, to know when they are tired, and to generally go to bed when their body tells them to, unless there is something important to them that they want to stay up for or get up early for.

That reconnection might happen in early or late childhood, or in their early or late teens. Each relationship is different. Healing has its own timing.

For example, my son has both a passion for, and a control pattern *with, screens, which has been part of a more complex sleep journey in his teen years. This is also related to the trauma he experienced when he was nearly five, when his dad and I separated. It was also influenced by my own* control pattern *with TV when I was a teen, which I share about later.*

I trust that any healing that you are wanting between yourself and your teen, and between themselves and their innate sleep wisdom, is possible. Even if that takes a while.

Belynda shares her experience:

"I didn't know about listening to children's feelings when my two children were young – I learned about this when they were four and one. But the approach I found (Hand in Hand Parenting – which has

many similarities to Aware Parenting) didn't have this overt focus on trusting children's own perception of their sleep needs, so in fact I still imposed 'bedtimes' (albeit in a connected, playful, and respectful way) right through until very recently. The idea of them being completely in charge of their own sleep needs is so radically different to what I had experienced or observed anywhere else!

They are now 14 and 11 and I'm often able to bring this trust to the process. I still find that I have some tension at times, that I talk to them about how tired they feel and question them about when they feel would be a good time to sleep, rather than quietly exuding confidence and trust in them. It is a work in progress. Adding in screens further complicates things!

But I love that I now have a map for how I'd like to proceed, and a clear and resonant process of reasoning as to why this way of doing things is most helpful for my children – because I want them to grow up trusting their own body-sensations, and I want them to build their own confidence and clarity about their decision-making and their needs. So when I stray from the way I want things to be, I have a space to reflect (Listening Partnerships) and a clear map to follow. I have lots of grief about not having this map earlier in their lives, but a lot of gratitude that I found it as they entered their teen years."

Self-Compassion Moment

I'm sending love to you and your feelings as you read this. It's very common for us all to be doing so much de-conditioning and new learning when we have teens. I invite us all to be deeply compassionate with ourselves and each other during this process.

Biological reasons for teens going to sleep later

We might find it helpful to hold in mind the research that suggests that once they reach puberty, melatonin production can occur later in the evening for teens. Let's also think about that from an evolutionary perspective. I love exploring possibilities about the original and wise reasons that our bodies have for doing what they do.

So, what might cause teens to naturally feel tired later at night once they reach puberty? Perhaps their burgeoning strength and maturity meant that, during the hunter-gatherer phase of our evolution, teens:

- Were out late finding a mate?
- Were out at night to take part in hunting?
- Played a more active role in keeping the community safe?

If we hold in mind these possibilities about the ancestral wisdom and wiring of their body, might it help us feel more comfortable when they want to go to bed later than us?

Whatever the evolutionary reasons, if we hold in mind that physiologically, many teens may feel tired a lot later than they used to, it can help us have a lot more compassion for them.

When they stay up late, remembering this information might help us be much less likely to respond to them in harsh, punitive, or otherwise unhelpful ways. We can also hold in mind the research on chronotypes. Our teen might be a night owl and we might be an early bird. Understanding our different sleep patterns can also help us trust their sleep choices more.

Self-Reflection Moment
I wonder how you feel and what you think when you read this? I'm sending love to all of your feelings. Learning to trust our teens can help us connect with all kinds of feelings in ourselves, often because we weren't trusted when we were teenagers. This can be incredibly painful. As always, I invite you to reach out for loving listening if you have uncomfortable feelings as you reflect on all of this.

Learning to trust them

With Aware Parenting, our aim is to support our teens to stay connected to their own body wisdom, and for them to make choices based on that deep self-connection. This is part of us learning to trust them and to support them to be connected with themselves. For example, if a teen goes to bed later several nights in a row and goes to school each day feeling tired, we can aim to trust that they will listen to that feedback from their body and choose to go to bed earlier. We might have compassionate conversations with them about how they feel, without judging, shaming, or coercing them to go to bed earlier. We might ask them if they want our help with listening to their sleepiness sensations or going to bed when they are tired.

The more we communicate to them that we trust that they will listen to their body and make choices based on that, the more they will experience being trusted and will be more likely to trust themselves.

Belynda shares more of her story here:

"My beautiful teen usually goes to bed later than I think he should – it is complicated and really hard for me to trust him (and 'let' the hard experiences happen)! When I sat with him and expressed this to him, I asked him what he needed to stay connected in with his own tiredness cues and sleep needs – he asked for some connection time before I head to bed (usually about 9.30pm) as he thinks that will help him be ready for sleep. We usually connect earlier (around 7.30pm) with some wrestling and chat. I love that he knew to ask for connection later in the evening.

I don't know if this situation will have a pretty bow and be resolved simply, but having a sense of wanting to trust him, and of knowing that he is learning through his experiences, along with having lots of **Listening Partnership** *support, means that we are muddling along together with a feeling of being on the same team. It is not neat, but it is connected, and that's the thing I'm really happy about."*

I love how Belynda talks about us not necessarily having a neat and simple resolution with a pretty bow, but focusing on the importance of connection and the sense of being on the same team.

This is key to practicing Aware Parenting – knowing that learning a whole different way of parenting within the **DDC** *is inevitably going to be challenging at times – and being deeply compassionate with ourselves about this.*

Offering our care and interest in our teenager and their lives, and our willingness to support them, without trying to coerce them into doing what we want them to do, dropping our 'should's', and even our subtle and gentle ways to try to make them do what we want them to do, can be a huge journey. Receiving lots of listening for ourselves is vital. When we were a teenager, we might have experienced not having much choice or autonomy at all around our sleep. Or, we may have experienced complete choice for when we went to sleep, but also a lack of the kind of connection and support that we actually wanted from our parents. Perhaps they had no idea of our sleep choices, or what we were doing, feeling, or thinking about in the evenings.

As a result, staying *connected* with our teen, showing our *interest*, our *care* about, and *compassion* for what they do in the evenings, how their bodies feel, and how tired or rested they might be, *but without telling them when to go to bed*, can be a big learning curve.

If you have come to Aware Parenting later and have used punishments or rewards, or have used coercion or power-over to get them to go to sleep when you want them to rather than when they feel tired, this process of them listening to their body's cues may take longer.

This is because they will initially be still learning to trust that they really *do* have choice now, followed by them actually listening in to their body's sensations and what those are communicating to them.

> ### Self-Compassion Moment
> If you did use punishments, rewards, coercion, or power-over to get your child or teen to go to sleep when you wanted them to, I'm sending you so much love and compassion. It's very common in the DDC that many of us might feel powerless in relation to getting our needs met as parents. It's when we feel powerless that we're most likely to turn to these power-over ways. This is why it's so important that we regularly have our own feelings heard.

Another effect of the *Disconnected Domination Culture* is how going to school can make things harder, because of the fixed and early times schools require teens to arrive at. Here's another opportunity to offer them empathy, have conversations, support them, and trust that they will make the best of this challenging situation. This might include conversations with them about the history of the culture they live in. It may include empathy if they feel tired and if they have painful emotions in relation to going to school. It might mean we lovingly ask them if they want any support from us in relation to when they go to sleep.

The more we can express our unconditional support and compassion for them, and our trust in their wisdom, along with our offers of guidance if they are willing to receive it, the more likely they will be able to connect in with their innate body knowledge about sleep.

As a homeschooling family, we found the mornings much easier as often there was no time that my daughter and son needed to be up by. However, I noticed that if my son really wanted to do something, especially where he would see his friends, he would jump out of bed, really willing to get up and start the day.

Self-Compassion Moment

I invite you to be compassionate with yourself and your teen, living in a culture that doesn't support people to listen to their bodies and their innate physiological needs and wisdom, and which doesn't trust teens and their own unique journey into independence.

From a teen: *Dad, remember when you used to threaten me that if I didn't go to bed when you said, you'd take away my phone and wouldn't give it back? I felt so mad when you did that, and I wanted to do all the things that you didn't want me to do even more. I really hated you for a while. I'm really happy that you stopped doing that. I like it now that we've connected back again, even going back to playing old school card games after dinner like we used to when I was a little kid. When I'm not fighting you, I can feel in more to what I want to do and don't want to do. I was reading that new manga series last week and I just wanted to read another chapter, and another, and I definitely felt tired in the mornings. Sometimes I don't really mind about being a bit tired, but I didn't like it when I played soccer and I missed that goal because I wasn't really with it after that really late night I had. I'm going to make sure I go to bed earlier on the nights before soccer training and matches. I guess that's what you talk about learning through experience, hey Dad?*

ii. To feel connected (*closeness creating a sense of safety*)

As parents, we can still be part of contributing to our teen's needs for connection and closeness. However, unlike when they were babies and young children, they now have so much agency and capacity to meet those needs in many ways. With Aware Parenting, it's still normal for teens to feel connected with their parents. Connecting before bed for a chat or a game, asking about their day, or being interested in what they are doing, reading, watching, or playing, can still be deeply nourishing for them. Many teens who have been brought up with Aware Parenting are still often open to hugs, physical affection, and rough and tumble type play with their parents.

However, this connectedness before sleep is not just about the in-the-moment connection with us. It's also about them having internalised the loving connection we've offered them in earlier years, so that they feel a sense of connection with themselves and their bodies.

If you didn't practice Aware Parenting earlier on, or if there was a rupture with your teen earlier on and they push away affection or closeness with you, it's absolutely possible for ruptures to be healed and reconnection to happen.

Having lots of our own feelings lovingly heard is central to this process.

> ### Self-Compassion Moment
> If your teen pushes away from connection and closeness with you because of ruptures between the two of you in the past, I'm sending so much love to you and your feelings.

I know how deeply painful that can be. I experienced a rupture with my daughter after her dad and I split up and I didn't always get there in time to protect her from her brother hitting her. After many years, that rupture eventually healed.

Even if ruptures happened between us a long time ago, it's still possible for them to heal and for us to become deeply connected with our teens again.

I so trust that any disconnection or rupture with your teen can heal. Their deep desire for healing is always calling them (and us). One of the most important ways to support that process is for us to receive lots of listening and empathy ourselves, from an empathy buddy and/or Aware Parenting instructor. That way, we can keep offering the kind of connection that is conducive to healing the rift.

Of course, many teens receive lots of their connection needs from their friends and, if they have one, a boyfriend or girlfriend. However, with Aware Parenting, it is possible that they can still enjoy connecting with their parents and siblings, and enjoy hugs and cuddles throughout their teen years.

> ### Self-Reflection Moment
> When you think of their connection needs, and see them messaging friends on their phone, does that help meet your need for understanding that they are aiming to get their needs for connection met? Do you find it easier to be calm and compassionate with them when you think this?

What this means in practical terms:

Offering connection

Even if a teen doesn't seem to want it, continuing to offer them connection can make a big difference to the bond between us and them. That might be by showing interest in what they're interested in, asking about how their day was, remembering to ask them about something significant that happened that day, such as that they always do that activity on Thursdays, or chatting about something that you know is meaningful to them. You might share about your day, or something that you're excited about, or are thinking about that you think might be interesting to them. You might offer affection, such as a hand on the centre of their back, or a hug, or to sit close with them. Some teens might be more willing to welcome physical contact if it's offered as a massage for their shoulders, head, or feet, or brushing or styling their hair.

At 18, my son sometimes asks me to give him shoulder massages, or to brush his curly shoulder-length hair and put it in a pony tail for him. It's a lovely way for us to connect.

When teens are going through more stressful times, they really need to know that we are still there, loving them and supporting them.

Offering connection to our teen may look quite different to connection with a child.

That generally means making the most of any connection they reach out for. If they want to chat with us, our being willing to prioritise that can make a difference, even if we're in the middle of doing something else. We can also make the most of connecting at other times of the day, such as offering them eye contact when we're close by, saying goodbye along with some conversation when they're going out somewhere, and warmly greeting them – alongside showing interest in what they've been doing – when they come home.

My daughter and I went through phases of connecting throughout the day via quizzes and word games that we'd play on our phones and send the results to each other. These were points of contact so when we connected in person, I could refer to something that had happened that day with the games we'd played. I learnt to be open to connecting in all kinds of different ways, including through screens. She also used to like dressing me up and putting make-up on me. The results were often very funny!

Maryanne shares how screens are also part of her connection with her son:

"I try to share little funny memes or videos with my teen son. Often he sends back his own choice of videos to make me laugh. My favourite are the short YouTube clips he sends that are focused on my interests (e.g. cooking)! And although I don't really watch YouTube, every now and then I spend an hour searching for a bunch of videos and memes which I then save, and share little by little over time. It has become a lovely way to feel connected when we aren't in the same place. Having a chuckle

together about what we've shared (once we are together again) adds to the feeling of connection."

It's those little moments of fun, understanding, care, and compassion that can make a huge difference to the ongoing sense of our teen feeling connected with us.

Joss Goulden, a Level 2 Aware Parenting instructor in Australia, whom you've already met, shares about her experience of this with her teens:

"The most important part for supporting my teens with sleep has been the connection aspect. Making time to offer moments of connection before I went to bed, as I was often sleeping before they did, finding lots of little ways to offer loving gestures during the day, having big chunks of time together, and lots of attachment play, particularly sharing laughter and fun together. It really helped to keep offering physical affection, showing genuine interest in what they were passionate about and a genuine desire to spend time together. Prioritising finding ways to show them my love. It has often been after moments of connection together that they have shared their feelings with me, and then they were so much more relaxed and able to sleep with more ease."

As part of trusting them and contributing to their needs for connection, we might let them know up until what time we're willing and available to connect with them before we go to sleep. If we go to bed at about the same time every night, that might mean telling them in general that we are available until whatever time that is. However, if we go to bed at a different time every night, we might let them know, say an hour before we go to bed, that we're available for chats or cuddles, watching things together, or helping them with homework.

Your teen might sometimes want to come and talk when you're tired and wanting to go to bed. If you can, prioritising that connection can make a huge difference to your relationship and to how they feel. Just as the childhood years go by quickly, so do the teen years, and it really is a golden opportunity to simply listen and be interested whenever they want to connect. However, it's also so important to listen to yourself. For example, if it's happening regularly, is there something you can do to encourage them to share earlier on, or can you have some rest so that you can stay up a bit later. One of my favourite phrases was, *"I'm willing for both of us to get our needs met."* I wonder if you find that helpful, too?

Joss continues:

"I noticed that so often my teens would invite connection in the evenings. They would want to chat and share later at night or want to play loud music and dance together before bed. Because I was familiar with Aware Parenting and understood why this was happening, I was able to join them in the connection and play and support releasing before I then went to bed."

From a teen: *Mum and Dad, I know I'm 14 and everything, but I do still need you. Since I had my 13th birthday, it's kind of like you think I don't really need you anymore. Sure, I've got lots of friends and I don't want to hang out with you all the time like I used to, but sometimes I think you don't really care about me. After dinner, I hear you and Sam and Dee all hanging out together and I don't really know how to join in nowadays. It sounds like you're having fun. I just sit here on my bed, listening to you all, wishing I was there with you too.*

What's this? You're sending me a text. It's got a lot of emojis! It's a picture of you all playing board games, and a piece of paper on a chair with my name and a question mark! Looks like you do want me to come and join in after all! I shut down the big smile on my face as I walk out of my room, cos I don't want you to know how much this means to me!

iii. To feel relaxed (*by releasing any healing-feelings present*)

There are certain elements of Aware Parenting that we would suggest practicing with younger children, but would not recommend using with teens to help them become deeply relaxed.

For example, we wouldn't recommend offering them a *Loving Limit* to get them to go to bed when we see that they might have accumulated feelings that are getting in the way of them going to bed when they are tired.

However, we can still support them in feeling more relaxed – through listening to them talking, bringing in humour and laughter together, and lovingly listening to them while they cry if they are wanting and willing for us to be with them.

Teens generally have less need to cry or express big angry emotions, although there may be times where they do have healing-feelings to release in this way. However, more of the time, their natural relaxation response is to talk about their experiences. They may also enjoy humour and fun, especially if it involves laughter, as a way to release tension. Offering little jokes and watching funny shows together can be a part of this process.

Some teens might have feelings bubbling up later on, after we've gone to sleep. It's important for us to listen in to whether we are willing for them to wake us up to share those feelings with us. Each of us will be different in our willingness for this, depending on all kinds of factors. You might have a big yes to that. Or you might not. If you are not willing to be woken up in the night for your teen to share feelings with you and they want to do that, you might want to have conversations with them to find other ways where you can both get your needs met. For example, that might include regular meet-ups, whether that's in the kitchen, or at a cafe, or on a walk, where you give them your undivided attention. There might be particular times when they need to talk to you, e.g. after a particular class at school, in which case you could schedule in those times. That way, you get uninterrupted sleep, and they have regular opportunities to share their feelings with you.

What this means in practical terms

Listening to what they want to share

Being interested in them, asking questions, and showing interest in what they're interested in are all ways to support teens to open up and share about what's going on for them. You might find that asking thoughtful and open-ended questions is really helpful, e.g. *"I always love hearing your perspective – what do you think about xyz?"* Or *"I noticed you've been hanging out with Y a lot lately, what do you enjoy about connecting with them?"*

Having fun together

If you find yourself in a fun mode, I invite you to share that with your teen. Yes, sometimes they might roll their eyes, but you might find that they smile or even join in. Perhaps as a family, you enjoy making music and singing together in ways that bring fun. If there are videos you enjoy watching together that help you both laugh, how about doing that in the evening? Or perhaps they're into playing fun games on whatever the latest new app is. Being goofy and joining in can go a long way to supporting them to feel more relaxed through laughter. You might find that they want to tell you jokes before sleep, or you might enjoy watching a comedy together. With practice, you might naturally get more goofy together when you're tired.

With teens, humour often replaces more specific attachment play games as a way to release tension.

I found that once my daughter and son became teens, my responding with humour and fun in the conversation often brought laughter, connection, and an easeful sense of release and relief. Even a few sentences expressed with humour changed the whole feeling tone of our conversations and helped us all feel connected and more relaxed, including in the evenings.

Joss, a Level 2 Aware Parenting instructor you've already met, shares her experience of doing *attachment play* with her teens:

"Attachment play *with my teenagers is such a central part of creating more connection and supporting healing when they have accumulated feelings. Finding ways to bring joy, fun, and laughter is so important for us all and I noticed so many times that their sleep was so much better after lots of play, just like when they were toddlers! I find it so helpful to remind myself to recognise their invitation to play and to find moments when their behaviour is suggesting that they would really benefit from some silliness and fun, so that they come back to being more relaxed and able to sleep. Some of my favourite games have been:*

Dancing together – following their lead or getting them to teach me silly TikTok dances, which they are always so much better at than I am.

Arm wrestles, pillow fights, and pushing games, with an element of nonsense, and again, they always win – I don't even need to let them win anymore!

Board games – collaborative and competitive ones, where we are joking and laughing and they are often winning.

Regular non-directive child-centred play, where they get to choose what we do and where we go and I just delight in being with them.

Role play and symbolic play where we act out their experiences – sometimes in jest and sometimes with more seriousness. E.g. My son has really enjoyed taking me through tunnels at water parks as part of healing his birth trauma.

The Masterchef game – when they are being demanding or I am sensing some disconnect, I love to bring in their favourite snack and pretend I am a contestant on a cooking show, asking for their feedback on my dish.

Joining them in their passions with enthusiasm – letting them choose a TV show to watch together or a movie, learning how to play a computer game with them, going to the gym together where they get to choose the workout plan.

Regression games, e.g. cuddling up next to them and trying to pick them up (which is not possible – they are so much bigger than me) and saying they will always be my baby, or playing games we used to play with them when they were little such as She's mine, no she's mine, where we pretend to fight over them.

Making our home a welcoming place for their friends and girlfriend/ boyfriend so that we can all still have fun together and so they choose to spend time with us still."

Vivian, an Aware Parenting instructor in Europe, shares:

"I personally find that attachment play with teens is very different compared to practicing it with young children. In my experience it is more personal, happens in the moment, and is very rarely pre-thought. We probably need to wait until the 'right' moment to include it. On

the other hand, it also invites us even more to deeply connect with the moment, with ourselves, our feelings , the energy in the room, or between us and our teen, and to trust our intuition and what comes up.

Here are a couple of examples:

Write or draw on each other's backs: Write simple words, or draw something, on each other's back with your finger. Guess what word, or drawing, it is.

Make up or hair styling: Let your teen do your make up and/or style or cut your hair."

> ### Self-Compassion Moment
> I'm sending love to any feelings you might feel when you read this. Many of us have lots of painful feelings in relation to how our parent/s were with us when we were teens. As usual, having those feelings heard can really help us be able to offer more of this kind of connection to our teens.

Listening to deeper feelings

If they do have some deeper and more painful feelings to express to you before bed, prioritising that, listening, and avoiding offering suggestions, advice or admonishment is really important.

If you want your teen to trust you, offering unconditional love when they're going through hard times is vital.

Sophie shares about her experience of listening to her teenage daughter:

"I try to remember to not judge my daughter when she expresses her feelings in the form of judgments. She sometimes calls one of her teachers a name that I really don't enjoy. Remembering that this is a time for me to listen to her with care, without offering any criticism or judgement of how she expresses herself, has been helpful. As she feels more and more supported by me (because I'm not lecturing her!) this has meant that she uses that language less and less."

The more you're willing to listen with empathy and acceptance, the more likely it is that they will ask for your support, perspective, and guidance. If you try to foist those on them, they're likely to shut down and stop telling you things. Sharing their concerns before bed can be another powerful way to help them feel more relaxed and to get that restorative sleep their body so deeply needs whilst they're growing and changing so much.

From a teen: *I actually can't believe how angry I'm feeling right now. Sabina was so out of line. I stomp around my bedroom, wanting to smash things. I'm a burning furnace of rage. I hear a knock on the door, and I want to throw something at it. You open the door, Mum, and straight away, my rage bubbles out at you. "What do you want?" I shout.*

"I heard some noise and wanted to see how you are, sweetheart," you reply. Well, that gets my back up straight away. "Can't you just leave me alone?!" I look up, and I see you looking at me. For some reason, that makes me angrier. "What do you care?" I snarl at you, and look back down at my phone. I'm surprised to see that you don't leave. I look up again. "What!?" I say.

"I care about you," you say, and if I wasn't so mad, I might see some care in your eyes, but all I see is red.

"Well, I don't care about YOU!" I shout. There's silence. But you still don't leave.

"I'm here. I'm listening," you say.

"OH MY GOD. Why don't you just SHUT UP!" I respond. "I have just about had it with you!" I'm so full of rage that I don't have the space to be scared about what you might do. But you don't go, and these feelings bubble out even more. "I am SOOOO MAD right now. I don't even know what to do." I feel this inferno of flaming rage inside of me. Somehow, even though I am super fed up with you being there, you being there is also helping me. I feel all this energy in my body, and each time I speak, I can feel it flowing out of me.

"I'm listening, and I'm going to keep on listening, sweetheart." Somehow, your words are a safe wall I can push up against.

"Aarrrrggghhh.... I am soooooo angry. How DARE she do that to me! I thought we were best friends. I am OUTRAGED. How could she have done that!" I'm pacing up and down my room, and out of the corner of my eye, I can still see you there, standing at the door.

"I hear you." And again, another swirl of rage bubbles up when you speak.

"She betrayed my trust. How can I ever speak to her again? That was just SO unfair."

"Oh, sweetheart," you say, and somehow, my heart breaks when I hear that word. The angry dam breaks, and all the sadness and hurt pours out. I start to cry. I'm literally like a dam full of water, as so many tears come out. I look up, and I can see the request in your eyes. I nod. You come close, and you put your hand on the centre of my back. I'm so glad that you knew that a hug would be too much. Somehow, the touch of your hand means I cry even more.

I can really feel that you're here with me, Mum, and that I'm safe. Wow. I keep crying and crying, all the hurt of the day pouring out of me. I am so sad. So sad. There's tears, and there's snot, and we're sitting on my bed now, and it's falling on my new jeans, and you don't even moan about the washing. I lean in to you, just a bit, to see how I feel. Yep, more tears. I didn't even know that I could cry this much. My heart actually hurts. I cry some more, like I'm right in the centre of the pain.

Finally, the snot and the tears dry up, and I'm doing this weird sighing thing. Quietly at first, I start to tell you what happened with Sabina, and you listen, and you nod, and somehow you know just the things to say and it's all helping. The pain is lessening and I'm starting to feel relieved. I tell you the whole story, and you say some lovely things to me. That means a lot, Mum.

You ask if I want a hug, and I say yes, even though we haven't hugged for quite a while. I lean in to you and you smell just as I remember you. We stay like that for quite a while. I feel even more relieved and relaxed. We break apart, and look in each other's eyes. "How are you now, sweetheart? You ask.

"Starving!" I say.

"It's late, so how about we just have beans on toast together and curl up on the sofa and listen to some music?"

"Sounds great, Mum," I respond. You make the food, and I get some pillows from my room. We eat together and I play some new songs to you. We chat about silly stuff, like bands, and remembering that concert we went to when I was 11. I talk a bit about what I'll do tomorrow if I see Sabina, and you listen. I yawn. "I'm so tired, Mum." We put the plates and stuff into the sink and both head off to bed. I'm shocked about how relaxed I feel. And my heart feels so open to you, Mum, it's lovely. I don't even feel worried about seeing Sabina tomorrow. Somehow I know that I'm going to be okay. I snuggle up into my bed. I don't think it'll take me long to go to sleep tonight. I won't need to play music on my earbuds to go to sleep like I usually do.

Helping them with *control patterns*

If our teen often overrides their sensations of sleepiness as well as painful feelings through *control patterns* such as screens or reading, it's important that we don't just leave them to it. There are many ways to support them. We might have conversations with them, asking them about whether *they want* to be able to sleep earlier, or how *they* feel and think about their screen use or reading. We might ask them if they want our help with it.

Our role is to support them to feel relaxed, rather than using power-over them to make them do what we want them to do.

If they're on screens late every night, we might explore whether they want some creative ideas from us to help them to get off when they want to.

Perhaps we might offer to see if they're willing to do an experiment such as not using screens for a day or an evening, and seeing how they feel, how they sleep, and how they feel the next morning.

Maybe they would like us to connect with them at a certain time each evening and have some fun conversations.

Perhaps they want us to set up a timer to remind them to watch a funny video every evening to help them release some feelings through laughter so they find it easier to go to sleep.

Joss, the Level 2 Aware Parenting instructor you've already heard from, shares about her experience with *control patterns* and her teenagers:

"Control patterns with my teenagers are hard to navigate at times because I am not wanting to bring in Loving Limits *like when they were younger. So I find it really helpful to just notice when they are using* control patterns *and to take a moment to connect with myself and tend to my feelings that are there and all the things I am making it mean that they are dissociating, both about them and about me.*

I am then able to move in with compassion and warmth and love, to offer them connection and care or attachment play. *Sometimes this supports them to come back to balance and sometimes they want to keep using the* control pattern, *in which case I need to support myself again with any feelings I am having and then come back to trusting their processing and their timing."*

From a teen: *I absolutely love gaming Dad, and sometimes I love staying up until 2am, when I'm right in the middle of it all. I've met so many people on this new game, and I feel so excited when I'm playing it. But sometimes I just know that I can't get off it, even though I really want to. That's when I'm still on at 3am or later. I wish I could talk to you about it, and tell you about it all, the bits that I love and the times that I just can't stop. But every time I try to tell you, you just start going on about how the companies deliberately create the games to make me an addict. I need your help, but when you go on about all that stuff, I just don't feel understood or heard. I want you to be able to meet me where I am. I'm a gamer, and I love it, but I also need help to find ways to get off when I know I'm tired and that I will feel rough the next day. I wish you could really listen to me. It's nearly midnight, and I see a message come in on my phone. It's from you.*

"Want to talk?" you ask.

"Maybe. Are you going to have a go at me again?"

"Sorry mate, I won't do that this time, I promise."

"Okay, come over," I say.

You come to my room and you apologise. I'm a bit shocked. You've never apologised to me about all the screen stuff. You tell me you've been thinking and that you realise that you haven't been listening to me, and you see our relationship deteriorating. Hmm. That's a turn up for the books. I wasn't expecting that.

I'm not going to dive in straight away to ask for your help about the 3am stuff, but I will tell you about this new level I'm on. You stay for half an hour, and you really listen this time, Dad. I get all enthusiastic, telling you about what I'm loving with this particular version, and for once, you're paying attention. You keep looking, and nodding so I know that you're actually taking things in. I'm starting to trust you a bit more. If this happens a few more times, perhaps I can ask for your help with the 3am thing. Let's see how it goes.

You leave, and I almost ask you for a hug. Maybe next time. I can feel this openness in my body and I feel almost joyful about it. I turn off my computer and strangely, I find it easy to go to sleep after our chat. Thanks, Dad.

CHAPTER SUMMARY

We now have a different relationship with our teens and the three ingredients that they require for restful sleep:

i.   to feel tired (sleepy);

ii. to feel connected (*closeness creating a sense of safety*); and

iii. to feel relaxed (*by releasing any healing-feelings present*).

Our aim is to give them responsibility to take action when they are tired, so that they feel relaxed and can sleep restfully. Our role is to observe whether they are connected with their own sensations of tiredness, their needs for connection, and their innate relaxation-through-release response. If they are, we can trust them to take responsibility for each of the ingredients.

However, if we observe on an ongoing basis that they are not connected with one or more of these, we are invited to support them in reconnecting with whatever that is, in a way that respectfully trusts that they still have that innate wisdom within them.

To feel tired

With teens, our role is no longer about taking actions once we notice their tiredness, but rather to trust them to be connected with the sensations that tell them they're tired, and to take action as a result. However, this doesn't mean not doing anything if we repeatedly see them overriding their sensations of sleepiness. We can still have a loving influence.

Whatever we did when they were younger in relation to sleep, it is possible to help them regain their accurate understanding of what their sensations are communicating to them, to know when they are tired, and to generally go to bed when their body communicates to them to.

The more we can express our unconditional support and compassion for them, and our trust in their wisdom, along with our offers of guidance if they are willing to receive it, the more likely they will be able to connect in with their innate body knowledge about sleep.

To feel connected (closeness creating a sense of safety)

If you didn't practice Aware Parenting earlier on, or if there was a rupture with your teen earlier on and they don't want to be affectionate or close with you, it's really possible for ruptures to be healed and reconnection to happen.

With Aware Parenting, teens can still enjoy connecting with their parents and siblings, and enjoy hugs and cuddles in the evenings throughout their teen years. Little moments of care and compassion can make a huge difference to their ongoing sense of connection with us.

To feel relaxed (by releasing any healing-feelings present)

I *don't* recommend *Loving Limits* for bedtimes with teens. We can still support them in feeling more relaxed through listening to them talking, using humour and laughter together, and listening to them crying if they are wanting and willing for us to listen to them. Listening to what they want to share, having fun together, and listening to deeper feelings are also still central to Aware Parenting at this age.

The more we are willing to listen with empathy and acceptance, the more likely it is that they will ask for our support, perspective, and guidance.

Helping them with control patterns

If our teen often overrides their feelings of tiredness (and other uncomfortable feelings) through screens or reading, we are also invited to support them. That might be through having conversations with them, asking them about how they feel and think about their screen use or reading. We might ask them if they want us to help them with this. Lovingly listening to them and offering connection and fun can help them need to use the *control pattern* less.

Your teen still really needs your loving support.

31. Your own inner work

Just like when we have babies and children, our painful experiences with sleep as teens may show up in our parenting, inviting us to do our own inner work.

A vital topic to explore is our feelings in relation to trusting our teen and their innate sleep wisdom.

If you find it hard to trust your teen's inherent wisdom about when to go to sleep, I invite you to receive some listening from your empathy buddy or an Aware Parenting instructor. Receiving loving empathy for our own feelings is vital.

Many of us will have been told when to go to bed as teens. We might have been punished, shamed, or judged if we didn't go to bed when our parent/s wanted us to. We may not have been trusted in relation to choosing when to go to bed as teens, and therefore find it hard to even let in the concept of trusting our teen, let alone doing so. Having lots of empathy for our own feelings is so important.

Alternatively, our parents might have 'left us to it' when we became teens, thinking that we no longer needed connection, support, and asked-for guidance from them. In which case, we might find it hard to know how to stay connected with our teen and offer helpful and timely support and asked-for guidance. This might also affect our willingness to ask for support in our parenting.

Most of us:

- weren't trusted in our own timing of increasing independence;
- were told what time we had to go to bed as teens;
- were punished, shamed, or threatened in relation to bedtimes;
- were given choice but offered no connection;
- were left on our own with screen or reading *control patterns*; or
- had our own internal clocks overridden and not supported as teens.

Because of this, any and all relevant feelings of our own can bubble up in relation to trusting, connecting with, and offering apt guidance and support where required and asked for with our teens.

If our teens need our help to reconnect with their sensations of sleepiness, their need for connection and safety, or to express painful feelings from the past, our own inner work will make all of those more possible.

Our feelings and thoughts from our teen years may show up in very different ways if we have more than one offspring. I found that my experiences with my daughter and her sleep as a teen were very different to those with my son in his teen years. This was caused by a combination of the specific support and stress I received as a child, as well as the support and stress they experienced.

With my daughter, I found it easy to trust her sleep as a teen. I'd helped her differentiate out hunger, tiredness, and healing-feelings when she was three, as I shared about before (after an earlier breast-feeding control pattern). That process, combined with my own experience of being trusted with choosing when to go to bed as a teen meant it was really easy to trust her. When I was a teenager, I experienced being trusted with my sleep by my parents.

When you reflect on your teen years, you might also find helpful elements in relation to sleep as well as painful ones.

From when I was about 10, I received a lot of trust from my parents about when I went to bed. I went to bed later than most of my peers, and I don't remember ever being shamed or punished in relation to going to bed at a particular time. When I started going out in the evenings when I was 17, my parents were also the least authoritarian of all my friends' parents in terms of when they wanted me to be home. I experienced being trusted around bedtimes, and I really saw how that affected me and my relationship with sleep, because I listened to myself. I did have a control pattern with watching TV, and I would have loved more help from my parents with that, but I am grateful that I grew into adulthood with a trust and ease in relation to my sleep.

I had a job as a waitress and bar person the summer I turned 18, after I finished school and before I went to University. On the weekends, after finishing work late, I would drive a group of us waitresses up to London, an hour-long drive, and we would go dancing in clubs until the early hours. I'd go to bed at 5 or 6 am in the morning, and then be up again in the early afternoon, ready for work in the early evening. It was a fun adventure for that short time, and I look back at it feeling glad that I had those experiences for a few months. I was living at home, and my parents didn't judge me or my choices with those late nights (actually, early mornings). They were humorous about it, without shaming me. Later that year, I lived in Australia and got up early several times a week to go ice skating before starting my waitressing job and went to bed early.

When I went to University the following year, I found it easy to make healthy choices about my sleep. I had lots of fun and went out a lot, but got up in time for lectures, as well as earlier than that several times a week to go ice skating beforehand. Just as I observed with my son decades later, that when he was interested in something, he was willing to get up super early, so was I willing to get up so I could skate, which was my passion at the time. I worked really hard at University, enough to get a First Class Honours Degree.

In retrospect, my parents' easeful attitude in relation to bedtimes really helped me to feel relaxed in relation to sleep, from my teen years in my twenties, then as a new mother, and with my daughter's sleep.

Each of us will have unique themes in relation to sleep and our own experiences as teens that will likely show up in different ways when we're relating to our own teens and sleep. That's one of the reasons why comparing ourselves with other parents and their teens is never helpful! Comparison is part of *DDC* conditioning and doesn't ever help!

I experienced a different theme that made things hard for me with my son's sleep as a teen, including my own screen control pattern *that I would have loved more help with when I was a teenager.*

I needed to receive lots of listening for my feelings when my son was in his early teenage years. So many feelings of powerlessness from my own childhood bubbled up to be lovingly heard when he wanted to go to bed much later than I did.

When I received Aletha Solter's edits of the first draft of this book, I received a really simple missing bit of clarity that helped me really understand about what had been going on for me with my son's sleep a few years ago. Had I had a session with her years ago, when I was having challenges, that would have saved me a lot of inner turmoil. That is why I so highly recommend getting support from an Aware Parenting instructor if you're finding things hard, or if things aren't changing, despite your understanding of Aware Parenting, or your swaps with your empathy buddy. Understanding the one element of Aware Parenting, teens, and sleep that I had missed would have transformed my experience. I see the importance of support and information day after day with my own mentees.

I'd love to share more about what happened with my son in his early teen years. He is a night owl and loves going to bed late and waking up late. He also has a screen control pattern. *If he was awake later than me, the layout of our house (he was sleeping in our living room, because we only had two bedrooms at the time) meant that the light from his computer would shine into my room and keep me awake. As a result, I would ask him to go to bed at the same time as me. Often, I would wake up again later on, and he would still be awake, and I would ask him again to go to bed, because the light was making it hard for me to sleep. Me not getting my need met to sleep when I wanted to led to lots of painful parenting moments. I often felt powerless and there were many times that the powerlessness bubbled out in unenjoyable ways towards my lovely son.*

When Aletha Solter edited this book, I realised that there were three key elements to what had been going on. The first was my need for sleep. Had I been clear about that being the issue, rather than trying to get him to go to bed when I did, I could have found some other way to meet my needs and block the light out. On reflection, that was obvious, because as soon as I had a new room built for him, where his being awake at night did not keep me awake, the tension I had felt dissipated. That was one of the key parts to my reactions all along.

One of the other reasons I found it hard was because I used to watch TV in my bedroom at night as a teenager back in the 80's; it was a big control pattern *for me, and I hadn't done as much inner work on my teenage years as I had on my childhood and infancy. This meant it was harder for me to support him with his* control pattern *with screens. I often felt huge feelings of powerlessness when I saw him on the screen in the evening.*

However, that wasn't the whole cause of the painful feelings that would often bubble up. The third element was because I felt scared when I imagined the neighbours judging me if they saw the lights on and knew that my son was up late. This invited me to do a lot of inner work so that I could get to the point of being unwilling to be affected by the judgments of others about his sleep. Once that happened, all the fear and powerlessness fell away.

Once he had his own room, and I'd received more listening, and had done more inner work in relation to my teenage years, and I was no longer willing to be affected by any judgments of others, I came to the point that if he was awake in the middle of the night chatting to a friend on the other side of the world, I would feel relaxed and happy. What a relief!

From a Marion Method *perspective, each of my reactions demonstrated one of the three types of feelings:* **needs-feelings** *of tiredness and frustration because of my need for sleep, unexpressed* **healing-feelings** *of overwhelm, loneliness, and confusion from my own teenage years, and* **thoughts-feelings** *of fear from what I was telling myself about what the neighbours might think.*

Nowadays (he's 18), I love observing how much he chooses his own sleep times. When he really wants to get up for things – like the farmers' market every Friday morning, so he can help his Dad and chat to his friends – he asks me to wake him up at 6 am or earlier. He jumps out of bed straight away. He will aim to go to sleep earlier the night before, or he will have a nap later on if he's tired. Or sometimes, he's just tired on Fridays, and I offer him empathy. I love seeing that whenever he really wants to do something, he is so willing to get up, whatever time that is, and aims to adjust his sleep accordingly.

However, he doesn't listen to his sleepiness sensations in the clear way that my daughter does. I believe that there is still some healing and connecting there to do from his earlier years and the effect of the separation that his dad and I went through. I trust that even though he is 18, there is still plenty of time and opportunity for more healing to happen. He and I, and he and his dad, are all really connected, so I know that we can still support him with this. He still comes to us for guidance and listens to what we say.

Self-Compassion Moment

I'm sending you lots of love here. Do you ever feel frustrated or powerless when your teen wants to stay up later than you would want them to? Do you ever feel scared, when you think painful thoughts about what will happen to them in the future if they don't go to bed when you think is healthy, or if they're awake reading or on a screen? Do you ever feel scared when you imagine other people judging you or your teen in relation to what time they go to bed? Do you receive enough empathy about this? The more listening we receive, the more we will be able to support them, trust them and help them trust themselves. We will also be a safer and more empathic space for them if they want support with a control pattern such as with screens.

Joss, who you've heard from before, shares her experience:

"The most important thing I have found to support my teens with sleep is to be getting regular non-judgmental, compassionate support and listening myself – whether that is listening to my worries about them and their sleep, or my younger teenage parts that had so many challenges without a safe place to share them. It might be in relation to my own unmet needs in the present, or unmet needs that have been an on-going theme in my life. Without regular listening and opportunities to heal for myself, I would not have been able to offer my teens much of what they needed."

Living and growing up in the *DDC*, it's really common that we learnt to judge ourselves, our parenting, or our teen, if they often go to bed late, or if they are up late reading or on a screen. Those judgments can get in the way of us being able to offer our teens connection and support, alongside the trust that they need.

In addition, we might have lots of fearful thoughts about their future. For example, *"If they keep on staying up late at night, how will they ever xyz?"* The more we're thinking these thoughts, the more scared we will feel, and the less likely we will be able to offer them warm connection, support, and trust. We're much more likely to start using power-over, threats, or judgements towards them. And although those are always repairable, they do get in the way of the kind of warm connection that our teens most need from us, to be more connected with their own sleep wisdom.

Self-Compassion Moment

I'm sending so much love to you as you read this. Do you tend to go into powerlessness when your teen stays up late, perhaps shifting into power-over, or harshness? Do you feel frustrated or angry? Perhaps you just go numb, dissociate, and avoid connecting with them – not even noticing what time they go to bed or what they do before bed? Perhaps you feel incandescent rage when you see them on their phone or computer late at night, and see them yawning or feeling tired the next morning? Perhaps you feel tempted to go in with judgments, shaming, coercion, or power-over? However you feel, I'm sending so much love to all of your feelings. The more your own emotions are felt, expressed, and lovingly heard, the more you'll be able to support your teen in a calm, present, and loving way.

In addition, you might be faced with judgment from other parents or family members once you do trust your teen. Those might emerge in the evenings after you've hung out with your teen, for example, if your partner or ex has a different approach to parenting.

A core part of *DDC* conditioning is the paradox of trying to get babies to be independent early, while also preventing teens from becoming independent in their own timing. Hence, 'Disconnected' and 'Domination'.

This judgment from others might be particularly strong if your teen has some big healing-feelings and they're coming out towards you, perhaps in the form of behaviour that other paradigms might call 'disrespectful' or 'rude' but you can clearly see are painful emotions that then need help to express in healing ways. Those feelings might be getting in the way of their innate body wisdom with sleep. Listening lovingly to their feelings, knowing that they need our help to release the feelings so that they can listen to what their body is telling them, requires us to feel calm and compassionate. Receiving empathy is so vital to being able to support them. We might also have a *Marion Method* phrase such as, *"I'm not willing to be affected by the judgments of others here,"* to help us stay calm and connected.

Belynda shares,

"The overwhelming negativity of society towards teens really impacts my ability to trust my sons. There is a real sense, and this is something that has been said in direct words more than once to me, that our teens are 'taking the mick' or 'getting one over us'. I feel so lucky that I have lots of Listening Partnerships where I can bring up my feelings if I find those thoughts creeping in.

My initial impulse in hard moments is often to move in with coercion or even threats. Having a space where I can reflect on this, and become clear about the direction I want to take, has been so helpful. I can't recommend Listening Partnerships highly enough, especially to parents of teens. It really provides such a safe haven to analyse and explore the way the broader societal judgements of teens impact us, as well as our own experiences and imprints of being a teen. This has allowed me, again and again, to come back to connection and trust, and to slowly work with my sons on their control patterns *and to build a strong sense of me as their ally rather than as their controller! Controlling their* control patterns *really doesn't get to the heart of things. Connection does."*

I love this phrase from Belynda! "Controlling their *control patterns* really doesn't get to the heart of things. Connection does."

Self-Compassion Moment

I wonder if this resonates with you? I'm sending so much love to you if you've felt tempted to coerce your teen or use threats. It's so common for us to feel powerless as parents, and to fall into power-over. The more we have our feelings heard, and tend to the source of them, the less likely it is that we will respond in these harsh ways.

Self-Reflection Moment

Increasingly trusting our teens in relation to sleep can help us connect with all kinds of painful feelings in ourselves. Doing our own inner work and receiving support for our own feelings can make a huge difference.

Here are some prompts for you to reflect on. I invite you to check in with yourself to see if you want to, and are willing to, do some reflections.

What happened for you with bedtimes when you were a teen?

Were you trusted to make your own choice about when to go to bed?

If so, how was that for you?

Were you made to go to bed at a certain time?

Did you experience threats, punishments, or rewards?

Did you have any particular control patterns that you used before sleep?

Did your parent/s notice that? If so, how did they respond?

What help would you have liked with that?

What would you have loved from them in the evenings?

What would you have loved for them to say to you about your sleep?

Did you ever try to express painful feelings before sleep as a teen?

If so, how were you responded to?

What sleep habits or nighttime control patterns did you notice in your other family members?

Is there anything else that jumps out at you as significant?

To your inner teenager:

I see how much more independent you're becoming.

And I will always be here to connect with you, however old you are.

You'll never be too old for a big hug, or a listening ear from me.

I deeply trust you.

I trust your amazing body.

I trust that you know exactly when you are tired, and what your body needs.

I love you unconditionally when you override those signals because you're loving doing what you're doing.

I love seeing you spread your wings out into the world.

I feel so happy seeing you connecting with your friends and making plans.

I support you in doing what you love in the evenings.

I'm always interested in what you are doing.

I'm always here to listen to whatever you're willing to share with me.

And if you ever need help, because you're finding it hard to stop reading, or get off the screen when you're tired, I will always be here to help.

I will never judge you or shame you.

I will never coerce you or tell you what to do.

But I'm always here to help, whenever you need me.

I love you unconditionally.

I love the person you're becoming.

I love seeing you follow your own path.

I love seeing you do what you love.

I see you.

I celebrate you.

I love you.

I'm sending love to you, and to your inner teenager.

32. The steps for supporting your teen to sleep restfully

1. Thinking: Hold the theory clearly in your mind

The three things needed for sound sleep:

- to feel tired (sleepy);
- to feel connected (*closeness creating a sense of safety*); and
- to feel relaxed (*by releasing any healing-feelings present*).

Many teens feel tired later in the evening than they did as children, and that may be later than us as adults.

Connection is vital at every age, and at this age, some or many of their connection needs may be met by their peers.

For teens, *talking* and *playfulness* often overtake crying and raging as a form of emotional release, but at times they will have bigger feelings that need to come out with tears or angry words.

The three ways teens heal from stress and trauma:

- laughter, humour, and playfulness;
- expression through talking; and
- crying and raging.

Teens commonly suppress their feelings through reading books and using screens.

2. Feeling: Have your own feelings heard

If you observe that your teen is not listening to their feelings of tiredness, and/or you see them mildly dissociating from their painful feelings before sleep, it's so understandable that you might feel painful feelings. Having an empathy buddy is so central to our parenting, especially if you see that your teen is really tired, and they're wanting to play a game to another level, want to finish watching a three-hour movie, or are having a two-hour-long conversation with their new love interest.

If you're about to explode, use power-over, get punitive, threatening, or shaming, leaving some voice notes with your empathy buddy about how you're feeling can help you feel calmer again so that you don't try to use power-over them about their bedtime. Us judging our teen or feeling powerless is likely to do the opposite of what we want. If we find ourselves experiencing these thoughts or feelings, that is a clear invitation to share our feelings with an empathic listener, such as our empathy buddy or Aware Parenting instructor.

3. Presence: Connecting in with yourself and helping yourself become present

That includes supporting yourself to being unwilling to judge them or yourself, offering yourself loving compassion, and moving in to focus on your feelings and sensations. I invite you to do something that helps you connect in with yourself before you offer them connection.

You might have more time for this now they are a teen! Perhaps you might want to do some yoga or meditation, go for a walk, or simply to connect with your breathing and look out the window at the trees. Sometimes presence is as simple as being present with what is present: noticing the sensations in your body as you stroke the dog, have a warm or cool drink, eat, do the washing up, or load the dishwasher.

This presence might help you deeply connect with them if they do want to chat, cuddle, or ask for help with homework before bed. But equally, it might help you avoid going into judgment or powerlessness in relation to their sleep choices, to offer them empathy and humour, and to stay calm, trusting, and equanimous if they are staying up later than you!

The more present you are, the more you can offer your loving presence.

That is going to be most helpful to support them to be connected with themselves and their needs and feelings in relation to sleep.

4. Preparation: Preparing yourself physically and emotionally

In contrast to when they were younger, your preparation once they are a teen is more likely to be in relation your thoughts and feelings about offering them connection, support, humour, and listening before you go to sleep, and trusting them and their own choices in relation to sleep.

You might connect with your empathy buddy for a few minutes on an app, telling them about how you are willing[68] for your interaction with your teen to go, so you feel more able to go and connect with your teen.

You might want to remember some particular moments in the past when you felt absolute adoring love for them, so you can offer that quality of unconditional love to them now.

You might watch five minutes of your favourite laughter video, so that you can go in and be humorous with them.

You might look up some information about something important to them, such as the latest song from their favourite band or the scores of the sports team they love to watch, so you can talk with them about those.

If they're learning a language, you might look up how to say a funny sentence in that language.

You might send them a funny meme or short video that you think they might enjoy.

You might read this book for a few minutes, to remind you of some theory, such as the aim to help them be connected with the three ingredients in themselves.

If they have a reading or screen *control pattern*, you might prepare yourself to support them with that by receiving lots of loving listening about your own experiences at their age, or about your own experiences of *control patterns*, or about your judgements and feelings about reading and screens. That way, you will be more likely to be able to ask them

---

68 The willingness work is from *The Marion Method*.

about their book or game, and show interest without moving into powerlessness, frustration, or judgement.

One of the things I found that made a huge difference with my son in his early teen years, when I was thinking fear thoughts about his future, or feeling frustrated or powerless, was to focus on unconditionally loving him. Even if things were going awry with screens or sleep, I found it possible to trust that if we stayed connected and I loved him unconditionally, things would work it. It was a life-saver at times.

You might want to remind yourself that offering your teen warmth, connection, and playfulness is part of melting the freeze, or dissociation, into the healing flowing of feelings.

5. Tired: Watching for tiredness signs

With teens, we might gently offer them empathy when they are clearly tired.

However, we don't recommend telling them to go to bed.

If they have a sense of us coercing them, they are likely to want to stay up later, just to meet their needs for agency and autonomy.

However, we might ask them if they want help in relation to listening to their sleepiness sensations and going to bed. If they've told us that they would like our help, then we might gently point out if we see tiredness signs as a way to lovingly support them to be connected with their innate body wisdom. Humour can be a powerful way to support them with this.

Belynda shares:

"I do find for my son that him telling me what time he plans to go to bed helps him –without a clear idea of what time he thinks makes sense, he tends to stay up very late and then the next day say, "Oops, I meant to go to bed earlier and now I'm tired". I think if it is done in a very non-power-over way, and if the teen requests it, these agreements can be a help."

From a teen: I'm not five, Mum. Why do you keep telling me when to go to bed? I felt so embarrassed when you said it in front of Roberta yesterday. Urgh. Just stop doing it! I just don't even want to talk to you when you treat me like a child. Hmm... what's this... you've texted me a word game. I remember when we used to do word games together. That was fun. Huh... what does this one spell out? Oh, you're saying sorry for telling me to go to bed when Roberta was here last night. Well, at last! And what's this? You've sent me some funny memes. They are actually quite funny. I laugh a bit. They are sort of fun for mum humour.

Then I hear a knock on my door. It's you, and wow, is that my favourite hot chocolate and a brownie? Yum, Mum! I let you in, and you don't even say anything about all my stuff everywhere. Phew. I'm a bit reluctant to talk at first, but I warm up a bit and start telling you about what Seb said today. After that, you tell me that you've been doing some thinking, and you are going to be changing some of the parenting things you do, including about bedtimes and telling me when to go to bed. You ramble on a bit about supporting me to listen to my body, and how important that is. I get it, Mum.

But I do feel relieved. But also a bit scared, because even though I'm 15 and I know a lot of stuff, I do still need your help. Oh, but then you go on to say that you are there to help me if I need help with going to bed, and actually, I find that I feel this openness and love in my heart towards you. I can literally feel my heart being more open and wanting to be closer with you. Some tears come to my eyes and I brush them away, wondering if you'll see. It turns out that you stay, and we decide to watch an old movie that used to be my favourite when I was little. We have pizza while we're watching. Afterwards, it's quite late, and you say goodnight, and I find that although I haven't texted Roberta yet, that I want to go to bed. It's so confusing being a teenager. I want you to trust me and I love to be independent, but sometimes I also need your support, Mum. Tonight was all of those. Thank you.

Our aim is to offer our teenagers empathy,
support, and trust, rather than judgment,
distance, and coercion.

6. Connected: Offer them closeness and connection

Being connected with yourself will help you be able to offer them connection.

You might be simply reminding them that you're available for connection for the next certain number of hours, or asking them if they'd like to connect with you, or whether they need any help from you. You may be going to their room with jokey playfulness, or with a funny meme to show them, or to tell them a joke. Or it may be remembering something significant about their day and asking them about it, for example, about how the soccer match went, or the art class. Offering eye contact, warm touch, a hug, some jokey playfulness, or sitting close to them can all bring about closeness.

Making requests about our own needs

Those needs might include the freedom for us to go to sleep when we want – and thus, for peace and quiet in the home at that time and afterwards. For example, we might ask them to avoid making loud noises after we have gone to bed, or to turn off lights that would keep us awake. Or, we might choose to be flexible about the latest time we say that we're willing to help them, so that if they have a stressful day and really need to talk, we will be willing to do that.

7. Relaxed

1a. Notice where you might be inadvertently distracting them from their innate relaxation processes

Teens might be trying to talk with us and share about how they're feeling, and instead of listening compassionately, we might be tempted to ask them about when they're planning on going to bed, or telling them that we don't want them to have as much screen time, or start talking about other things we're concerned about, rather than listening to them and what's going on for them.

Even though they're older, it's still part of our role to offer them emotional support.

Teens may still need to cry and express anger at times, and they might still want to be playful and laugh to release feelings before sleep.

In thinking that our teens don't need us as much, we might unwittingly distract them from these healing processes.

1b. Notice where they might be using *control patterns*, and be available to offer support

In non-coercive and respectful ways, we might go and offer loving connection when we see them reading or watching screens to dissociate from feelings.

We can remember that warmth is the antidote to freeze – at any age.

2. Instead of distracting them, follow their lead

This might be simply sitting down and listening to them talk if they share about something that was hard for them that day. Or that might mean joining in if they find something funny and want to share it with us. This is part of trusting them and that they know what they need. However, we might find this harder as they get older, as they might not so clearly communicate about what they need from us.

3. Keep following their lead

If they want to keep talking, or laughing together, or sharing feelings, or watching funny videos together, staying with that process can create a profound sense of connection.

4. Noticing whether they're becoming more relaxed and present

This can still be relevant with teens, because it can help us continue offering connection and listening. Perhaps we notice that they are warming up with us, making more eye contact, smiling more and sharing more. This can help us understand that the connection we're offering them is helpful for them. Noticing that can support any parts of us which might be judging ourselves or them, or feeling doubtful that what we are doing is making a difference.

From a teen: I am so angry. What a sh*t show of a day that was today. Could anything else have gone wrong? I get home and go straight to my room, shut my door, and turn on my computer to start gaming. I want to go and shred some dudes right now. After a few levels, I still feel fed up, but I'm really into this new game. It takes all my concentration, which also helps me forget about what happened today.

There's a knock on the door, and it's you, Dad. Uh oh, lecture time. That's all I need. You come in, and I keep gaming. Huh, but here's a surprise. I look up, and see that you turn towards my screen and smile, and ask me about it. Okay, let's go with that. I share a bit, thinking that you will soon start with the lecture about my homework, or too much gaming, or going to bed too late. Boring. But no, you just keep on listening. You ask if you can join in.

Well, Dad, this game is obviously too complex for you, but we can start with another game that I've just come across which is pretty new to me too. You pull up a stool and sit beside me, and you ask me how to play it. I keep thinking you're going to go into punishment mode, but the opposite happens. You start being goofy, and over the top when you keep missing the goal. "It's NOT FAIR that you're so ace at this game," you say. I laugh a bit. Well, bro, of course I'm better at it than you. You never play. We keep going and going, and we both laugh a bit, and Mum brings in some dinner. We stop the game and watch some videos about the creators while we eat. I'm surprised to find that I'm enjoying hanging out with you.

When we've finished eating, you find some old toy swords that are still hanging up behind my door, and start a sword fight with me. But you keep on falling over, or pretending to die and landing on top of me. You really are a goofball, Dad! But despite myself, I find myself laughing more. We end up slouching on the big beanbag together, and you tell me about the computer game you played when you were my age. So old school! We have actually laughed a lot. I feel so much more relaxed.

I try telling you about what happened today, and wow, Dad, you actually listen. You don't lecture me, you don't tell me what I should do, you actually listen to me. You nod, and I keep sharing. I raise my voice when I get to the angry bit. I am still so mad about it. I'm shouting now. You don't react. You just keep on looking at me, and listening. I've been avoiding looking you in the eyes, but then I do. I see that you see me. I actually feel a bit tearful. Huh. I don't think I've shared my feelings with you for years.

Once I've told you the whole story, you offer me a hug, and you hold me for a long time. A couple of tears run down my face. I feel how solid you are. And that you do love me. After what seems like hours, we move apart, and somehow we both just know that we're tired and will be going off to bed soon. We head to the bathroom together, making more jokes. When I get into bed a bit later on, I can really feel the softness of the sheets and my pillow. I don't feel angry any more. I actually feel more calm than I've felt in a long time. Wow. Dad really showed up for me tonight.

8. Your feelings

It's so common for lots of our own feelings to bubble up when we are being invited to trust our teens, while also staying connected with them, and also being a support and guide if they clearly want and need it, e.g. in relation to reading and screens before bed. So, after being with our teen and seeing the choices they make, it's very likely that more of our own feelings might bubble up again.

If you don't have a life partner to share your feelings with, and haven't yet instigated an empathy buddy agreement, you might find that journalling is a powerful and helpful way to explore and express your feelings in the evenings, after talking with your teen.

9. Conversations with your teen at other times

The connection we have with our teens in the evenings is a microcosm of our connection the rest of the time.

Having conversations, discussing feelings, needs, and values, finding ways for everyone to get their needs met, doing activities together, going places together, playing sport or music together, playing cards or board games, or being silly and goofy together can all create a warm context which the evenings are a part of.

If there's a rift between you and your teen, it really is possible for that rift to heal.

The first step of healing a rift is usually having our own feelings heard by a loving listener so we can go to our teen as the parent, from a place of compassion and a willingness to heal the rupture, rather from the hurt places, which are often our inner children.

CHAPTER SUMMARY

To support your teen with sleep, you can focus on thinking (holding the theory clearly in your mind), feeling (having your feelings heard), presence (connecting in with yourself), preparing yourself physically and emotionally, watching for tired signs, offering closeness and connection, and supporting them to feel relaxed through being humorous and listening to them sharing about their experiences.

I trust that whatever is going on with your teen and sleep, that your own inner work can bring about more harmony and trust between the two of you, and that in the long term, that will help their relationship with themselves, their body, and their sleep.

33. Specific suggestions for particular situations

Your teen wants to stay up later than you

In Aware Parenting, our aim is to trust our teen to listen to their body, so that they adjust their own behaviour through listening to themselves and their own experiences.

If our teen wants to stay up later than us, from an Aware Parenting perspective, we would aim to support them to stay up and trust them to go to sleep when they need to.

If we are concerned that our own needs for sleep might not get met, we might then make requests of them, e.g. that they are quiet once we've gone to sleep, that they don't turn lights on that would wake us up, etc. In order to trust our teens like this, many of us will need to have a lot of our own feelings lovingly heard.

If you've only recently started practicing Aware Parenting, there may be a process of adjustment. For example, if a teen hasn't had much agency or autonomy, they may choose to stay up later than their body is telling them, while they catch up on getting those agency needs met and learn to trust that they really do get to choose now.

However, if they regularly override their sensations of sleepiness or regularly use *control patterns* which mean that they are often tired the next day, we can lovingly support them to connect with, and trust, their needs and feelings. We can do this through conversations, empathy, and humour.

Our teens need a beautiful balance of trust and support, and we can explore how much of each they require.

Self-Compassion Moment

I'm sending love to however you feel when you read this. It's normal for most of us to have big feelings when we think of trusting teens in this way. Most of us were not trusted in these ways when we were teens. We might also feel concerned that other parents or family members will judge us or our parenting if our teen stays up late.

Your teen is on a screen in the evening and doesn't want to get off

Joining in and showing interest in what our teen is doing can be helpful. That could be asking if they're willing for you to join them and sitting next to them and watching. That could be asking questions and really listening. If they're gaming, you might ask if they can teach you, and regularly play together in the evenings as a way of connecting.

The more you understand what they're doing and the more they experience you being interested in what they're doing and understanding them, the more likely it is that they will ask for your help if they need it.

For example, you might be concerned that them being on a screen means that they're not listening to their body's tiredness signals. The more they experience you listening to them, valuing their feelings, thoughts, and needs, the more likely it is that they will be willing to listen to your supportive information.

Being playful and funny can help bring about connection, leading to them being more likely to be willing to have conversations with you and receive your support. For example, you could give them information about the effect of screens on eyesight (studies have shown that too much screen use can lead to myopia), or you could help them notice when they are sleepy. Or you could also ask if they would be willing to try an experiment, such as no screens after 10pm for a few days (which they monitor for themselves) followed by another conversation.

Your teen reads for hours and stays up really late

Again, Aware Parenting invites you to connect with and trust your teen. That includes showing interest and curiosity about what they're reading and why they love it. The more they experience you trusting them and not judging them, the more that will support them to be connected with what their body is telling them. If we frequently judge our child for reading for hours, or try to coerce them to stop, the judgment and coercion will be more likely to get in the way of them being able to hear what their bodies are telling them.

From a teen: *Mum, I am really loving reading this series of books. I love this whole fantasy genre and how I imagine that I'm actually there. I feel excited and energised and intrigued and all kinds of feelings. It's inspired me to start writing some stories of my own. But I've noticed that now school has got so stressful, what with exams and stuff, I'm reading for hours and hours at night. I'm starting to feel tired at school now. Yesterday, I nearly fell asleep in history. It was so boring. I didn't like how I felt in my body and how hard it was for me to stay awake, even if Mr. Perkins is the ultimate bore. I think I'd like to talk to you about it.*

You used to tell me what time to go to bed, and you'd get all judgy when you saw me awake late, but I've noticed that you've stopped doing that recently. It's why I'm trusting you more to ask for help about this. I did ask Rebecca about it, because she loves reading this series too, but she said she finds it easy to stop reading when she can feel her eyes wanting to close. I just push past it and read another chapter, and another. I know you love reading too, so I think you might be able to help me with it. Hmm... perhaps I will come out with you next time you invite me out for a coffee on a Sunday morning. I hope you do ask me again. I do still need you, you know.

Your teen wants to go to bed much later than you want them to

Being on their side and on their team will mean you have way more influence rather than if you try to coerce them, judge them or use power over them to 'make them' go to bed when you want them to do. It's normal for teens to want a lot of agency, autonomy, and choice, and it's important for us to support their needs for autonomy and choice about when to go to bed.

However, the more connection there is between the two of you, the more they will be willing to receive support from you if they need it because their going to bed later is coming from them overriding their sensations of sleepiness and/or any accumulated feelings.

Supporting teenagers generally requires us to receive lots of emotional support. Trusting them can be a challenge for us, but the more we are able to get free from our *DDC* conditioning and have our feelings heard, the more we will be able to support their sleep with compassion, connection, and consideration. That is always going to lead to more enjoyable and helpful interactions compared to if we start with judging them, fearing about their future, and having set ideas about what they 'should' do regarding sleep!

Self-Compassion Moment
I'm sending you so much love and compassion in this process. If you ever want to imagine me standing next to you, reminding you of the phrase, "I trust you," please do! You might find that saying those words to your teen is also helpful for them. Being trusted is powerful medicine.

I'm so willing for there to be even more trust and harmony between you and your teen.

34. Common sleep questions and answers for parents of teenagers (ages 13-19)

Two-home-family with different beliefs

Q ~ We are a two-home family. The other parent is not on board with Aware Parenting. Do you have any tips on supporting teens with sleep, especially regarding the coercion and shame used in the other household around sleep?

A ~ My heart goes out to you and the situation you're in. Being the household where there isn't coercion and shaming can also mean you provide the safe space to let out all of the painful feelings from what happens in the other home. I invite you to make sure that you have lots of listening when your teen is at their other home, so that you are at your most spacious for offering lots of empathy and listening when they come back to you. For teens, having conversations to name the differences they experience in each home, and acknowledging how hard that can be to come back and forth, can make a big difference.

You may find that it's even more important for them to know that they have choice in relation to their bedtimes, and that you're not shaming them for their bedtime choices. Bringing humour in to the situation so you can both release some of the tension through laughter might also be helpful. Perhaps you could find a TV show to watch together which has funny sketches about teens and sleep. Helping them know that you're on their team, and that you're supporting them to deeply listen to what their body needs, rather than for their choices to be a reaction to what happens at the other household might also be supportive. And then back to lots more listening for yourself.

13-year-old keeps reading when tired

Q ~ My 13-year-old daughter loves reading, and will clearly often keep reading when she's tired. I've been telling her that she shouldn't do that, and I'm noticing that my responses are getting more charged, and she's taking no notice of me. What can I do?

A ~ I'm sending love to you and how you feel when you see her reading when she's tired. I invite you to receive lots of empathy so you can have your feelings heard about this. I invite you to explore all the experiences that seeing her do this help you connect with, including your own experiences of reading when you're tired, or not listening to your tiredness cues in other ways, both in the present, and when you were her age. You might also enquire into what you're telling yourself about this situation, and whether you might like to change your thoughts about this. In *The Marion Method*, the willingness work can be really helpful for these kinds of situations.

The more connected you are to your own compassion and power, the more you will be able to connect with her in ways that support the bond between the two of you. Being interested and curious about what she's reading might be one way to rebuild the connection. You might even read the book that she is reading, so you can have conversations about it. The more genuinely interested you are, and the more she feels your care and interest in her, the more she is likely to be influenced by you. That might include you sharing about your own experiences of reading or doing other things that you love, even when you're tired.

15-year-old finds it hard to get up for school

Q ~ I like the whole thing about trusting teenagers, but my 15-year-old son is a night owl and finds it hard to get up the next morning for school. If I don't threaten him with taking away his screen time, he stays up late and is tired in the morning. What can I do?

A ~ I so acknowledge how much you care about your son and his need for sleep, and your concern about what might happen if you don't threaten him with taking away his screen time. It can be so hard to see our teens make choices that we really don't want them to make, can't it? My first invitation would be to do some journalling, or have some listening time with an empathy buddy or Aware Parenting instructor, to express all your feelings about this. You might find that what's going on with him is helping you connect with experiences you had with sleep and trust when you were 15, for example. You might have noticed that you threatening him with taking away his screen time may be bringing a wedge of disconnection in between the two of you. Once you've had some listening, you might feel called to have a conversation with him where you tell him that you've been concerned when he stays up late on his screen and is tired in the morning, and that you don't want to threaten him with taking away his screen time, but you're worried about what would happen if you didn't.

Having respectful, heartfelt, and honest conversations with him are likely to lead to clarity about the next steps for you both here.

16-year-old loves gaming late in the evening

Q ~ I have a gamer in the house! My 16-year-old daughter absolutely loves gaming. I hate it. I just don't understand what she sees in it. If we let her, she would probably stay up until 2am every night. My husband and I just can't trust her. We've told her she can have an hour after dinner for gaming, as long as she's done her homework. But nowadays she just won't talk to us, and the battles are getting bigger and bigger. It got so bad that we said she could only have screen time on the weekends, so that she goes to bed on time during the week, and now she's hardly talking to us. What can we do?

A ~ I'm sending you so much love. I really hear how much you hate gaming, and how you don't understand what she sees in it, and are concerned that she would stay up until 2am every night if you let her. I also hear how big and painful the battles are getting, and my heart goes out to you all. The first step is always your own feelings, so I invite you to receive plenty of listening where you can share about all your painful feelings. Imagine sharing over and over again how much you hate seeing her gaming, and being unconditionally loved! The more your feelings are heard, the more you will be able to think clearly, and the more you'll be able to listen to your daughter and her experiences and feelings.

I'm imagining that you might find that a breakthrough could happen if you got to the point where you could ask her with interest about her gaming, and even ask her if she's willing to play a game with you. The more connected you feel with her, and the more you understand why she loves gaming, the easier you will find it to ease in to trusting her more. And the more she knows that you are actually interested in what she loves, the whole house is likely to be more harmonious. She will likely be more willing to hear about your values, while staying connected with her own. From there, her sleep choices are likely to have way less charge for everyone and to be much more likely to be coming from her own innate wisdom rather than her reactions to what is happening between the three of you. Remembering that your aim is to support her to be connected with her own body wisdom around sleep might be really helpful too. Are you willing for that?

I'm so willing for you and your teen to experience even more connection, trust, and harmony, as well as restful and restorative sleep!

SUMMARY OF SECTION FOUR

I wonder how you're feeling, having read this section? The Aware Parenting perspective to sleep and teens is so different from most other paradigms, and so different to the *DDC* way of seeing things, so it's so normal if you're feeling lots of feelings.

I'm here to remind you that this is a journey, and as Belynda so beautifully expressed, that parenting is often not neat and tied into a bow.

However, holding the context that your teen experiences you as on their team, that the two of you are connected with each other, and that your aim is to help them become an adult connected with their innate body wisdom around sleep, can really help.

If you have a teenage son or daughter, and this is the first section you've read, after you have read it you may want to go back and read the sections focused on babies and children, to help you understand your teen and their earlier stages of life even more. It's never too late to offer reparative experiences of closeness, *attachment play,* and listening to unexpressed feelings with Aware Parenting.

35. Trust

And now we come to the end of this tome of a book, full circle, back to trust.

I wonder if you now have more trust in your baby, child, or teen's sleep wisdom?

Aware Parenting invites us to get free from our *Disconnected Domination Culture* conditioning about sleep and return to a deep trust in the innate wisdom of our children's bodies. In that process, we are invited to see parenting in relation to sleep in a very different way.

Together, we've reflected back on the huge journey we've made as human beings, and the profound changes that have happened in the last several centuries, and particularly the past 200 years, since the Industrial Revolution and the advent of electricity and lighting at night. Even more so in more recent years with the advent of social media, blue light technology and powerful gaming apps. We have been enticed to move far away from our evolutionary blueprint.

Connection is our birthright and our expectation, and the challenges with our children's sleep can invite us to see how far we have strayed from what is innate in us, in terms of sleeping arrangements, beliefs about sleep, and perceptions of children.

In a mechanistic and information age, babies can often be seen in a machine-like way, sleeping like 'clockwork', with complex sleep timings to remember. Children and teens might be portrayed as robotic beings who need to be trained to be compliant, including with sleep.

But babies, children, and teens thrive on connection, and they have innate wisdom. They know how to feel deeply relaxed, they know how to heal from stress and trauma, and they know how to sleep in restful and restorative ways.

It is our own cultural conditioning and childhood hurts that get in the way of seeing their intrinsic wisdom and cooperating with it. We are invited to get free from our cultural conditioning, so that we stop getting in the way of those natural processes. Doing our own inner work to attend to our own unexpressed feelings, so we can see our children clearly, makes a huge difference to them.

> As parents, our big picture invitation is to support our babies, children, and teens, so that they not only have restful sleep at each age, but so they also grow up into adults deeply connected with their *own* innate wisdom in relation to sleep.

Tiredness: The more we can *read* and *respond* to their cues of *tiredness* when they are younger, the more they will internalise our responses. This means that they know what their cues of tiredness are, and they will generally listen to, and act on those sensations and needs. Modelling that we listen to our own tiredness can also have a significant effect on them listening to theirs as they get older.

Closeness: The more that we *offer* them *closeness* and *connection* before sleep for as long as they need it, the more that they also internalise that closeness and the sense of safety that comes with it. This means they are likely to move into independence with sleep when they are truly ready. It also means it's likely that they will be connected with their needs for closeness as adults, and to be willing for closeness when they want and need it. They're also likely to know if they don't feel safe to sleep, such as after a stressful or traumatic event, and what they need if that's the case, including having extra closeness.

Relaxation: The more that we can *cooperate* and *collaborate* with their *innate relaxation-through-release responses* when they are younger, the more they will stay connected with their capacity to do that when they are adults. It's likely that they will be more present in their body as a result. It also means they are more likely to reach out to their partner or friend to share their feelings in the evenings rather than turning to alcohol, food, screens, or whatever other options will be around when they are adults.

So, Aware Parenting affects their sleep during their childhood and adult years, but it goes even beyond that, into the next generation (if they go on to have children).

With these experiences internalised, they are likely to find it much easier to respond to their own babies' and children's three requirements for restful sleep. With an embodied trust in their own bodies in relation to sleep, they will probably easily and deeply trust their children's innate wisdom with sleep.

The changes we make in relation to sleep beliefs and practices can have very long-term effects.

Self-Compassion Moment

I'm here to remind you that if you are just beginning Aware Parenting now, that whatever age your child is, it's never too late to make changes. Most of us didn't start our own inner journey of healing and transformation until adulthood. Humans are wired for healing, and that innate desire for healing is strong in every child.

Change is possible, at any age.

If your *baby* uses *control patterns* to get to sleep every night and is waking up every hour, you have so much time over the coming years to support them to express the healing-feelings that are probably waking them up.

If your *toddler* has slept in a cot since birth and you think they are not securely attached and want to start co-sleeping with them, it is so possible to support a change in their attachment status.

If your *young child* sucks their thumb to go to sleep, lots of *attachment play* will help unfreeze those healing-feelings so they can flow out.

If your *older child* has their nose glued in a book for hours every evening before sleep, you really can bring about more connection and support them to express their feelings to you.

If your *young teen* wants to be on screens every night, it's possible to be on their team and bring in loads of warmth, interest, and playfulness, so that they come to you if they need help in getting off the screen at night.

If there's been a rupture between you and your *older teen* and you're fighting over bedtimes, it really is possible to heal the rupture and feel deeply connected with each other, so you can rebuild the trust together, supporting them to also trust themselves and their body more.

However, for us to be able to offer support in each of these, we are generally going to be invited to do a whole load of inner work.

This is likely to include the following from an Aware Parenting perspective:

- having someone else, or multiple people regularly listen to our painful feelings;
- diving in deep to the theory and practice of Aware Parenting so that it becomes second nature;
- reflecting back on our own experiences of sleep;
- exploring what happened with sleep for us when we were the age our child is now; and
- noticing when we're judging them, and replacing those thoughts with an Aware Parenting understanding of why they're doing what they're doing.

From a *Marion Method* perspective, we might:

- notice when we're judging ourselves or our parenting, and put down the sticks;
- hear loving responses from our *Inner Loving Mother*;
- replace inner harshness with deep self-compassion;
- go back in time to create healing with the *Inner Loving Presence Process*;
- receive loving compassion when we're thinking fearful thoughts about the future; and
- replace those with what we are *willing for* instead.

As Belynda so beautifully said, we may not tie everything up with a neat bow.

We *might not* be able to listen to as many of our baby's healing-feelings as we'd really love to, and we may see that still affect their sleep.

However, perhaps we do listen to their healing-feelings often, and see how much more relaxed they are while they're sleeping and awake, and that they wake up much less than they used to.

Our toddler *might still* have a thumb-sucking *control pattern* that they use before sleep when they've had a more stressful day, or we haven't had as much presence in ourselves to offer them support.

However, now we understand exactly what is going on for them, we know what we can do to help them feel more connected with their body and feelings, and release that stress from their body.

We *may not* always have the emotional resources to respond with *attachment play* when our four year old wants that before sleep.

However, we know how to notice when that happens, and what we can do so we are more likely to be able to respond with a big yes the next evening.

Our six-year-old *might ask* for lots of things before bed, and sometimes we might forget about *Loving Limits*, and feel resentful or frustrated.

However, we will know how to repair, help them heal from any effects of that, and will be more likely to remember the need for *Loving Limits* the next time it's happening.

Our eight-year-old *might frequently* want to share feelings with us before bed, and sometimes we might wish that they would just stop talking and crying and just go to sleep.

However, we will know that this is a sign that our own feelings need to be heard, and perhaps that we also have some unmet needs that need tending to.

Our child *might want* to co-sleep with us for way longer than any of our friend's children, and sometimes we might subtly shame them or try to coerce them to sleep alone.

However, we can then come back to enquiring in to what's going on for us and what's going on for them, what they need, and what their innate timing is, and repair any rupture in our connection.

We *might find* it really hard to trust our teen in relation to sleep, and to be unsure about whether they're needing help from us.

However, we can come back to receiving empathy about it all, so we can get clear about what's going on and what they need.

Our teen *might have* a big *control pattern* with screens that is affecting their ability to listen to their tiredness, and we might be responding in unhelpful ways to them.

However, if we return to the theory, and enquire into our own feelings and thoughts, we can go back to being on their team, willing to believe that they will reconnect with their body, offering lots of playfulness and laughter, and being a powerful and loving support and ally to them.

And sometimes, there will be apparent miracles.

Your baby might sleep really restfully after you've regularly listened to lots of healing-feelings before sleep.

You may find you don't need to tiptoe around your baby when they are sleeping.

Your baby might cry in your arms before sleep and after completing a whole cycle, may be the most present they've ever been, gazing in to your eyes for what seems like eternity.

Your toddler might sleep through the night most of the time, while still co-sleeping and breastfeeding during the day.

You may feel so much more connected with your little one after implementing more connection and listening before sleep.

Your child may easily sleep through the night without being in the same one position underneath your shoulder.

You may fall back in love with your child when you do *attachment play* with them before bed, seeing the delight and joy in their eyes.

You might find that *you* feel much more relaxed and sleep more restfully yourself after doing *attachment play* with your child before sleep.

You might discover that your child really does want to share their deepest feelings with you before bed, and that in the process, your bond deepens in a way that you didn't know was possible.

They might now mostly have a deep sense of relaxation and peace in their body when they are sleeping.

Your child might start freely expressing their feelings with you, after never having done so before.

Your tween might have a big explosion and rage towards you before sleep, and you find that you can stay lovingly present with them all the way through. Afterwards, you might find that the disconnection you've sensed between you for years has gone, and it's as if all your birthdays have come at once.

Your teen might start seeking out connection with you in the evenings, and you may find that you return to feeling the love for them as much as you did when you felt most loving towards them when they were younger.

Your teenager might start responding to their sensations of tiredness more often, and asking you for help if they're finding that hard.

You might find deep closeness with your teen through playing an online game in the evenings, or sending each other funny memes, and then chatting about them in the kitchen together before you go to bed.

You may clearly see that as they move into adulthood, they are deeply connected with themselves and their body, trusting their own innate sleep sensations and wisdom, willing to reach out for connection when they need it, and unwilling to be harsh with themselves when stress is making sleep harder.

You might find that you understand your own sleep more, and that your relationship with the three ingredients lead to you sleeping more restfully, and listening lovingly to yourself if you wake up in the middle of the night.

Miracles really can happen, however painful the past has been in relation to sleep and connection. You are so powerful and can create profound change.

This is a huge journey, to free ourselves from **DDC** *conditioning and reconnect with trust in the innate wisdom of our children's bodies.*

I invite us to be deeply compassionate with ourselves in that process, however it looks in our specific family, with each unique child.

> ### Self-Reflection Moment
> *I wonder how you're feeling, having just read this?*

I am so willing for you to have found so much more clarity and peace in relation to sleep.

I am so willing for you and your child/ren to be deeply connected and to get lots more lovely, restful sleep. It really is possible!

Sleep is the ultimate physical and emotional barometer. It's sleep that brings so many parents to Aware Parenting, but along the way, the barometer becomes an invitation for deep connection and transformation.

I wonder if you're seeing it that way now?

In attending to whatever is going on for your child in relation to sleep, you are actually attending to their long-term emotional wellbeing.

In offering them plenty of closeness, you're helping them be securely attached, which means they know that they can rely on support, and that they can reach out for help.

In responding compassionately to their play or crying, you are helping them to deeply trust themselves and their own innate healing processes.

In listening to their crying and raging, you are not only helping them heal from stress and trauma, you're also helping them be freer from accumulated feelings, which will help every area of their life. You are also supporting them to have fewer *control patterns*, which will also affect their adulthood too.

You are helping them become more present and more relaxed, which will profoundly affect their experience of themselves, their relationships, and their life.

In trusting their timing and pacing of independence in relation to sleep, you are helping them deeply trust themselves.

CHAPTER SUMMARY

Aware Parenting invites us to get free from our *Disconnected Domination Culture* conditioning about sleep and return to a deep trust in the innate wisdom of our children's bodies.

Connection is our birthright and our expectation, and the challenges with our children's sleep can invite us to see how far we have strayed from what is innate in us, in terms of sleeping arrangements, beliefs about sleep, and perceptions of children.

Babies, children, and teens thrive on connection, and they have innate wisdom. They know how to feel deeply relaxed, and they know how to heal from stress and trauma.

In the big picture, our invitation as parents is to support our babies, children, and teens, so that they not only have relaxing and restorative sleep, but that they also grow up into adults deeply connected with their own innate wisdom in relation to sleep.

Aware Parenting affects their sleep during their childhood and adult years, but it goes even beyond that, into the next generation (if they have children). The changes we make in relation to sleep beliefs and practices have very long-term effects. Change is possible, at any age.

And yet, as Belynda so beautifully said, we may not tie everything up with a neat bow. However, apparent miracles really can happen, however painful the past has been in relation to sleep and connection. You are so powerful and can create profound change.

This is a huge journey, to free ourselves from *DDC* conditioning and reconnect with trust in the innate wisdom of our children's bodies. I invite us to be deeply compassionate with ourselves in that process, however it looks in our specific family, with each unique child.

Sleep is the ultimate physical and emotional barometer. It's sleep that brings so many parents to Aware Parenting, but along the way, the barometer becomes an invitation for deep connection and transformation. In attending to whatever is going on for your child in relation to sleep, you are actually attending to their long-term emotional welling.

Attending to sleep issues with Aware Parenting is certainly not an easy path, nor a magic wand. And yet, it can be one of the most deeply fulfilling processes – helping your child to feel deeply relaxed in their body, being there for them in their biggest feelings, and giving them a deep sense of unconditional love.

I am sending *you* so much love.

I so appreciate all that you are doing, and all that you will do.

It really is making a difference.

Lots of love,
Marion
xoxoxo

October 2024

QUICK REFERENCE GUIDE

The steps of supporting your baby to sleep summary

1. Thinking: Hold the theory clearly in your mind

The three things needed for sound sleep:

- to feel tired (sleepy);
- to feel connected (*closeness creating a sense of safety*); and
- to feel relaxed (*by releasing any healing-feelings present*).

The two reasons for crying:

- for communication; and
- for healing.

The two types of feelings:

- needs-feelings; and
- healing-feelings.

The two ways babies heal from stress and trauma:

- crying with our loving support while they make vigorous movements; and
- *attachment play* (less common for young babies).

2. Feeling: Have your own feelings heard

Even leaving a minute or a few minutes of messages, knowing that we are going to be lovingly heard, can make a huge difference to how we feel and how much emotional energy we have to support our baby in the going to sleep process.

3. Presence: Connecting in with yourself
and helping yourself become present

To help our baby feel connected with us and with their healing-feelings, we need to be relatively present and connected to ourselves and our own body.

4. Preparation: Preparing yourself physically and emotionally

This might mean going to the toilet, having a snack and a drink, and setting up the environment if you know that you're going to offer your little one your presence to express their healing-feelings.

5. Tired: Watching for tiredness signs

If you haven't done the things you wanted to do before helping them sleep, like changing their clothes, you might find that they want to cry whilst doing those things.

6. Connected: Offer them closeness and connection

The more connected and present you are with yourself, the more they will feel deeply connected when you're with them.

7. Supporting them to feel relaxed

1. Notice where you might be inadvertently distracting them from their innate relaxation-through-release processes
2. Instead of distracting them, follow their lead
3. Keep following their lead
4. Notice whether they're becoming more relaxed and present

8. Keep connected: Stay close with them as they fall asleep

If your baby is in your arms, or you're lying down next to your toddler, you might want to wait for about 10-15 minutes after they've fallen asleep before placing them down or leaving (or stay close, if you want to rest, or sleep, or enjoy the cuddle!).

9. If they wake up soon after

If they wake up soon after falling asleep, it tells you they probably had more feelings to express.

10. Your feelings

If painful feelings came up for you during the process, perhaps you'd like to talk to your partner if you have one, message/phone/video call your empathy buddy, message the Aware Parenting instructor you're working with, or do some journalling.

11. Observation

The more of a difference you see in their muscle relaxation and sleep, and in their daytime eye contact, melting cuddles and presence, the more it will give you reassurance that what you are doing is helping them feel more relaxed and thus sleep more peacefully.

The steps of supporting your child to sleep summary

1. Thinking: Hold the theory clearly in your mind

The three things needed for sound sleep:

- to feel tired (sleepy);
- to feel connected (*closeness creating a sense of safety*); and
- to feel relaxed (*by releasing any healing-feelings present*).

The three ways children heal from stress and trauma:

- *attachment play*;
- crying/raging with vigorous movement and loving support; and
- talking (less effective for younger children, more helpful and important with older children).

Children have unexpressed feelings bubbling up when they are:

- playing rambunctiously;
- asking for lots of things;
- wanting us to read to them or play with them more[69];
- suppressing feelings, e.g. with thumb-sucking or a dummy; and/or
- wriggling or antsy.

2. Feeling: Have your own feelings heard

The more your feelings are welcomed, the more spaciousness you will have to welcome your child's feelings.

3. Presence: Connecting in with yourself and helping yourself become present

The more connected with yourself and present you are, the more likely it is that your child will feel connected with you and will release healing-feelings.

4. Preparation: Preparing yourself physically and emotionally

Comfortable clothes, ready for *attachment play.*

A voice note with your empathy buddy.

Dancing around the kitchen to feel powerful if you think *Loving Limits* will be required.

5. Tired: Watching for tiredness signs

Supporting them to notice their own tiredness signs so they can increasingly take responsibility for their own going to sleep process.

---

69 However, please hold in mind that if they haven't had much connection with you during the day, their need for connection might override their need for sleep.

6. Connected: Offer them closeness and connection

Being close during dinner, offering endearments, closeness while brushing teeth, chatting on the sofa, singing songs, or rough and tumble.

7. Relaxed

1a. *Notice* where you might be inadvertently distracting them from their innate relaxation processes (more likely to be for younger children).

They might be trying to find a pretext to have a big cry over a small thing. You might be offering them a snack, or a dummy, or a screen, or a story.

1b. *Notice* when they are distracting themselves with *control patterns*.

i. Our own ongoing *inner* work e.g. sharing our feelings and thoughts about their *control pattern* to our empathy buddy;

ii. Moving in with warmth and compassion (thinking about the warmth melting the freeze);

iii. Offering *attachment play* that's related to the *control pattern* in some way;

iv. Offering a *Loving Limit*.

2. *Instead* of distracting them, follow their lead. If they're trying to distract themselves, move in with *attachment play* or *Loving Limits*.

If they invite play, join in with them. Do what they're doing, or add in *attachment play*, such as:

- *power-reversal play* (by being less powerful and mock-surprised about how much bigger, faster or more powerful they are); or

- *nonsense play* (by being silly and goofy and incompetent); or

- *separation games* (by bringing in elements like hide and seek).

If they are trying to distract themselves with one more toy, you could offer a *Loving Limit*.

If they are wanting you to distract them from their feelings such as by asking you to read them more stories, you could also offer a *Loving Limit*.

If they're trying to find a pretext – an **emotional coat hanger** *to find a reason to have a big cry or rage*, offer them empathy and stay with their feelings.

If they're using a *control pattern* **to dissociate**, offer *attachment play*, followed by a *Loving Limit* if necessary.

If they start trying to cry, simply be with them and their feelings.

3. *Keep* following their lead or doing what they really need to feel truly relaxed.

It's normal and natural for all children to have a lot of big feelings sitting inside them.

Focus on keeping connected with yourself, staying present if you can, through:

- *connecting* in with your *breathing*;
- *noticing* the *details* about their face or hair; and
- *feeling* the *sensations* of your sitting bones on the chair.

If you do feel concerned that they have an unmet need, you can always stop and offer them what you think will meet that need, and then observe them afterwards.

If you keep listening to the end of the release process, the crying will eventually taper off and come to a natural completion.

4. *Notice* whether they're becoming more relaxed and present

This will help you with reassurance that expressing these big feelings has been helpful for them.

8. Keep connected: Stay close with them as they fall asleep

Follow their lead on the timing of when they no longer need this.

9. If they wake up soon after

If they wake up soon after, it's likely that they have more feelings to express. Saying, *"I'm here with you,"* and offering a soft touch can help them express more.

10. Your feelings

If we are going to be able to consistently listen to our child's healing-feelings, it's vital to have our emotions own lovingly heard.

11. Observation

Noticing differences will give you reassurance that what you are doing is helpful for them. Increased relaxation can be seen through relaxed muscles, meeting hugs, and eye contact.

The steps of supporting your teen to sleep summary

1. Thinking: Hold the theory clearly in your mind

The three things needed for sound sleep:

- to feel tired (sleepy);
- to feel connected (*closeness creating a sense of safety*); and
- to feel relaxed (*by releasing any healing-feelings present*).

The three ways teens heal from stress and trauma:

- laughter and playfulness;
- expression through talking; and
- crying and raging.

2. Feeling: Have your own feelings heard

Especially exploring our feelings in relation to trusting our teen.

3. Presence: Connecting in with yourself and helping yourself become present

The more present you are, the more you can offer your loving presence.

4. Preparation: Preparing yourself physically and emotionally

E.g. in relation your thoughts and feelings about offering them connection before you go to sleep, and trusting them and their own choices in relation to sleep.

5. Tired: Watching for tiredness signs

We might gently offer them empathy when they are clearly tired. I don't recommend telling them to go to bed.

6. Connected: Offer them closeness and connection

Going to their room with jokey playfulness, or with a funny meme to show them, or to tell them a joke. Remembering something significant about their day and asking them about it.

7. Relaxed

1a. *Notice* where you might be inadvertently distracting them from their innate relaxation processes, e.g. they want to share with us and we ask them about what time they will go to bed.

1b. *Notice* where they might be using *control patterns*, and be available to offer support.

We might go and offer loving connection when we see them reading or watching screens to dissociate from feelings. Warmth is the antidote to freeze.

2. *Instead* of distracting them, follow their lead

Listening to them talk or joining in if they find something funny and want to share it with us.

3. **Keep** following their lead

If they want to keep talking, or laughing together, or sharing feelings, or watching funny videos together, staying with that process can create a profound sense of connection.

3. **Noticing** whether they're becoming more relaxed and present

This can still be relevant with teens, because it can help us continue offering connection and listening if we see it's making a difference.

8. Your feelings

It's really common that we might judge ourselves, our parenting, or our teen. We might have fearful thoughts about their future. Receiving empathy, and doing our own inner work to put down the guilt sticks and connect with what we are willing for in the future can make a huge difference.

9. Conversations with your teen at other times

Having conversations, discussing feelings, needs and values, finding ways for everyone to get their needs met, and being silly together can all create a warm context.

LOVING PHRASES FROM ME TO YOU

I'm sending you so much love.

I invite you to put down the guilt stick.

I invite you to be deeply compassionate with yourself.

My heart goes out to you.

Changing our cultural conditioning is designed to be hard.

I understand how hard it is.

You can do this.

Your needs are so important, sweetheart.

Everyone needs support.

We're not meant to live without community support.

You are doing the job of a whole community.

I so acknowledge all that you're doing.

I so appreciate all that you're doing.

All of your feelings are natural and normal.

Your feelings are beautiful gifts.

I welcome all of your feelings.

All of your feelings are welcome.

I'm right here with you.

I'm listening.

LANGUAGE SUGGESTIONS

Please note that there is no official language in Aware Parenting. These are my suggestions, but the most important thing is *you* finding language that resonates with you and that helps you feel loving and powerful, and which helps them feel loved and safe.

Language in relation to crying

What we can say when our baby is crying in our arms:

"I'm here and I'm listening, sweetheart."

"I'm right here with you."

"You're letting it all out."

"I love you."

I invite you to find words that help you feel most loving and calm.

What we can say when our child or teen is crying with us:

"I'm here with you, sweetheart. I love you. I'm listening."

Language in relation to playing

What can we say when we want to stop playing *attachment play*:

If you start getting tired or just don't want to play any more, you can offer them a *Limit*[70], *"I've so enjoyed playing with you, and I'm going to put a timer on for five minutes, and I'm not willing to play any more after that, because I'm tired. Then, I'm going to help you go to bed.[71]"*

And when the timer goes off, *"I'm not willing to play any more sweetheart. Let's go to the bedroom now."*

---

70 It's a *Limit*, not a *Loving Limit*, because it's from your own unwillingness to play for longer, rather than to support them to express feelings that are causing them to want to keep playing.

71 This is for younger children who are still needing our support to go to sleep. Once they are older and no longer need that support, we wouldn't recommend a *Loving Limit* telling then when to go to sleep.

You might want to do some *attachment play* to get into bed – *"Let's pretend we're sloths and we're moving reallllllllyyyy slooooowwwwly to the bed."*

If they have feelings in response, we can listen lovingly to those. *"I hear that you wanted to play more, sweetheart. I understand. I'm listening."*

What we can say when they want to keep playing but are clearly tired and have feelings:

If you sense that there are deeper feelings underneath that are preventing them from feeling relaxed enough to be able to go to sleep, or if you think a cry is bubbling, you might offer a *Loving Limit.* *"I'm going to put a timer on for five minutes, and I'm not willing to play any more after that, because I don't think it's the most helpful thing for you."*

And when the timer goes off, *"I'm not willing to play any more sweetheart, becuase I don't think that's the most helpful thing for you and I'm right here and listening."* If this brings forth tears, listen lovingly, offering empathy.

If the crying intensifies when you offer warmth or empathy, that tells you that you're helping them express the feelings that have been sitting inside them. *"You really wanted to play more, sweetheart. I hear you. I understand. I'm listening."*

What we can say if they start getting rough in the play:

You can offer a *Loving Limit,* starting with doing the minimum to stop the roughness, and then something like, *"I'm not willing for you to do that, sweetheart, because I'm here to keep everyone safe. And I'm right here and I'm listening."*

Language in relation to dissociation, distraction, and *control patterns*

Loving Limits in response to distraction or *control patterns*

I would generally go for connection and attachment play before *Loving Limits* with *control patterns*. I love to express *Loving Limits* using phrases such as, *"I really hear that you want me to get you another toy, sweetheart, and I'm not willing to get another toy because I don't think that's most helpful for you right now, and I'm here and I'm listening."*[72]

If they are trying to distract themselves with one more toy, and you clearly see that this isn't about here and now needs (because they're not happy with anything), you could offer a *Loving Limit. "I hear that you want to get another toy from the living room, and I'm not willing for you to do that, sweetheart, because I don't think that's the most helpful thing for you right now. And I'm right here and I'm listening,"* and then listen to the feelings that they've been trying to distract themselves from.

If they are wanting you to distract them from their feelings such as by asking you to read them more stories, you could also offer a *Loving Limit, "I hear that you want me to read you more stories, and I'm not willing to read you any more, sweetheart, because I don't think that's the most helpful thing for you right now, and I'm right here and I'm listening,"* and then listen to those feelings that they were trying to distract themselves from.

If they're trying to find a pretext – an emotional coat hanger to find a reason to have a big cry or rage, once you realise that that's what they're doing, you could simply offer them empathy and stay with their feelings, *"Oh sweetheart, I really hear that those pyjamas aren't the ones you wanted tonight, and the other ones are all wet in the washing machine. I hear you. I'm listening. I'm right here with you."*

Language in relation to aggression

Loving Limits in response to aggression:

I love the phrase, *"I'm not willing for you to hit me, sweetheart, because I'm here to keep everyone safe, and I'm right here, and I'm listening."*

I don't recommend saying, *"It's not okay to hit,"* because this is a judgment and is likely to lead to more painful feelings such as shame or guilt and is less likely to create a sense of emotional safety.

---

72 Please note that this language is my preferred way to express a *Loving Limit*, but there are other possible phrases to use. There is no set language for *Loving Limits* in Aware Parenting.

Likewise, saying, *"Be gentle!"* is not likely to stop the hitting, nor to help them feel and express the feelings underlying the hitting.

Thirdly, I also don't recommend, *"We don't hit in our family,"* because if they have, what does that mean for them?

Please note that there is no specific language in Aware Parenting for *Loving Limits*. I invite you to choose language that helps you feel safe, loving, and truly powerful, and which helps your child feel safe and loved.

I specifically choose, *"I'm not willing,"* because I find that it helps me connect deeply with my true power, and can help a child feel safe and connected with us and with themselves. The *"... and I'm listening,"* can help them feel our loving presence.

I invite you to create your own phrases that you most enjoy for common scenarios in your family, and to make a note of them.

ACKNOWLEDGEMENTS

I am so grateful to Aletha Solter, PhD, Founder of The Aware Parenting Institute and Aware Parenting, for her profound work, her books, her deeply clear thinking, and her wise guidance and support, including editing this book (twice!) and making many editorial suggestions. My understanding of Aware Parenting deepened yet again in receiving her sage counsel during the editing process. If you haven't already read her books, I highly recommend reading all of them several times. You can find them on her website: **www.awareparenting.com**

I so appreciate my amazing book publishing consultant, Julie Postance, for helping my book dreams come into form, and to wonderful Sophie White, for her beautiful typesetting and cover editing. I've said it twice, and I'll say it again (and again, and again), you two really are the dream team!

I love the cover and am again so thankful to Jelena Mirkovic for creating a design that I find so beautiful.

Editing is always wonderful with my lovely Editors, Belynda Smith and Jenny Exall (Jenny edited the first version that I wrote last year). Thank you again, dear Belynda and Jenny. Belynda, I particularly appreciate your willingness to share your touching stories in the teens section. In addition, your ongoing support through the editing process has made it all so enjoyable.

I'm so grateful to everyone who was a beta reader, including Joss Goulden, Eirini Anagnostopoulou, Kimberley Cousins, Meg Rankin, Jasmine Prescott, and Maru Rojas. Your notes and warm words of support and celebration mean so much to me.

Big thanks go to all the parents and Aware Parenting instructors who were willing to share their stories in the book. Words cannot express my gratitude to you for helping bring this book to life.

I'm so appreciative of everyone who gave me suggestions and inspirations, including my Marion's Books Support Team. Special thanks to Eirini Anagnostopoulou, Joy Borish, Ann Ett, Linde Lambrechts, Anna Haberfield, India Farr, Jacqy Pen, Theodoria Plantaria, Joss Goulden, Sheryl Stoller, Clare Peace, and Lynda Silk. A very special thank you goes to Eva Gandrudbakken for researching the history of baby sleep in Norway for me.

I'm also so appreciative of all the parents I have mentored over the years, and who have joined my workshops, groups, and online courses. Walking beside you has been such an honour. I've learnt so much from you.

Many thanks go to all the people who shared their sleep questions for the Q and A's which bring specific details and richness to the book.

Thank you to Michael, the father of my children, for the beautiful photo of our children on the front, and for his wise support throughout the book writing and editing process, as well as for actually putting Aware Parenting into practice together.

My deepest gratitude is always to my daughter and son, who taught me so much about sleep and trust, and highlighted the parts of me that needed tending to so that I could offer them the most helpful support. I so appreciate their willingness for their photo to be on the cover and for me to share our sleep stories. A big thank you to my daughter, for creating the beautiful crying in arms diagram on the next page.

I'm forever thankful of my Dad and of all his support in my earlier years, so I could be doing this now.

And to my incredible Mum, thank you for being willing to transform so that we now have my dream mother-daughter relationship. You have shown me the power of reparenting, and how we are never too old to heal and grow. Thank you beyond all thank you's, including for all that you do around the house so that I have had way more time for writing and editing!

An additional furry thank you to Buddha and Koyo, my Frenchie friends, who have kept me company during all of the writing and editing process!

POSSIBLE PHYSIOLOGICAL CAUSES OF SLEEP CHALLENGES

In the book, I offered detailed information about what causes – and prevents – relaxed and restful sleep, in terms of both innate needs and intrinsic body wisdom.

Here is a list of possible physiological causes of sleep challenges. I invite you to read through this list and to enquire into whether any of the things might be affecting your child's relaxation levels and sleep.

Please note that where I state that information is not from Aware Parenting, that neither the information nor the recommendations are endorsed by Aletha Solter, nor by Aware Parenting.

I invite you to trust yourself if you think any of them might be relevant. If you do sense that one or more may be, I invite you to listen in to yourself and whether you are called to reach out for information and support from a relevant and trusted health practitioner.

Aware Parenting acknowledges these influences

Noise

Even a child who is deeply relaxed might find it harder to go to sleep and stay asleep if there's lots of noise.

(However, the more relaxed a child is, through being supported with Aware Parenting, the less they are affected by noise while going to sleep and when sleeping).

Illness or pain

When babies, children or teens have physical symptoms, this can clearly affect their sleep. If we trust the wisdom of their bodies, we might also be curious about whether there might be important reasons for them to sleep less, or be awake in the middle of the night when they have physical symptoms.

Children can suffer from headaches, stomachaches, earaches, itchy rashes, and many other uncomfortable ailments caused by illnesses, accidents, or surgery.

If you're ever concerned about your child's wellness, please reach out to your usual health practitioner. I invite you to deeply trust your intuition here.

Teething

It's normal for babies and children to be more restless and to wake up more when they have teeth coming through.

It is also possible to help many of them feel more comfortable when they are teething, with Aware Parenting.

Children can feel agitated when they have a loose or wobbly tooth. If tweens or teens have braces, they can also feel discomfort, which can affect their sleep.

Temperature

If babies, children or teens are too hot or too cold, this can affect their sleep.

Feeding challenges

If a baby has feeding challenges, this may affect their sleep.

Food intolerances

If a baby or child is being breastfed, they may be affected by what their mother is eating, particularly by foods such as dairy, wheat, onions and spices, and this can affect their sleep. Some babies, children and teens may have food intolerances that influence their sleep.

In addition, some non-Aware Parenting modalities suggest that there may be connections between food intolerances and stress.

Aware Parenting supports the natural release of stress through innate healing and relaxation processes.

Physical tension from their birth

Babies and children can feel physical tension or pain because of how they were born – which can affect their sleep. This can be very common if their birth was very long or very quick, if they were posterior, or if they were born with ventouse or forceps.

The practice of Aware Parenting can also help children release physical tension that was caused by their birth.

This information is not from Aware Parenting:

Effects of caffeine or artificial food additives

Caffeine and artificial additives in food can create agitation in some children and can thus affect their sleep.

Gut biome and digestive issues

Digestive and gut issues can affect sleep for some children.

You might also want to hold in mind that hyperarounsal and dissociation affect digestion, and that supporting children to heal from stress or trauma, through practicing Aware Parenting, may also help bring about more ease with digestion.

Jordan said: *"After listening to my baby with Aware Parenting, I feel like I've cracked a code to parenting no one talks about. My son is three months old and all of a sudden he sleeps better, feeds better and his digestive system is working better since being present and allowing him to release any emotion and tension from his body. I'm honestly so amazed and thankful. I feel so much calmer as a mother. I'm incredibly thankful for your work, as is my husband who can finally hold our baby while he is asleep without him jolting awake every time! Thank you again."*

Mouth breathing

Other modalities suggest that if children mouth breathe, this may lead to more unsettled sleep as well as bed wetting in children. Snoring can be an indication of mouth breathing.

Artificial chemicals in washing powder, soap, shampoo, etc.

Some children can be affected by the artificial chemicals in products such as washing powder, soap, shampoo, etc., which can affect how relaxed they feel, and thus their sleep.

Bedding or pyjamas made with artificial fibres or treated with chemicals

Some children might find it harder to relax and sleep restfully if their nightwear and/or bedding is made of artificial fibres or if they were made or processed with chemicals. Some people recommend products made from organic fibres.

Blue light and bright lights

Some people believe that blue light in the evenings may influence sleep by affecting the production of melatonin. If you think this might be affecting your child, you might consider getting some blue-blocking light bulbs that are either amber or red light. If your child or teen watches screens in the evening, you might choose to get them blue-light blocking glasses or screen protectors.

EMFs, wi-fi, dirty electricity, etc.

Some people believe that children may be affected by electro-magnetic fields such as wi-fi, and by what is known as 'dirty' electricity. For example, if they are sleeping close to a wi-fi modem or utility smart meter, or a fridge or oven is backed up next to a wall where they're sleeping.

Mould

Some parents have told me they think that mould affects their child's sleep. A building biologist can measure mould in a home.

I'm sending you so much love as you read, listen to or watch this information. And again, please trust yourself if you're called to attend to one or more of these things.

I invite you to go through the same process of research that I discussed at the beginning of the book – to trust what resonates with you, to experiment, and to observe whether the changes you make lead to any differences in their sleep.

> ### Self-Compassion Moment
> *I invite you to pause for a moment. Perhaps you might even want to put your hand on your heart. If you're feeling overwhelmed, confused or frustrated, I'm sending you lots of love. I also want to let you know that with Aware Parenting, many children sleep peacefully without being affected by any of these elements in the list above.*

DIAGRAM OF THE CRYING IN ARMS
POSITION I PREFERRED

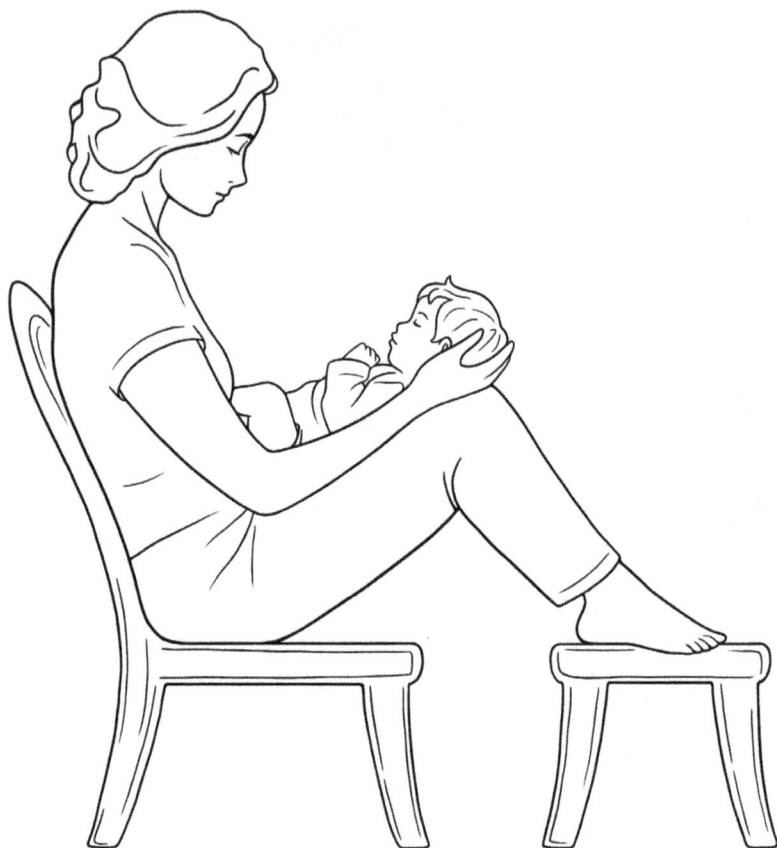

GLOSSARY

Aware Parenting terminology

Attachment play

Nine specific kinds of play between parents and children as described in Aletha Solter's book *Attachment Play*. This type of play creates connection, elicits cooperation, and supports children to both prepare for, and heal from, stressful or traumatic events.

Balance of attention

A state in which a child feels physically and emotionally safe while revisiting past stress or trauma. The *balance of attention* is necessary for emotional release and healing to occur (crying, play, laughter, etc.).

Classical Attachment Parenting

This term refers to the original attachment parenting paradigm, which was first described by William and Martha Sears. The Aware Parenting version of attachment parenting has several key differences from this original version. (This term was created by Marion Rose and has been adopted by Aletha Solter.)

Control pattern

Repetitive or compulsive behaviours which are usually acquired during infancy and childhood to suppress crying and strong emotions. A typical *control pattern* is thumb-sucking. *Control patterns* can put babies and children into states of mind dissociation. They are also called emotional suppression habits and self-soothing behaviours. They are sometimes called 'repression mechanisms'.

Dissociation ('freeze or surrender')

This is one of two primary physiological reactions to real or perceived threats or trauma. (The other is hyperarousal.) During dissociation, the parasympathetic nervous system is dominant, and children are quiet, passive, compliant, inattentive, unresponsive, and numb. They are often using a *control pattern*.

Emotional release

Any behaviour which helps restore homeostasis by releasing tension from the nervous system that was acquired during stressful or traumatic experiences. Forms of emotional release in children include crying, raging, trembling, laughter, certain kinds of therapeutic play, and body movements, as well as therapeutic talking. These are also called healing mechanisms and tension-release processes and are often shortened to the term, 'release.'

Hyperarousal ('fight or flight')

This is one of two primary physiological responses to real or perceived threats or trauma. (The other is dissociation.) During hyperarousal, the sympathetic nervous system is dominant, and children are agitated, distractible, impulsive, hypervigilant, defiant, reactive, aggressive, or destructive.

Loving Limits

These are the combination of a verbal or physical limit paired with empathy to create a pretext for a baby or child to cry to release pent-up stress. *Loving Limits* say no to a behaviour or a child's request and yes to the underlying feelings causing the behaviour. (This term was developed by Marion Rose and adopted by Aletha Solter.) We may offer a *Loving Limit* in response to a child's behaviour, such as if they are hitting or biting. We might also offer a *Loving Limit* in response to a child's requests, such as if they are asking for the breast and we don't think that they are hungry. As Aletha Solter says, in this second situation, this is essentially a limit on our own behaviour.

Suppression

This is when children are disconnecting from their feelings or using a *control pattern* so that they stop feeling their feelings, either when they move their attention to something else, or when we distract their attention away to something else.

Terminology and concepts not used in Aware Parenting

'Overtired'

In Aware Parenting, a child who is tired and connected but isn't going to sleep, and who is crying and arching their back isn't 'overtired' but is utilising their innate healing and relaxation response to release stress and trauma from their body before sleep.

'Fighting sleep'

In Aware Parenting, rather than fighting sleep, we see that parents are more often fighting a baby's/child's natural processes to feel relaxed enough to sleep, often through crying with our loving support. Babies and children need to feel tired, connected, and relaxed to be able to sleep peacefully and restfully.

See chapter 13 for more sleep terms that aren't used in Aware Parenting.

Marion Method terminology

Disconnected Domination Culture

The culture that has been in place since industrialisation and has spread around the world through colonisation, but has its roots thousands of years before. The core tenet of disconnection is disconnecting babies from families, and disconnecting us from our bodies, feelings, wisdom, nature, seasons, and traditions. From that disconnection comes domination – force, coercion, guilt, should and have-to, power-over and authoritarianism.

Emotional sticks

These are ways we learn to judge or shame ourselves in *The Disconnected Domination Culture*. Examples of emotional sticks include guilt and shame and all other forms of self-judgement.

Healing-feelings

Feelings that are caused by stress or trauma and when expressed through crying and raging with vigorous movement in loving arms or with loving support, or through therapeutic play or talking, help a child release that stress or trauma and move back into homeostasis.

Needs-feelings

Feelings that are caused by immediate needs in the present moment and which go away when the need is met.

Thoughts-feelings

Feelings that are caused by thoughts, including harsh thoughts learnt from living in the *DDC*. Thoughts-feelings become more relevant as children get older, and are particularly helpful for parents to understand in themselves so that we can replace them with a deeply compassionate inner dialogue.

RECOMMENDED READING & RESOURCES

Aletha Solter's Aware Parenting Institute website

www.awareparenting.com

Books by Aletha Solter PhD

Attachment Play: How to solve children's behavior problems with play, laughter and connection

Cooperative and Connected: Helping children flourish without punishments or rewards

Healing Your Traumatized Child: A parent's guide to children's natural recovery processes

Raising Drug-Free Kids: 100 tips for parents

Tears and Tantrums: What to do when babies and children cry

The Aware Baby

For more information: **http://www.awareparenting.com/books.htm**

Books by Marion Rose PhD

I'm Here and I'm Listening: Empathic and empowering responses to needs, feelings, and behaviours with Aware Parenting

Raising Resilient and Compassionate Children: A parent's guide to understanding behaviour, feelings, and relationships
(Co-authored with Lael Stone)

The Emotional Life of Babies: Find closeness, presence, and sleep for you and your baby with this compassionate approach to crying

Marion Rose's website

www.marionrose.net

Aware Parenting courses by Marion Rose PhD

https://marionrose.net/aware-parenting-courses/

Sound Sleep and Secure Attachment with Aware Parenting Course 2.0

https://marionrose.samcart.com/products/sound-sleep-and-secure-attachment-with-aware-parenting-course/

Marion Method courses by Marion Rose PhD

https://marionrose.net/marion-method-courses/

Podcasts by Marion Rose PhD

The Aware Parenting Podcast

This was co-hosted with Lael Stone until episode 124.

https://podcasts.apple.com/au/podcast/the-aware-parenting-podcast/id1455772681

The Aware Parenting and Natural Learning Podcast

This is co-hosted with Joss Goulden.

https://podcasts.apple.com/au/podcast/the-aware-parenting-and-natural-learning-podcast/id1643837590

The Marion Method Podcast: The Psychospiritual Podcast

https://podcasts.apple.com/au/podcast/the-psychospiritual-podcast/id1344385341

Aware Parenting Community

The Aware Parenting (based on the work of Aletha Solter, PhD.) Facebook group. This is a free Facebook group facilitated by a team of Aware Parenting instructors.

REFERENCES

Aron, E. (2014) *The Highly Sensitive Child: Helping our children thrive when the world overwhelms them.*

Barry, Elaine. S. (2020) *What Is "Normal" Infant Sleep? Why We Still Do Not Know.* **https://journals.sagepub.com/doi/abs/10.1177/0033294120909447?journalCode=prxa**

Everett, D. (2009). *Don't Sleep, There are Snakes: Life and language in the Amazonian jungle.*

Grille, R. (2013). *Parenting for a Peaceful World.*

Hewlett, Barry S. (2017). *Hunter-gatherer Childhoods: Evolutionary, developmental, and cultural perspectives (Evolutionary Foundations of Human Behavior Series).*

King, Suvi Pilvi (2022). The Secret of Arctic "Survival Parenting". **https://www.bbc.com/future/article/20220105-the-arctic-parenting-style-that-fosters-resilience**

Lawlor, R. (1991) *Voices of The First Day: Awakening in the Aboriginal Dreamtime.*

Liedloff, J. (1975). *The Continuum Concept.*

The Baby Historian. **https://thebabyhistorian.com/**

AWARE PARENTING INSTRUCTORS

To find an Aware Parenting instructor in Australia, New Zealand, or Indonesia, you can visit my website here: **https://marionrose.net/aware-parenting-instructors-in-australia-and-new-zealand/**

To find an Aware Parenting instructor in another country, I invite you to visit the Aware Parenting Institute at: **http://www.awareparenting.com/instruct.htm** and click on your country. If you live in a country with a regional coordinator, you will find further links to click on.

CO-SLEEPING

If you choose to co-sleep, please make sure you do so safely. You can read more about safe co-sleeping in *The Aware Baby* by Aletha Solter.

I also recommend James McKenna's work on co-sleeping:
https://cosleeping.nd.edu/safe-co-sleeping-guidelines/

WAYS YOU CAN WORK WITH ME

If you enjoyed this book, and would like to work with me, here are some of the ways you can do that.

Articles on my website
https://marionrose.net/articles/

Free Aware Parenting Courses
https://marionrose.net/aware-parenting-courses/#free-intro-courses

Aware Parenting Courses
https://marionrose.net/aware-parenting-courses/#specific-topics

Aware Parenting Instructor Mentoring Training
https://marionrose.net/aware-parenting-courses/#aware-parenting-instructor-mentoring-course

1:1 Mentoring
https://marionrose.net/mentoring/

IF YOU ENJOYED THIS BOOK

If you enjoyed this book, I'm so glad! I would love for Aware Parenting and *The Marion Method* to spread to even more people and I wonder if you are willing to consider letting others know about this book as part of that.

Here are some ways you can do so.

Please share your review on Amazon – it helps people see if this book might resonate with them.

Please leave a review on Goodreads.

Are you willing to tell your friends about it via your blog, podcast or YouTube channel, or on Facebook, Instagram, X (formerly known as Twitter), Pinterest, or Linkedin?

Are you willing to share about it with your friends and family members or colleagues?

I so appreciate your support!

AUTHOR CONTACT PAGE

Email:
marion@marionrose.net

Website:
https://marionrose.net/

Instagram:
@_marion_rose_
@awareparenting
@theawareparentingpodcast

Facebook:
https://www.facebook.com/MarionRosePhD

www.ingramcontent.com/pod-product-compliance
Lightning Source LLC
Chambersburg PA
CBHW031934090426
42811CB00002B/175